Current Cancer Research

Series Editor

Wafik El-Deiry
Brown University Cancer Center
Providence, RI, USA

More information about this series at http://www.springer.com/series/7892

Anne C. Chiang • Roy S. Herbst

Editors

Lung Cancer

New Understandings and Therapies

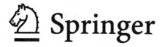 Springer

Editors
Anne C. Chiang
Yale Comprehensive Cancer Center
Yale University
New Haven, CT, USA

Roy S. Herbst
Yale Comprehensive Cancer Center
Yale University
New Haevn, CT, USA

ISSN 2199-2584   ISSN 2199-2592   (electronic)
Current Cancer Research
ISBN 978-3-030-74030-6   ISBN 978-3-030-74028-3   (eBook)
https://doi.org/10.1007/978-3-030-74028-3

This Humana imprint is published by the registered company Springer Nature Switzerland AG
The registered company address is: Gewerbestrasse 11, 6330 Cham, Switzerland

Contents

Chapter 1
Tumor Microenvironment: Immune Effector and Suppressor Imbalance

Kelsey Sheehan and Kurt A. Schalper

Abstract Despite the broad clinical use of immune checkpoint inhibitors (ICI), prominent questions remain relative to their mechanism of action and optimal patient selection strategies. Enhanced understanding of tumor/immune cell interactions in the tumor microenvironment (TME) and identification of dominant immune evasion pathways in the context of individual patients will be required to expand the impact of immunostimulatory anti-cancer therapies. This chapter summarizes current evidence about immune stimulatory and suppressor signals in the TME focusing on their dynamic interplay in human non-small cell lung cancer, expected tumor tissue/cell location and potential for therapeutic targeting. We also discuss the role of molecular TME immune features as biomarkers and their potential impact in future cancer therapeutics.

Keywords Lung cancer · Tumor microenvironment · Immunostimulatory therapies · Biomarkers

1 Introduction

During the last decade immunostimulatory therapies targeting the immune inhibitory receptors PD-1 and CTLA-4, collectively called immune checkpoint inhibitors (ICIs), have shown prominent clinical activity and demonstrated the power of the immune system against cancer. These therapies changed the paradigm of anti-cancer treatment by producing for the first time prominent anti-tumor responses

K. Sheehan
Department of Medicine (Medical Oncology), Yale School of Medicine/Yale Cancer Center,
VA Connecticut Medical Center,
West Haven, CT, USA

K. A. Schalper (✉)
Departments of Medicine (Medical Oncology) and Pathology, Yale School of Medicine,
New Haven, CT, USA
e-mail: Kurt.schalper@yale.edu

© Springer Nature Switzerland AG 2021
A. C. Chiang, R. S. Herbst (eds.), *Lung Cancer*, Current Cancer Research,
https://doi.org/10.1007/978-3-030-74028-3_1

through targeting non-tumor cells. By blocking inhibitory T-cell signaling, T-cells become re-activated to recognize and destroy malignant cells. These treatments have been approved for use in multiple tumor types and brought hope to many patients. However, the proportion of patients deriving sustained benefit is dissimilar across tumor types. Targeting these pathways has led to dramatic clinical responses; for example, in patients with metastatic melanoma where survival benefit has been shown for single agent CTLA-4 blockade with ipilimumab [1], anti-PD-1 therapy with nivolumab [2, 3], and an even greater survival benefit for nivolumab in combination with ipilimumab [4]. The clinical benefit is not restricted to melanoma, and ICIs are now standard first and second line therapies for many tumor types including lymphoma, renal cell cancer (RCC), head and neck cancer, bladder urothelial carcinomas, primary liver malignancies, and gastro-esophageal adenocarcinomas [5]. Despite these significant advances, there remains a large unmet clinical need as the majority patients who are treated with ICIs fail to derive sustained clinical benefit. For example, the response rate to single-agent PD-1 blockade in patients with advanced non-small cell lung cancer (NSCLC) is ~20% and higher activity is achieved using combination treatments [6]. However, clinical responses in multiple other high impact malignancies such as pancreatic, colorectal and prostate adenocarcinomas are extremely uncommon and clustered in a relatively small fraction of tumors harboring mismatch repair deficiency and/or high nonsynonymous mutational burden [7–9]. The determinants for the striking differences in the activity of ICI across different tumor types remain uncertain.

In addition to primary resistance to ICIs, most patients who initially respond develop secondary/acquired resistance during treatment and ultimately succumb to the disease. To reduce mortality, it is imperative to: (i) Identify robust biomarkers for selection of patients for treatment; (ii) Develop biologically supported treatment combinations to break tumor immune tolerance in the tumor bed; and (iii) Uncover dominant immunotherapy targets beyond PD-1/CTLA-4 that may serve to treat patients with refractory tumors.

Efforts have been undertaken to identify determinants for sensitivity and resistance to PD-1 axis blockers that can be used as predictive biomarkers. Diverse tumor and immune-cell factors have been recognized including the expression of PD-L1 protein, pre-existence of adaptive anti-tumor immune responses (e.g. tumor infiltrating lymphocytes [TILs] or IFNγ-based RNA signatures), increased number of nonsynonymous somatic mutations, mismatch repair deficiency and the presence of deleterious variants in individual genes. However, few biomarkers are approved for clinical use and their performance is suboptimal. Together, most available literature supports a prominent role of the tumor microenvironment (TME) in the regulation of anti-cancer immune responses and treatment resistance. It is therefore expected that detailed studies of this compartment and of tumor/immune-cell interactions will support the development of novel biomarkers and identification of dominant immune evasion pathways with actionable potential (Fig. 1.1).

Conceptually, the TME is comprised of two major compartments: one formed by malignant tumor cells and another composed of the surrounding non-malignant stromal cells such as infiltrating immune cells, fibroblasts, and vasculature. In

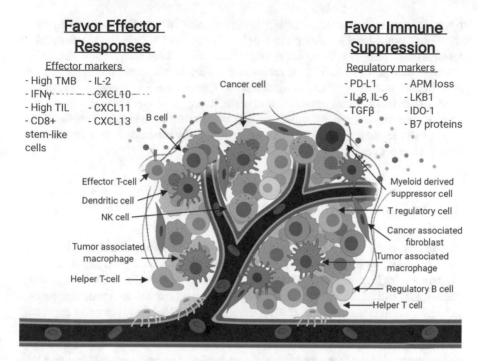

Fig. 1.1 Imbalance between pro- and anti-tumor signals in the tumor microenvironment (TME). Schema showing representative interactions between tumor and stromal/immune cells in the tumor niche. The TME in NSCLC is characterized by the presence of dominant immune suppressive signals that outweigh the pro-inflammatory effector responses against malignant cells and lead to tumor growth and dissemination. Multiple tumor-cell, immune-cell and stromal cell factors are expected to be in play simultaneously and some of these have a biomarker role. Identification of the dominant immune defects in specific tumors could support development of biologically driven immunostimulatory therapies. TMB = tumor mutational burden, IFNγ = interferon gamma, TIL = tumor infiltrating lymphocytes, CXCL10 = C-X-C motif chemokine ligand 10, CXCL11 = C-X-C motif chemokine ligand 11, CXCL13 = C-X-C motif chemokine ligand 13, PD-L1 = programmed death-ligand 1, TGFß = transforming growth factor beta, APM = antigen processing machinery, LKB1 = liver kinase B1, also known as serine/threonine kinase 11 (STK11), IDO1 = Indoleamine 2, 3-dioxygenase 1, NK cells = natural killer cells. Created with BioRender.com

aggressive cancers, tumor cells develop potent immune evasion mechanisms and overcome immunosurveillance allowing for unchecked expansion of the tumor compartment (e.g. tumor growth) and eventual metastatic dissemination. Immunostimulatory anti-cancer therapies are able to counteract this and restore anti-cancer immune cells in the TME with enhanced tumor cell killing. While these compartments are physically and chemically interconnected and tumor-immune cell responses most likely mirror each other, differences in cell properties and spatial distribution between transformed and surrounding immune cells are expected. In addition, continuous cycles of immune activation and regulation are likely to occur in tumors during cancer development and progression. Sustained T-cell activation can trigger multiple immunoregulatory mechanisms that can ultimately override and repress effector anti-cancer responses. Consistent with this notion, multiple studies have identified effector T-cells in the TME displaying features of terminal differentiation/exhaustion and dysfunction. This interplay is key to the development of tumors and their metastatic potential, and it ultimately determines how tumors will respond to immunotherapy. The purpose of this chapter is to provide a foundational immunobiological understanding of the TME of human lung cancer, describe the role of individual cell compartments and their functions; and explore the clinical potential of this information for biomarker development and cancer therapeutics.

2 The Tumor Compartment

Tumor cells are integral components of the TME and they represent a variable, and most likely dynamic, part of most solid malignancies. Despite presumably originating from a single clonal population, tumor cells can display dissimilar morphology, phenotypes and functional profiles, a phenomenon referred to as intratumor heterogeneity. In general, tumor cells contain mutant neopeptides and aberrantly expressed or modified antigenic proteins that can be recognized as non-self by the adaptive immune system. However, malignant cells are also commonly equipped with multiple suppressive mechanisms to evade or counteract immune recognition and killing. These include: (i) the expression of immune inhibitory signals (e.g. PD-L1, IDO-1, FGL1, etc.), (ii) upregulation of immune suppressive cytokines/chemokines (e.g. IL-6, IL-8, TGFβ, etc.) which can affect neighboring immune and non-immune cells and enable further tumor growth; (iii) defective antigen presentation machinery; and (iv) altered intracellular signaling and differentiation programs.

2.1 Immune Inhibitory Signals

NSCLC cells can express PD-L1 in their surface, which serves as a ligand for the PD-1 immune inhibitory receptor commonly present on antigen-activated T-cells. Blockade of the PD-L1/PD-1 interaction with monoclonal antibodies is associated with T-cell reinvigoration and anti-tumor responses. As expected, this effect is more prominent in tumors with elevated PD-L1 levels. Notably, expression of PD-L1 in tumor cells is most commonly a consequence of adaptive pro-inflammatory responses in the TME and is potently induced by IFNγ. Interferon signaling in malignant cells occurs through the JAK/STAT pathway and is believed to serve as a hard-wired response from epithelial cells to balance sustained local immune activation and prevent potential tissue damage [10].

Additional immune inhibitory molecules have been identified in NSCLC and could mediate immune evasion. For example, B7-H3, also known as CD276, is a membrane protein from the B7-family of immunoregulatory ligands and has been detected in a large proportion of lung malignancies [11, 12]. Although the receptor mediating the inhibitory effect of B7-H3 remains unidentified, its expression has been shown to inhibit T cell activation and proliferation [13]. B7-H4 is another transmembrane protein from the B7-family expressed in a relatively small fraction of NSCLCs which inhibits TCR-mediated T cell proliferation, cell cycle progression and IL-2 production [13–15]. VISTA is a third immune regulatory protein from the B7 family expressed in NSCLC that can interact with the receptor PSGL-1 on T-cells in a pH-specific manner to suppresses T cell activation [13, 16, 17].

Immune regulatory enzymes can also be upregulated by cancer cells. For example, a fraction of NSCLCs express IDO1 in tumor cells, an enzyme that catabolizes tryptophan [14]. Tryptophan catabolism is an important mechanism of tumor cell immune evasion. Depletion of tryptophan leads to the accumulation of Trp-tRNA, which activates the stress-response kinase GCN2. In effector T-cells, activated GCN2 leads to cell cycle arrest and/or apoptosis, thereby contributing to an immune suppressive TME [18]. Another example of important immune regulatory enzyme upregulation is CD73. It is highly expressed on multiple cell types in the TME. CD73 dephosphorylates extracellular ATP, leading to an accumulation of adenosine. Extracellular adenosine has immune dampening effects, like the suppression of effector cell function and stabilization of immunosuppressive regulatory cells [19].

Understanding the interplay and functional interaction of different immune suppressive signals in lung tumors could help define which of them are exerting a dominant biological effect in favoring tumor growth. This information could be used to design optimal therapeutic interventions.

2.2 Immune Suppressive Cytokines

After T-cell activation in the TME and local production of IFNγ and TNFα, potent immune suppressive cytokines/chemokines can be upregulated to counteract local inflammation such as IL-6 and IL-8 [20, 21]. Notably, these cytokines can both suppress immune responses and also favor tumor-cell growth. IL-6 signaling through interaction with the IL-6 receptor (CD126) is involved in tumor development and progression. In lung cancer, high levels of IL-6 have are associated with poor outcomes. IL-6 is produced by tumor cells as well as some immune cells and fibroblasts. It leads to the release of angiogenic factors, including VEGF, which promotes tumor development, and contributes to an immune suppressive environment by supporting the development of myeloid-derived suppressor cells (MDSCs) and macrophages. Through the STAT3 pathway, IL-6 leads to expression of anti-apoptotic proteins, which ultimately supports tumor growth [22].

IL-8 is another chemokine which plays a role in the TME through interaction with its receptors CXCR1 and CXCR2. Tumor-derived IL-8 promotes the chemoattraction of immune suppressive neutrophils and MDSCs into the TME, which leads to defective effector CD8+ T-cell responses and reduced sensitivity to ICI [23, 24]. Additionally, TME-derived IL-8 can favor tumor angiogenesis and mediate epithelial-to-mesenchymal transition, a process which leads to increased metastatic potential and tumor resistance to immune cell killing [21].

2.3 Antigen Presentation Machinery Alterations

Local pro-inflammatory cytokines such as IFNγ released after immune activation can increase the expression of antigen presenting proteins in cells such as human leukocyte antigens (HLA) class-I and class-II molecules to favor immune surveillance. However, tumor cells can harbor defects in antigen presentation proteins or in intracellular antigen processing pathways mediating reduced antigen exposure. These alterations can occur in both immunotherapy naïve patients and after treatment with ICI [25, 26]. Recent studies have identified deleterious mutations in the invariant HLA class I chain β-2 microglobulin as mediators of acquired resistance to ICI in melanoma and NSCLC [26–28]. Defective antigen presentation of HLA class-I peptides could occur as a consequence of defects in multiple proteins (e.g. HLA-A, -B, -C, TAP1, TAP2, LMP2, LMP7, LMP10, calnexin, calreticulin, tapasin, etc.); and specific protein alterations can be genomic and non-genomic [29]. The frequency and magnitude of antigen presentation protein alterations in most cancers are not fully elucidated since most studies have analyzed only genomic alterations. Defects in intracellular peptide processing or signaling pathways responsible for the expression or upregulation of antigen presenting molecules in response to cytokines could also alter the immune recognition of tumor cells.

2.4 Altered Intracellular Signaling and Differentiation

Activation of the wnt/ß catenin pathway in tumor cells has been identified as a mechanism of resistance to ICIs [30]; this has been shown specifically in melanoma, but the importance of wnt signaling and its association with immune exclusion in tumors has also been demonstrated in many tumor types, including lung cancer [31]. Activation of this pathway ultimately results in the suppression of *Ccl4* transcription and secretion. *Ccl4* is a chemoattractant for myeloid cells, and decreased production leads to decreased dendritic cell recruitment and an unfavorable TME which promotes tumor growth [32]. In lung cancer, *CTNNB1* mutations, which promote ß catenin stabilization, have been specifically identified [33].

Alterations in genes encoding proteins involved in immune related intracellular signaling pathways such as LKB1/STK11 and FBXW7 have also been shown to limit adaptive anti-tumor responses and sensitivity to ICI through defective activation of cytosolic DNA sensing pathways and associated innate immune signals [34, 35].

3 The Stromal Compartment

The stromal compartment composition is also variable across malignancies and is comprised of a complex network of non-tumor cells. Conceptually, stromal cells in the TME can be divided into two major categories: immune cells (e.g. innate and adaptive immune system) and non-immune cells forming the supportive connective tissue. These cell types interact with one another and with malignant cells, and these interactions can influence the local progression, metastatic spread or eradication of the tumor. The balance of immune activating and suppressing signals produced by various immune and non-immune cells of the TME is key to these changes in tumors. Stromal cells are also the target of approved and experimental therapeutics. An additional non-cellular component of the stroma involved in tumor progression and immune evasion is the extracellular matrix (ECM).

Notably, stromal cells and ECM are uncommonly the focus of genomic analysis of tumor samples since they are expected to generally lack detectable somatic genomic alterations. In addition, large scale transcriptomic studies have focused mostly on the analysis of samples enriched in malignant tumor cells with relative underrepresentation of stromal elements.

3.1 *Immune Cells in the Stroma*

The analysis of the immune cells in the TME has prognostic implications in various malignancies, and modulating immune activating and suppressing signals has become the focus of novel anti-cancer therapeutics. In general, CD8+ cytotoxic T-cells and CD4+ Th1 helper cells mediate anti-tumor responses while other cells including regulatory T-cells (Tregs) and myeloid derived suppressor cells (MDSCs) can limit the adaptive immunity and favor tumor growth [36]. Notably, immune cell subpopulations in human tumors exist in a continuum of functional states and in many cases can have intermediate phenotypes. Cells of both the innate and adaptive immune system play distinct and prominent roles in the tumor niche. This section will provide an overview of these various immune cells of the TME and their role in tumor biology.

3.1.1 Adaptive Immune Cells: T Lymphocytes

Cytotoxic T-cells in the TME are key players in the recognition and elimination of malignant target cells displaying foreign antigens. In normal conditions, most nucleated cells express HLA molecules on their surface, which present intracellularly derived short peptide sequences, epitopes, to CD8+ T-cells. In the case of malignancy, tumor-derived epitopes, known as *tumor neoantigens* or tumor-specific antigens, are recognized by CD8+ T-cells as foreign, which results in T-cell activation, expansion and cytotoxic killing. Tumor neoantigens originating from mutant sequences or aberrantly expressed/modified proteins are thought to play a key role in T-cell mediated anti-tumor activity and are being used as targets for therapeutic vaccines [37]. CD8+ T-cells include multiple functional subsets that may be at different proportions in cancer such as naïve cells, progenitor/stem cell-like effector cells (e.g. PD-1$^+$/TCF-7$^+$), central memory, effector memory and effector. Recently, a role of terminally differentiated/exhausted CD8+ T-cells expressing multiple co-inhibitory receptors and a unique transcriptional program (e.g. TOX$^+$/TCF-7$^-$) has been identified as a dominant population in tumors and associated with resistance to PD-1 axis blockers [38–42].

CD4+ T helper cells are another broad class of immune cells which perform multiple functions in the TME. They are in general classified based on their differentiation, function and predominant cytokine production into Th1, Th2, Th9, Th17, Th22, T-regs and Tfh. T_H1 cells produce IFNγ, a cytokine which leads to effector responses and the elimination of cancer cells. T_H2 cells activate B-cells and produce an immunosuppressive cytokine, IL-10. In general, high numbers of T_H2 cells is associated with aggressive tumors [43] and a higher T_H1:T_H2 ratio correlates with a better prognosis [44]. *Th9* cells are characterized by the secretion of IL-9 and IL-10, and they have been demonstrated to have both anti-tumor properties and pro-metastatic effects [45, 46]. Their anti-tumor activity is correlated with CCL20, derived from bronchial and alveolar epithelial cells, and they can lead to dendritic cell recruitment and increased antigen presentation [47]. *Th17* cells produce IL-17, an inflammatory cytokine which may lead to tumor growth or tumor rejection depending on the host's immune status. In lung cancer, Th17 cells are associated with poor prognosis [43]. *Th22* cells produce IL-22, a tumor-promoting cytokine which has downstream effects including tumor proliferation, anti-apoptosis, and recruitment of anti-inflammatory immune cells [48]. T-follicular helper cells (Tfh) produce CXCL13 and migrate to B-cell zones in lymphoid tissue. Elevated Tfh levels in lung cancer tissue correspond with increased mutational burden and immunogenic antigen expression. PD-1 is highly expressed on Tfh cells, and the effects of anti-PD1 therapy on Tfh function is under active investigation [49].

T-regulatory cells (Tregs) are CD4+/CD25+/FOXP3+ immune suppressive cells which help to maintain tissue homeostasis through inhibition of other immune populations. In the context of the TME, their suppression of effector T cells is through secretion of inhibitory cytokines, including TGF-β and IL-10, as well as direct suppression via PD-1, CTLA-4 and other cell to cell signaling pathways [50, 51]. Increased levels of intratumoral and peripheral Tregs in NSCLC correlates with poorer prognosis, increased metastatic risk [52], and a higher risk of recurrence of resected tumors [53, 54]. It has been proposed that Treg depletion is the major mechanism of action of CTLA-4 blocking antibodies and high numbers of Tregs could make tumors less sensitive to ICIs [52].

3.1.2   Adaptive Immune Cells: B Lymphocytes

B-cells are part of the humoral immunity component of the adaptive immune system. They represent a relatively smaller proportion of TILs, produce antibodies and can also present antigens. B lymphocytes play a role in anti-tumor immunity against cancer and are the subject of ongoing research for both prognostic and therapeutic purposes.

It has been demonstrated that all major subsets of B lymphocytes can be found in lung tumors and that they primarily reside in *tertiary lymphoid structures* (TLS), lymphoid aggregates within the peritumor stroma which are structurally similar to secondary lymphoid tissues [55]. High densities of TLS have been correlated with improved patient survival across several tumor types including NSCLC [56]. A primary function of B cells in the TME is the production of tumor-specific antibodies, and the presence of tumor infiltrating plasma cells has been correlated with better survival in lung cancer patients. The role of immunoglobulins secreted by B cells in anti-tumor responses is an area of active investigation [55]. High CD20 expression has also been correlated with longer survival in a NSCLC patient cohort [57]. In addition to antibody production, B-cells interact with T-lymphocytes in the TME and can promote T-cell activity. Some studies done with human/murine tumor models demonstrate that certain populations of B cells correlate with an effector T-cell response in NSCLC and that B cells induce T-cell secretion of IFNγ [55]. B cells can also promote tumor destruction by NK cells, thereby limiting tumor growth [58].

However, some B cell populations, referred to as *regulatory B cells* (Bregs) have been found to have pro-tumor effects [59]. The significance of Bregs in human cancers is not fully elucidated, but they are thought to have the capacity to suppress Th1 and cytotoxic T cells, thereby promoting tumor growth [58].

3.1.3   Innate Immune Cells: NK Cells

NK cells are CD3−/CD56+ innate cytotoxic lymphocytes with the ability to kill tumor cells and account for 10–20% of immune cells in lung cancer tissue [60]. Questions about the capacity of NK cell responses to build memory are currently being addressed. NK cells found in NSCLC tumors have been shown to have altered receptor expression patterns, impaired IFNγ production, and a pro-angiogenic phenotype compared to NK cells from non-tumor tissues, suggesting a role in shaping the TME [61]. Although the role of NK cells in anti-tumor effect induced by ICIs is not fully understood, high baseline intratumor CD56+ immune cells were associated with longer survival in patients with advanced NSCLC treated with PD-1 axis blockers, suggesting the potential for this cell type as a predictive marker [62].

3.1.4   Innate Immune Cells: Myeloid Cells

Myeloid cells comprise multiple cell types originating from common bone marrow precursors differentiating into functionally distinct subsets including macrophages, dendritic cells, MDSCs and neutrophils. These cells and their subsets are found in variable proportions across malignancies.

Tumor associated macrophages (TAMs) are recognized as a prominent component of the TME in most solid malignancies, with both tumor-promoting and anti-tumor roles. TAMs are expected to be derived from several cell types: blood myeloid-derived suppressor cells, blood monocytes and tissue-resident macrophages. TAMs are distributed over a complex functional spectrum, the extremes of which have been clustered into two different forms of macrophage activation states: M1-like, or classic phenotype, and M2-like, or alternative phenotype. M1-like macrophages are generally polarized by IFNγ and have anti-tumor functions. M2-like macrophages are polarized by IL-4 or IL-13 and are, conversely, immunosuppressive [63]. After differentiation, TAMs have been shown to influence vastly diverse components of cancer biology from angiogenesis to cell proliferation, genetic instability and provision of a protective niche for cancer stem cells [63]. One specific way by which TAMs promote tumor growth is by producing cytokines that can suppress T-cell activation, which is thought to be one mechanism of resistance to T-cell based therapeutics such as ICIs [64]. However, they have also been shown to provide synergy in tumor killing after radiation and play a role in the abscopal effect [63]. TAMs are the target of some new investigational therapeutic approaches, intended to be used alone or in combination with other classes of therapy [63].

Importantly, it has been shown that macrophages express PD-L1 significantly more than other immune cells, and high PD-L1 expression in macrophages correlates with high PD-L1 expression in tumors. Additionally, high PD-L1 expression in macrophages is associated with longer overall survival (OS) in lung cancer patients treated with anti-PD1 therapy [65].

The overall potential prognostic value of TAM density in a tumor has been investigated and ten studies included in one meta-analysis which included lung cancer patients had mixed results [66].

Myeloid derived suppressor cells (MDSCs) are inhibitory cells of the innate immune system which have been found to play a role in multiple diseases. A primary function of these cells is inhibiting T cell function, which can promote tumor growth [67]. They can also differentiate into TAMs and favor the development of Tregs, thereby further promoting immune suppression [50]. Two discrete subsets of MDSCs have been identified: monocytic (mMDSC) and granulocytic (gMDSC), which have both been demonstrated to be immune suppressive [68].

Dendritic cells (DCs) are professional APCs which can mediate expansion and activation of effector CD8+ responses via presentation of exogenous antigens. They can also activate B-cell responses via cytokine stimulation. However, there is evidence that defective DCs in the TME can induce T-cell tolerance which prevents malignant cell recognition and ultimately leads to tumor growth [69]. Research suggests that tumor cells themselves suppress DC function or lead to the recruitment of immune-suppressive DCs rather than immune-activating DCs. Manipulating DCs for therapeutic benefit is an area of active research [70].

Tumor associated neutrophils (TANs) can also accumulate in the TME, and they are most commonly associated with worse outcomes in several different types of cancer, though both tumor suppressive and tumor promoting functions of these cells have been elucidated [71]. One mechanism by which TANs have been demonstrated to be tumor-promoting is via the production of neutrophil extracellular traps (NETs), which coat tumor cells, protecting them from cytotoxicity [24]. IL-8 plays an important role in regulating neutrophil chemotaxis and formation of NETs. It has been shown that early increases in serum IL-8 levels is a strong predictor of poor outcome in retrospective cohorts of advanced melanoma or NSCLC patients treated with ICIs [72], and a larger analysis of patients treated in phase 3 clinical trials also showed that elevated baseline serum IL-8 levels are associated with increased TANs and poor outcomes after ICI in multiple tumor types [23]. These data support the possible value of serum IL-8 levels as a biomarker and create a link between TANs and immune regulation in the TME.

3.2 Non-immune Cells in the Stroma

There has been increasing interest in the role of non-immune cells which make up the TME and the role these cells play in cancer development as well as their potential as therapeutic targets. One research group used single cell RNA sequencing technology to catalog the TME transcriptome in human lung tumors and compared these tumors to matched non-malignant lung samples in an effort to characterize both the stromal and tumor cells. Using this technique, they identified 52 subtypes of stromal cells, some of which were novel, and investigated the correlation of stromal cell distribution with patient survival [73]. Their work demonstrates the vast diversity of stromal cell subtypes and highlights the fact that we are just beginning to understand the clinical significance of many of these cell types.

3.2.1 Non-immune Cells in the Stroma: Cancer Associated Fibroblasts (CAFs)

Cancer associated fibroblasts (CAFs) have been implicated in the development and growth of tumors via angiogenesis, cancer cell proliferation and invasion, and they are thought to contribute to an immune suppressive TME. These cells are derived from multiple different precursor cells, including smooth muscle cells, myoepithelial cells and mesenchymal stem cells. It is thought that the differentiation of these various cell types into myofibroblasts, or CAFs, can lead to organ fibrosis, which increases the risk of developing cancer [50]. When fibroblasts are indolent, they are referred to as resting fibroblasts. Once activated, they can also differentiate into adipocytes and can be programmed into pluripotent stem cells [74].

CAFs secrete growth factors like hepatocyte growth factor (HGF), fibroblast growth factor (FGF) and insulin like growth factor 1 (IGF-1), which favor cancer growth [50]. It has been demonstrated in vitro that CAFs influence the metabolism of NSCLC cell lines specifically through the production of reactive oxygen species and TGF-β signaling pathways [75].

CAFs have also been demonstrated to mediate tumor growth and development. One group demonstrated that a pro-inflammatory gene signature in CAFs from dysplastic skin was consistently maintained in CAFs from skin carcinomas in a mouse model. In addition, fibroblasts from mouse models of mammary and pancreatic tumors as well as human skin expressed this pro-inflammatory CAF gene signature. The NF-kappa B signaling pathway participates in CAFs' role in recruiting macrophages, enabling neovascularization and contributing to cancer growth [76]. It was also demonstrated that mixing normal skin fibroblasts with cancer cells led to greater tumor growth than tumor cells alone. This work demonstrates the fluidity of the TME and the cross talk between tumor cells and stromal cells [76].

CAFs are also generally thought to have an immunosuppressive effect on the TME, although most of the data on CAF immune modulatory effects are from in vitro studies. CAF-secreted IL-6 can restrict dendritic cell maturation and disable T-cell activation, but it is unclear to what degree other sources of IL-6 in the TME as well as other cytokines or growth factors are required to have these downstream immunosuppressive effects [74].

There has been interest in the potential prognostic implications of CAFs in tumors. In NSCLC, CAF activation markers are associated with poor survival and an increased mortality risk [77].

3.2.2 Non-immune Cells in the Stroma: Vascular Cells

Pericytes are perivascular stromal cells. They stabilize blood vessels but more recently have been shown to participate in various disease states. Pericytes can function as stem cells and regulate the behavior of other progenitor cells. They also play a role in tumor angiogenesis, although clinical efforts to block pericyte activity have not had promising results [78].

There is increasing evidence that pericytes play a role in the formation of a "premetastatic niche," the collection of hematopoietic cells, stromal cells and extracellular matrix which harbors the ultimate development of metastases. One group demonstrated that pericytes lose the expression of traditional markers in response to tumor secreted factors, then proliferate, migrate and increase extracellular matrix synthesis. The resultant environment is rich in fibronectin, which could favor the metastatic process [79].

Lymphatic vessels are a route by which tumors metastasize, and the interaction between *lymphatic endothelial cells* and cancer cells is another component of the TME which is under active investigation. One study demonstrated that medium with ELK3-suppressed lymphatic endothelial cells (LECs) was unable to promote the migration and invasion of breast cancer cells, suggesting that ELK3-dependent pathways in LECs are important components of a pro-metastatic TME [80]. Further elucidation of the pathways underlying the pro-metastatic cross-talk between tumor cells and LECs could lead to the development of therapeutic options targeting these pathways.

Vascular endothelial cells are another stromal component of the TME. In addition to allowing the exchange of oxygen and metabolic substrates, these cells regulate the migration of leukocytes from blood vessels into peripheral tissues, including tumors. However, it has been demonstrated that the activation of pro-inflammatory pathways in tumors does not result in the expression of vascular adhesion molecules which would be needed for the entry of lymphocytes into the tumor bed, a phenomenon termed endothelial anergy [81]. Bevacizumab, the anti-VEGF antibody used in lung cancer treatment, targets the tumor vasculature. It is thought that this agent works by both starving the tumor of blood supply while also normalizing the tumor vasculature, thereby enabling immune cell migration and favoring anti-cancer responses [82].

3.3   Non-Cellular Elements of the TME: The Extracellular Matrix (ECM)

The ECM is a complex network of proteins, proteoglycans and glycoproteins which form aggregates of fibrils and sheet-like structures and provides the scaffolding of mature tissues. There is increasing appreciation for the importance of both the biochemical and biophysical characteristics of the dynamic ECM, like its molecular density, rigidity and tension [83]. A wide variety of ECM proteins release bioactive peptides when cleaved by specific enzymes. A multitude of these proteins, proteases and peptides are being investigated for their potential role in cancer metastasis [83].

The ECM is being constantly remodeled, and it influences cell adhesion and migration, which support a role in growth of malignant tumors [84]. A prominent way this remodeling occurs is through matrix metalloproteases (MMPs); MMPs process and degrade ECM proteins. They are secreted by malignant cells, TAMs, and CAFs, so they represent one mechanism by which the ECM is in constant communication with the surrounding cells, including tumor cells. ECM remodeling can also be influenced by the local production of chemokines, growth and angiogenic factors [50]. One pathway by which this occurs is the TGFβ pathway activation of quiescent fibroblasts [85]. In general, activation of this pathway leads to upregulation of collagen and stiffening of the ECM which subsequently influences the motility and proliferation of TME cells. The FGF pathway cooperates with TGFβ signaling and ultimately results in acquisition of a stem cell-like phenotype. The Rho/ROCK pathway is implicated in remodeling focal adhesions which affects the migration and adhesion of malignant cells. These various pathways are examples of how the cross talk between tumors and the ECM can lead to tumor survival and expansion [85].

The ECM is also relevant in metastasis. Migrating cancer cells must infiltrate the ECM, so both the biochemical and biophysical characteristics of the ECM can influence the ability of tumors to spread. As noted previously with regard to pericytes, different characteristics of the ECM are thought to be more conducive to the establishment of metastatic tumors, so it is theorized that the ECM is an important component of a "premetastatic niche." However, our understanding of the specific qualities of the ECM which make it more conducive to metastatic disease is limited, so there are not yet opportunities for therapeutic intervention [83].

ECM protein networks can also limit the access of immune cells to the tumor niche, thereby promoting cancer development and growth. One study used live cell imaging to evaluate the migration of T-cells into and within human NSCLCs. Purified T-cells added to lung tumor slices behaved like TILs, and they migrated along fibers that were excluded from the tumor-stroma boundary more than into islets of tumor cells, thereby suggesting a role of the ECM in limiting access of T-cells to the tumor foci. Unsurprisingly, given these interactions of the ECM with tumor cells and T-cells, a dense stroma has been shown to correlate with a poorer prognosis in lung adenocarcinoma [86].

4 Biomarkers

Features of the TME have been adopted as predictive immunotherapy biomarkers to guide optimal patient selection for treatments. Predictive biomarkers have been identified originating from tumor cells, immune and non-immune cells. Markers in the tumor compartment comprise DNA alterations or expression of immune inhibitory ligands. Stromal- or immune-cell biomarkers are more generally phenotypic and involve changes in the level of cell populations or their functional profiles. A summary of current and potential future TME biomarkers are shown in Table 1.1. Efforts are ongoing to expand the biomarker repertoire from the TME and integrate non-redundant, independent metrics to achieve increased performance [42, 87, 88].

4.1 Validated Biomarkers in the Tumor

4.1.1 PD-L1 Expression

Expression of PD-L1 has long been considered as a biomarker for susceptibility of tumors to ICIs, and it has been investigated at great length since the advent of PD-1 axis blockers (see earlier sections of the chapter for detailed discussion of the PD-L1 pathway). There are multiple approved immunohistochemistry assays and scoring systems to detect PD-L1 expression in NSCLC. The anti-PD-1 agent pembrolizumab was approved in conjunction with a companion diagnostic test, the PD-L1 IHC 22C3 pharmDx test (Agilent Technologies). There are also FDA-approved

Table 1.1 Current and potential TME-based Immunotherapy Biomarkers for NSCLC

	Biomarker	Significance
Tumor	PD-L1 expression	Associated with increased clinical benefit to ICI
	Oncogenic driver mutations (EGFR, ALK, ROS)	Associated with reduced benefit to ICI
	Tumor mutational burden (TMB)	Associated with increased sensitivity to ICI
	Loss of function mutations in IFNγ-signaling genes	Associated with acquired resistance to ICI
	ß-2 microglobulin mutation	Associated with reduced HLA class-I expression and acquired resistance to ICI
	Wnt/ß catenin activation	Decreased *Ccl4* secretion and resistance to ICI
	LKB1 inactivation mutations	Associated with co-mutations in KRAS, low TILs and reduced sensitivity to ICI
Stroma	Increased TILs or IFNγ-related mRNA signatures	Associated with increased sensitivity to ICI
	B-cells and tertiary lymphoid structures	Associated with increased sensitivity to ICI
	Stem-like effector CD8+ TILs	Associated with increased sensitivity to ICI
	Terminal T-cell exhaustion	Associated with reduced sensitivity to ICI
	TGFß pathway upregulation	Associated with reduced sensitivity to ICI
	Alternative immune inhibitory pathways: IDO, CD73/CD39, B7-family members	Associated with reduced sensitivity to ICI

drug-specific diagnostic assays for nivolumab (Agilent PD-L1 IHC 28–8 pharmDx), atezolizumab (Ventana PD-L1 [SP142] Assay) and durvalumab (Ventana PD-L1 [SP263] Assay) [89]. PD-L1 positivity varies by assay, but is generally accepted that NSCLCs with PD-L1 expression in tumor cells benefit more from PD-1 blockade than PD-L1 negative cases [89].

PD-L1 expression is not a perfectly sensitive or specific biomarker. High PD-L1 expression is generally a marker of greater sensitivity to ICIs, but there are patients whose tumors have low or undetectable PD-L1 expression who respond to check-point inhibitor therapy and, conversely, patients with high PD-L1 expression who do not respond well to these therapies. This apparent inconsistency can be at least partially explained by technical challenges for detection/scoring of PD-L1 protein in clinical specimens. In addition, the PD1/PD-L1 pathway may be only one of many interdependent immune evasion pathways that determine the ultimate immune system response to a tumor, as described prior sections of this chapter. PD-L1 can be heavily glycosylated and one study developed a method of de-glycosylation which leads to increased detection of PD-L1 and better correlation with clinical outcomes [90]. Additionally, as noted above, multiple assays have been developed to detect PD-L1 expression levels as companion diagnostics for different ICIs; these multiple diagnostic tests make implementation of testing difficult [91]. Notably, some PD-L1 assays score only tumors cells (e.g. TPS) and other include immune cells (TC and IC). Despite these limitations, PD-L1 expression is clinically used to stratify lung cancer patients for treatments and pembrolizumab is approved for use as monotherapy in the front line setting for metastatic NSCLC with tumor PD-L1 expression $\geq$50% and as monotherapy in the second line setting for tumors with PD-L1 expression $\geq$1%. Additionally, nivolumab/ipilimumab combination therapy is approved as frontline treatment in cases with PD-L1 TPS > 1% using the 28-8 assay [92] and atezolizumab for cases with TC/IC > 10% using Sp142 [93].

4.1.2 Oncogenic Drivers

A fraction of lung adenocarcinomas harbor activating and actionable mutations in driver oncogenes, including EGFR, ALK and ROS1. It has been consistently shown that the presence of mutations in these oncogenes render tumors less sensitive to ICIs. Tumors harboring these mutations are generally associated with lower number of somatic mutations/neoantigens and T-cell infiltration [42, 94], which could explain the clinical observation. Regardless of PD-L1 expression status, patients whose tumors are EGFR mutant or ALK rearranged are not recommended in the first line setting; the use of ICIs in the second line setting for these patients is controversial [33].

4.1.3 Tumor Mutational Burden

Tumor mutational burden (TMB) has emerged as a genomic biomarker for predicting response to ICIs in multiple tumor types. TMB is defined as the total number of nonsynonymous mutations in the coding regions of genes or area of DNA covered by a specific test and is typically expressed as the number of mutations per megabase. Tumors with high TMB express large numbers of abnormal proteins, which in turn serve as neoantigens which can be recognized by the immune system [95]. The utility and optimal use of TMB as a biomarker for response to immunotherapy in lung cancer is an area of active investigation and some debate (see prior chapter for more details).

4.2   Validated Biomarkers in the Stroma

Discovery and implementation of biomarkers originating from stromal cells has been hindered by the lack of standardized methods to study these cells and the high intra-tumor variation of these signals. Emerging metrics from TILs and other immune cells have emerged as candidate biomarkers.

4.2.1 Tumor Infiltrating Lymphocytes (TILs)

TILs can be identified using multiple methods, the most common of which has been immunohistochemistry. TILs have prognostic implications in NSCLC and higher CD8 levels are consistently associated with longer survival [96]. One meta-analysis including 8600 patients demonstrated that high levels of CD8+ cells in the stroma or tumor nest was associated with improved OS in NSCLC [97]. In addition, increased levels of TILs in pre-treatment tumor samples is strongly associated with better outcomes after ICI in NSCLC and melanoma [96, 98]. It has been proposed that immune cell infiltrates be integrated into a tumor-node-metastasis-immunoscore (TNM-I) system in a clinical setting, similar to the fields of colorectal cancer and breast cancer [99]. However, the predictive value of these proposed scores for ICI has not been demonstrated. The possible role of TILs as an independent predictive immunotherapy biomarker is also somewhat limited by its positive association with PD-L1 expression.

4.2.2 T-Cell RNA Signatures

Integration of T-cell and IFNγ-related signals using bulk tumor RNA profiling has been pursued as predictive ICI biomarker. Multiple signatures including different numbers and types of markers have been explored. One study has developed a method to analyze targeted gene expression profiles to quantify the T-cell "richness" of a TME. The assay was developed using data from various clinical trials of patients treated with PD-1 axis blockers and a commercial RNA analysis platform for clinical-grade implementation [100]. To date, mRNA-based immune-related assays have not been validated prospectively or approved for clinical use. T-cell inflamed gene expression profile has also been combined with TMB to stratify patients and predict clinical response to pembrolizumab with higher accuracy [88].

4.2.3 Developing Biomarkers

Interferon Gamma Response Pathway

The IFNγ pathway is integral to the immune response. As described earlier in this chapter, T-cells produce this cytokine as part of the anti-tumor response. IFNγ then binds to cell surface receptors which activate the JAK/STAT pathway, leading to antiproliferative responses in tumor cells and immune regulatory adaptations such as PD-L1 expression. Therefore, integrity of the pathway is considered as important for response to PD-1 axis blockers. Consistent with this notion, mutations in the JAK/STAT pathway have been identified in tumors from patients with acquired resistance to ICIs [33]. A defective JAK/STAT pathway in tumor cells could also limit antigen presentation and reduce the activity of immunostimulatory therapies relying on T-cell recognition and killing.

Beta-2-Microglobulin Alterations

Previous studies have identified 27–49% of NSCLCs lack HLA-I expression; another 47% were found in one study to have focal HLA-I downregulation [101, 102]. Beta-2-microglobulin is the invariant chain of the MHC class-I complex, and alterations in this protein can lead to resistance to ICI [33]. The prominent role of antigen presentation in NSCLC is also supported by the fact that HLA class I heavy chain down regulation and lack of beta-2 microglobulin expression is associated with a statistically worse prognosis even in the absence of immunotherapy [101]. Notably HLA class-I defects in tumor cells can occur as a consequence of both genomic and non-genomic mechanisms, which makes their assessment in clinical specimens difficult. The potential clinical role of HLA markers as predictive markers for immunotherapy in NSCLC is under investigation.

DNA Sensing Alterations: LKB1

LKB1/STK11 plays a role in the regulation of cellular metabolism and growth. Inactivating mutations in this gene have been demonstrated to confer an "immune cold" TME characterized by reduced infiltration of CD8+ T cells and lower PD-L1 expression. Clinically, it has been demonstrated that co-mutations in *KRAS* and *LKB1* are associated with low response rates to ICIs in lung cancer. In a mouse model, *LKB1* deletion was shown to induce resistance to PD-1 blockade, supporting a causal relationship [34]. The relative low frequency of cases with LKB1/KRAS co-mutation and the strong association with TILs and PD-L1 could potentially limit its use as an independent immunotherapy biomarker.

FBXW7

FBXW7 is a tumor suppressor gene which is mutated in ~6% of tumors, including lung cancer. It is located at chromosome 4q32, which is deleted in >30% of human malignancies [103]. Inactivating mutations in this gene lead to dysfunction of a ubiquitin ligase complex; the downstream result of this change is increase in cell proliferation proteins including MYC, cyclin D1 and JUN [35]. FBXW7 loss has been recently demonstrated to confer resistance to anti-PD-1 therapy in animal models and is associated with an altered immune environment [35]. Although not yet ready for integration into routine clinical practice, these results suggest a promising role for this biomarker in the future.

TGFß Pathway

Overexpression of TGFß has been demonstrated to be one mechanism by which tumor cells evade immune system recognition and killing [104], and it is hypothesized that some of these effects are due to its effect on CAFs [105]. Since TGFß can suppress T-cell activation and differentiation, immune checkpoint therapy combined with TGFß inhibition is being investigated for potential synergy [105]. It is also being investigated as a potential prognostic biomarker. One meta-analysis found that TGFß overexpression is associated with lower survival rates in NSCLC [104], but this biomarker needs further validation before integration into standard clinical practice. Recent studies suggest a negative predictive role of a TGFß RNA signature in patients with advanced urothelial carcinoma treated with the anti PD-L1 agent atezolizumab [106]. Expansion of the use of this signature to other tumor types, including NSCLC is expected.

Activation of Alternative Immune Pathways

It is expected that a fraction of NSCLCs evade immunity through alternative pathways unrelated to PD-1/PD-L1 or CTLA-4 and would therefore be insensitive to clinically approved ICIs. Upregulation of alternative immune suppressive molecules serving as the dominant immune escape mechanism could potentially be used as predictive biomarker. In this regard, IDO-1 expression in tumors has been proposed as a candidate biomarker of resistance to anti-PD-1 treatment in NSCLC [107]. Upregulation of additional B7-family members with immunoregulatory functions, described earlier in the chapter, is also expected and could serve as biomarkers in the future [15].

Microbiome

There has been increasing emphasis on the role of the microbiome in a multitude of diseases, and cancer is no exception. There is evidence that gut bacteria can affect the response to immunotherapy, and patients treated with antibiotics have decreased benefit of ICIs. Analysis of NSCLC patient stool samples at the time of diagnosis showed that there is a correlation between response to ICIs and the level of *Akkermansia muciniphila* in the stool, suggesting that the gut microbiome plays a role in this effect. The same group transplanted fecal microbiota from patients who responded to ICIs and those who didn't into germ-free mice. The mice were then inoculated with tumor cells and treated with anti-PD-1 therapy. Notably, mice who had been inoculated with fecal microbiota from ICI responders were sensitive to treatment, and those inoculated with fecal microbiota from non-responders were not [108]. Although these, and other, results are thought-provoking, further research is necessary to elucidate the role of the microbiome in the TME and its potential for use as a non-invasive biomarker.

Immune Heterogeneity

Another area of active investigation and potential impact for the development of biomarkers is the degree of immune heterogeneity within an individual's tumor. It has been found that the TME can vary widely in different parts of a tumor and that much of this heterogeneity is non-genetic [109]. One group analyzed surgical biopsies from NSCLC patients using whole exome sequencing, transcriptome profiling, and T-cell repertoire analysis and found that the TME was as varied within a single patient as it was between patients [110]. These findings suggest that analyses of tumor/immune-cell metrics such as PD-L1, TILs or TMB performed on biopsy specimens may not be reflective of the larger unsampled TME in other parts of the patient's tumor. Deciphering the contribution and clinical significance of tumor immune heterogeneity will be key to support progress in this field.

5 Conclusions

Understanding the TME is one of the most prominent challenges in immune-oncology and is likely to support new clinical developments. Immune activation against cancer is inevitably linked with multiple immune suppressive processes that can occur in more than one cell type and tumor tissue compartment. Identification of the dominant mechanisms mediating immune evasion in a particular tumor and context will be required to inform optimal therapeutic decisions and enhance patient outcomes. Emerging technologies and platforms for quantitative tumor tissue visualization using multiple markers/analytes, non-invasive diagnostics and molecular imaging/radiology allow for more detailed studies and assessment of dynamic features that can report on biologically relevant tumor molecular and immune adaptations. Development of molecular biomarkers for immunotherapy based on the TME is a rapidly evolving field, and incorporation of this information into clinical research will support making informed interventions and realizing the full potential of anti-cancer immunotherapy.

References

1. Hodi FS et al (2010) Improved survival with ipilimumab in patients with metastatic melanoma. N Engl J Med 363:711–723. https://doi.org/10.1056/NEJMoa1003466
2. Ascierto PA et al (2019) Survival outcomes in patients with previously untreated BRAF wild-type advanced melanoma treated with Nivolumab therapy: three-year follow-up of a randomized phase 3 trial. JAMA Oncol 5:187–194. https://doi.org/10.1001/jamaoncol.2018.4514
3. Robert C et al (2015) Nivolumab in previously untreated melanoma without BRAF mutation. N Engl J Med 372:320–330. https://doi.org/10.1056/NEJMoa1412082
4. Wolchok JD et al (2017) Overall survival with combined Nivolumab and Ipilimumab in advanced melanoma. N Engl J Med 377:1345–1356. https://doi.org/10.1056/NEJMoa1709684

5. Gong J, Chehrazi-Raffle A, Reddi S, Salgia R (2018) Development of PD-1 and PD-L1 inhibitors as a form of cancer immunotherapy: a comprehensive review of registration trials and future considerations. J Immunother Cancer 6:8. https://doi.org/10.1186/s40425-018-0316-z

6. Berghmans T, Durieux V, Hendriks LEL, Dingemans AM (2020) Immunotherapy: from advanced NSCLC to early stages, an evolving concept. Front Med (Lausanne) 7:90. https://doi.org/10.3389/fmed.2020.00090

7. Schizas D et al (2020) Immunotherapy for pancreatic cancer: a 2020 update. Cancer Treat Rev 86:102016. https://doi.org/10.1016/j.ctrv.2020.102016

8. Golshani G, Zhang Y (2020) Advances in immunotherapy for colorectal cancer: a review. Ther Adv Gastroenterol 13:1756284820917527. https://doi.org/10.1177/1756284820917527

9. Vitkin N, Nersesian S, Siemens DR, Koti M (2019) The tumor immune contexture of prostate Cancer. Front Immunol 10:603. https://doi.org/10.3389/fimmu.2019.00603

10. Garcia-Diaz A et al (2017) Interferon receptor signaling pathways regulating PD-L1 and PD-L2 expression. Cell Rep 19:1189–1201. https://doi.org/10.1016/j.celrep.2017.04.031

11. Altan M et al (2017) B7-H3 expression in NSCLC and its association with B7-H4, PD-L1 and tumor-infiltrating lymphocytes. Clin Cancer Res 23:5202–5209. https://doi.org/10.1158/1078-0432.CCR-16-3107

12. Carvajal-Hausdorf D et al (2019) Expression and clinical significance of PD-L1, B7-H3, B7-H4 and TILs in human small cell lung Cancer (SCLC). J Immunother Cancer 7:65. https://doi.org/10.1186/s40425-019-0540-1

13. Ni L, Dong C (2017) New B7 family checkpoints in human cancers. Mol Cancer Ther 16:1203–1211. https://doi.org/10.1158/1535-7163.MCT-16-0761

14. Schalper KA et al (2017) Differential expression and significance of PD-L1, IDO-1, and B7-H4 in human lung cancer. Clin Cancer Res 23:370–378. https://doi.org/10.1158/1078-0432.CCR-16-0150

15. Zang X et al (2003) B7x: a widely expressed B7 family member that inhibits T cell activation. Proc Natl Acad Sci U S A 100:10388–10392. https://doi.org/10.1073/pnas.1434299100

16. Villarroel-Espindola F et al (2018) Spatially resolved and quantitative analysis of VISTA/PD-1H as a novel immunotherapy target in human non-small cell lung cancer. Clin Cancer Res 24:1562–1573. https://doi.org/10.1158/1078-0432.CCR-17-2542

17. Johnston RJ et al (2019) VISTA is an acidic pH-selective ligand for PSGL-1. Nature 574:565–570. https://doi.org/10.1038/s41586-019-1674-5

18. Liu M et al (2018) Targeting the IDO1 pathway in cancer: from bench to bedside. J Hematol Oncol 11:100. https://doi.org/10.1186/s13045-018-0644-y

19. Leone RD, Emens LA (2018) Targeting adenosine for cancer immunotherapy. J Immunother Cancer 6:57. https://doi.org/10.1186/s40425-018-0360-8

20. Tsukamoto H et al (2018) Immune-suppressive effects of interleukin-6 on T-cell-mediated anti-tumor immunity. Cancer Sci 109:523–530. https://doi.org/10.1111/cas.13433

21. David JM, Dominguez C, Hamilton DH, Palena C (2016) The IL-8/IL-8R Axis: a double agent in tumor immune resistance. Vaccines (Basel) 4. https://doi.org/10.3390/vaccines4030022

22. Fisher DT, Appenheimer MM, Evans SS (2014) The two faces of IL-6 in the tumor microenvironment. Semin Immunol 26:38–47. https://doi.org/10.1016/j.smim.2014.01.008

23. Schalper KA et al (2020) Elevated serum interleukin-8 is associated with enhanced intratumor neutrophils and reduced clinical benefit of immune-checkpoint inhibitors. Nat Med 26:688–692. https://doi.org/10.1038/s41591-020-0856-x

24. Teijeira A et al (2020) CXCR1 and CXCR2 Chemokine Receptor agonists produced by tumors induce neutrophil extracellular traps that interfere with immune cytotoxicity. Immunity 52:856–871 e858. https://doi.org/10.1016/j.immuni.2020.03.001

25. Leone P et al (2013) MHC class I antigen processing and presenting machinery: organization, function, and defects in tumor cells. J Natl Cancer Inst 105:1172–1187. https://doi.org/10.1093/jnci/djt184

26. Gettinger S et al (2017) Impaired HLA class I antigen processing and presentation as a mechanism of acquired resistance to immune checkpoint inhibitors in lung cancer. Cancer Discov 7:1420–1435. https://doi.org/10.1158/2159-8290.CD-17-0593

27. Zaretsky JM et al (2016) Mutations associated with acquired resistance to PD-1 blockade in melanoma. N Engl J Med 375:819–829. https://doi.org/10.1056/NEJMoa1604958
28. Sade-Feldman M et al (2017) Resistance to checkpoint blockade therapy through inactivation of antigen presentation. Nat Commun 8:1136. https://doi.org/10.1038/s41467-017-01062-w
29. Seliger B, Ferrone S (2020) HLA class I antigen processing machinery defects in cancer cells-frequency, functional significance, and clinical relevance with special emphasis on their role in T cell-based immunotherapy of malignant disease. Methods Mol Biol 2055:325–350. https://doi.org/10.1007/978-1-4939-9773-2_15
30. Trujillo JA et al (2019) Secondary resistance to immunotherapy associated with beta-catenin pathway activation or PTEN loss in metastatic melanoma. J Immunother Cancer 7:295. https://doi.org/10.1186/s40425-019-0780-0
31. Luke JJ, Bao R, Sweis RF, Spranger S, Gajewski TF (2019) WNT/beta-catenin pathway activation correlates with immune exclusion across human cancers. Clin Cancer Res 25:3074–3083. https://doi.org/10.1158/1078-0432.CCR-18-1942
32. Zhan T, Rindtorff N, Boutros M (2017) Wnt signaling in cancer. Oncogene 36:1461–1473. https://doi.org/10.1038/onc.2016.304
33. Blons H, Garinet S, Laurent-Puig P, Oudart JB (2019) Molecular markers and prediction of response to immunotherapy in non-small cell lung cancer, an update. J Thorac Dis 11:S25–S36. https://doi.org/10.21037/jtd.2018.12.48
34. Skoulidis F et al (2018) STK11/LKB1 mutations and PD-1 inhibitor resistance in KRAS-mutant lung adenocarcinoma. Cancer Discov 8:822–835. https://doi.org/10.1158/2159-8290.CD-18-0099
35. Gstalder C et al (2020) Inactivation of Fbxw7 impairs dsRNA sensing and confers resistance to PD-1 blockade. Cancer Discov 10:1296–1311. https://doi.org/10.1158/2159-8290.CD-19-1416
36. Taube JM et al (2018) Implications of the tumor immune microenvironment for staging and therapeutics. Mod Pathol 31:214–234. https://doi.org/10.1038/modpathol.2017.156
37. Jiang T et al (2019) Tumor neoantigens: from basic research to clinical applications. J Hematol Oncol 12:93. https://doi.org/10.1186/s13045-019-0787-5
38. Sade-Feldman M et al (2018) Defining T cell states associated with response to checkpoint immunotherapy in melanoma. Cell 175:998–1013 e1020. https://doi.org/10.1016/j.cell.2018.10.038
39. Wherry EJ, Kurachi M (2015) Molecular and cellular insights into T cell exhaustion. Nat Rev Immunol 15:486–499. https://doi.org/10.1038/nri3862
40. Philip M, Schietinger A (2019) Heterogeneity and fate choice: T cell exhaustion in cancer and chronic infections. Curr Opin Immunol 58:98–103. https://doi.org/10.1016/j.coi.2019.04.014
41. Datar I et al (2019) Expression analysis and significance of PD-1, LAG-3, and TIM-3 in human non-small cell lung cancer using spatially resolved and multiparametric single-cell analysis. Clin Cancer Res 25:4663–4673. https://doi.org/10.1158/1078-0432.CCR-18-4142
42. Gettinger SN et al (2018) A dormant TIL phenotype defines non-small cell lung carcinomas sensitive to immune checkpoint blockers. Nat Commun 9:3196. https://doi.org/10.1038/s41467-018-05032-8
43. Fridman WH, Pages F, Sautes-Fridman C, Galon J (2012) The immune contexture in human tumours: impact on clinical outcome. Nat Rev Cancer 12:298–306. https://doi.org/10.1038/nrc3245
44. Ganguli P, Sarkar RR (2018) Exploring immuno-regulatory mechanisms in the tumor microenvironment: model and design of protocols for cancer remission. PLoS One 13:e0203030. https://doi.org/10.1371/journal.pone.0203030
45. Rivera Vargas T, Humblin E, Vegran F, Ghiringhelli F, Apetoh L (2017) TH9 cells in anti-tumor immunity. Semin Immunopathol 39:39–46. https://doi.org/10.1007/s00281-016-0599-4
46. Salazar Y et al (2020) Microenvironmental Th9 and Th17 lymphocytes induce metastatic spreading in lung cancer. J Clin Invest 130:3560–3575. https://doi.org/10.1172/JCI124037

47. Chen T et al (2020) Th9 cell differentiation and its dual effects in tumor development. Front Immunol 11:1026. https://doi.org/10.3389/fimmu.2020.01026
48. Voigt C et al (2017) Cancer cells induce interleukin-22 production from memory CD4(+) T cells via interleukin-1 to promote tumor growth. Proc Natl Acad Sci U S A 114:12994–12999. https://doi.org/10.1073/pnas.1705165114
49. Ng KW et al (2018) Somatic mutation-associated T follicular helper cell elevation in lung adenocarcinoma. Onco Targets Ther 7:e1504728. https://doi.org/10.1080/2162402X.2018.1504728
50. Balkwill FR, Capasso M, Hagemann T (2012) The tumor microenvironment at a glance. J Cell Sci 125:5591–5596. https://doi.org/10.1242/jcs.116392
51. Kotsakis A et al (2016) Prognostic value of circulating regulatory T cell subsets in untreated non-small cell lung cancer patients. Sci Rep 6:39247. https://doi.org/10.1038/srep39247
52. Neeve SC, Robinson BW, Fear VS (2019) The role and therapeutic implications of T cells in cancer of the lung. Clin Transl Immunol 8:e1076. https://doi.org/10.1002/cti2.1076
53. Petersen RP et al (2006) Tumor infiltrating Foxp3+ regulatory T-cells are associated with recurrence in pathologic stage I NSCLC patients. Cancer 107:2866–2872. https://doi.org/10.1002/cncr.22282
54. Shimizu K et al (2010) Tumor-infiltrating Foxp3+ regulatory T cells are correlated with cyclooxygenase-2 expression and are associated with recurrence in resected non-small cell lung cancer. J Thorac Oncol 5:585–590. https://doi.org/10.1097/JTO.0b013e3181d60fd7
55. Wang SS et al (2019) Tumor-infiltrating B cells: their role and application in anti-tumor immunity in lung cancer. Cell Mol Immunol 16:6–18. https://doi.org/10.1038/s41423-018-0027-x
56. Sautes-Fridman C et al (2016) Tertiary lymphoid structures in cancers: prognostic value, regulation, and manipulation for therapeutic intervention. Front Immunol 7:407. https://doi.org/10.3389/fimmu.2016.00407
57. Schalper KA et al (2015) Objective measurement and clinical significance of TILs in non-small cell lung cancer. J Natl Cancer Inst 107. https://doi.org/10.1093/jnci/dju435
58. Yuen GJ, Demissie E, Pillai S (2016) B lymphocytes and cancer: a love-hate relationship. Trends Cancer 2:747–757. https://doi.org/10.1016/j.trecan.2016.10.010
59. Zhang Y, Gallastegui N, Rosenblatt JD (2015) Regulatory B cells in anti-tumor immunity. Int Immunol 27:521–530. https://doi.org/10.1093/intimm/dxv034
60. Gentles AJ et al (2015) The prognostic landscape of genes and infiltrating immune cells across human cancers. Nat Med 21:938–945. https://doi.org/10.1038/nm.3909
61. Cong J, Wei H (2019) Natural killer cells in the lungs. Front Immunol 10:1416. https://doi.org/10.3389/fimmu.2019.01416
62. Zugazagoitia J et al (2020) Biomarkers associated with beneficial PD-1 checkpoint blockade in Non-Small Cell Lung Cancer (NSCLC) identified using high-Plex digital spatial profiling. Clin Cancer Res 26:4360–4368. https://doi.org/10.1158/1078-0432.CCR-20-0175
63. Mantovani A, Marchesi F, Malesci A, Laghi L, Allavena P (2017) Tumour-associated macrophages as treatment targets in oncology. Nat Rev Clin Oncol 14:399–416. https://doi.org/10.1038/nrclinonc.2016.217
64. Pathria P, Louis TL, Varner JA (2019) Targeting tumor-associated macrophages in cancer. Trends Immunol 40:310–327. https://doi.org/10.1016/j.it.2019.02.003
65. Liu Y et al (2020) Immune cell PD-L1 Colocalizes with macrophages and is associated with outcome in PD-1 pathway blockade therapy. Clin Cancer Res 26:970–977. https://doi.org/10.1158/1078-0432.CCR-19-1040
66. Zhang QW et al (2012) Prognostic significance of tumor-associated macrophages in solid tumor: a meta-analysis of the literature. PLoS One 7:e50946. https://doi.org/10.1371/journal.pone.0050946
67. Veglia F, Perego M, Gabrilovich D (2018) Myeloid-derived suppressor cells coming of age. Nat Immunol 19:108–119. https://doi.org/10.1038/s41590-017-0022-x
68. Gabrilovich D, Myeloid-Derived I (2017) Suppressor Cells. Cancer Immunol Res 5:3–8. https://doi.org/10.1158/2326-6066.CIR-16-0297

69. Fu C, Jiang A (2018) Dendritic cells and CD8 T cell immunity in tumor microenvironment. Front Immunol 9:3059. https://doi.org/10.3389/fimmu.2018.03059
70. Tran Janco JM, Lamichhane P, Karyampudi L, Knutson KL (2015) Tumor-infiltrating dendritic cells in cancer pathogenesis. J Immunol 194:2985–2991. https://doi.org/10.4049/jimmunol.1403134
71. Shaul ME, Fridlender ZG (2019) Tumour-associated neutrophils in patients with cancer. Nat Rev Clin Oncol 16:601–620. https://doi.org/10.1038/s41571-019-0222-4
72. Sanmamed MF et al (2017) Changes in serum interleukin-8 (IL-8) levels reflect and predict response to anti-PD-1 treatment in melanoma and non-small-cell lung cancer patients. Ann Oncol 28:1988–1995. https://doi.org/10.1093/annonc/mdx190
73. Lambrechts D et al (2018) Phenotype molding of stromal cells in the lung tumor microenvironment. Nat Med 24:1277–1289. https://doi.org/10.1038/s41591-018-0096-5
74. Kalluri R (2016) The biology and function of fibroblasts in cancer. Nat Rev Cancer 16:582–598. https://doi.org/10.1038/nrc.2016.73
75. Cruz-Bermudez A et al (2019) Cancer-associated fibroblasts modify lung cancer metabolism involving ROS and TGF-beta signaling. Free Radic Biol Med 130:163–173. https://doi.org/10.1016/j.freeradbiomed.2018.10.450
76. Erez N, Truitt M, Olson P, Arron ST, Hanahan D (2010) Cancer-associated fibroblasts are activated in incipient neoplasia to orchestrate tumor-promoting inflammation in an NF-kappaB-dependent manner. Cancer Cell 17:135–147. https://doi.org/10.1016/j.ccr.2009.12.041
77. Alcaraz J et al (2019) Stromal markers of activated tumor associated fibroblasts predict poor survival and are associated with necrosis in non-small cell lung cancer. Lung Cancer 135:151–160. https://doi.org/10.1016/j.lungcan.2019.07.020
78. Paiva AE et al (2018) Pericytes in the premetastatic niche. Cancer Res 78:2779–2786. https://doi.org/10.1158/0008-5472.CAN-17-3883
79. Murgai M et al (2017) KLF4-dependent perivascular cell plasticity mediates pre-metastatic niche formation and metastasis. Nat Med 23:1176–1190. https://doi.org/10.1038/nm.4400
80. Kim KS et al (2019) ELK3 expressed in lymphatic endothelial cells promotes breast cancer progression and metastasis through exosomal miRNAs. Sci Rep 9:8418. https://doi.org/10.1038/s41598-019-44828-6
81. Hendry SA et al (2016) The role of the tumor vasculature in the host immune response: implications for therapeutic strategies targeting the tumor microenvironment. Front Immunol 7:621. https://doi.org/10.3389/fimmu.2016.00621
82. Jain RK (2005) Normalization of tumor vasculature: an emerging concept in antiangiogenic therapy. Science 307:58–62. https://doi.org/10.1126/science.1104819
83. Eble JA, Niland S (2019) The extracellular matrix in tumor progression and metastasis. Clin Exp Metastasis 36:171–198. https://doi.org/10.1007/s10585-019-09966-1
84. Walker C, Mojares E, Del Rio Hernandez A (2018) Role of extracellular matrix in development and cancer progression. Int J Mol Sci 19. https://doi.org/10.3390/ijms19103028
85. Poltavets V, Kochetkova M, Pitson SM, Samuel MS (2018) The role of the extracellular matrix and its molecular and cellular regulators in cancer cell plasticity. Front Oncol 8:431. https://doi.org/10.3389/fonc.2018.00431
86. Salmon H, Donnadieu E (2012) Within tumors, interactions between T cells and tumor cells are impeded by the extracellular matrix. Onco Targets Ther 1:992–994. https://doi.org/10.4161/onci.20239
87. Rizvi H et al (2018) Molecular determinants of response to anti-programmed cell death (PD)-1 and anti-programmed death-ligand 1 (PD-L1) blockade in patients with non-small-cell lung cancer profiled with targeted next-generation sequencing. J Clin Oncol 36:633–641. https://doi.org/10.1200/JCO.2017.75.3384
88. Cristescu R et al (2018) Pan-tumor genomic biomarkers for PD-1 checkpoint blockade-based immunotherapy. Science 362. https://doi.org/10.1126/science.aar3593
89. Velcheti V et al (2018) Real-world PD-L1 testing and distribution of PD-L1 tumor expression by immunohistochemistry assay type among patients with metastatic non-small cell

lung cancer in the United States. PLoS One 13:e0206370. https://doi.org/10.1371/journal.pone.0206370

90. Lee HH et al (2019) Removal of N-linked glycosylation enhances PD-L1 detection and predicts anti-PD-1/PD-L1 therapeutic efficacy. Cancer Cell 36:168–178 e164. https://doi.org/10.1016/j.ccell.2019.06.008

91. Kerr K, The M (2018) PD-L1 immunohistochemistry biomarker: two steps forward, one step Back? J Thorac Oncol 13:291–294. https://doi.org/10.1016/j.jtho.2018.01.020

92. Hellmann MD et al (2019) Nivolumab plus Ipilimumab in advanced non-small-cell lung cancer. N Engl J Med 381:2020–2031. https://doi.org/10.1056/NEJMoa1910231

93. Herbst RS et al (2020) Atezolizumab for first-line treatment of PD-L1-selected patients with NSCLC. N Engl J Med 383:1328–1339. https://doi.org/10.1056/NEJMoa1917346

94. Toki MI et al (2018) Immune marker profiling and programmed death ligand 1 expression across NSCLC mutations. J Thorac Oncol 13:1884–1896. https://doi.org/10.1016/j.jtho.2018.09.012

95. Berland L et al (2019) Current views on tumor mutational burden in patients with non-small cell lung cancer treated by immune checkpoint inhibitors. J Thorac Dis 11:S71–S80. https://doi.org/10.21037/jtd.2018.11.102

96. Fumet JD et al (2018) Prognostic and predictive role of CD8 and PD-L1 determination in lung tumor tissue of patients under anti-PD-1 therapy. Br J Cancer 119:950–960. https://doi.org/10.1038/s41416-018-0220-9

97. Geng Y et al (2015) Prognostic role of tumor-infiltrating lymphocytes in lung cancer: a meta-analysis. Cell Physiol Biochem 37:1560–1571. https://doi.org/10.1159/000438523

98. Wong PF et al (2019) Multiplex quantitative analysis of tumor-infiltrating lymphocytes and immunotherapy outcome in metastatic melanoma. Clin Cancer Res 25:2442–2449. https://doi.org/10.1158/1078-0432.CCR-18-2652

99. Donnem T et al (2016) Strategies for clinical implementation of TNM-Immunoscore in resected nonsmall-cell lung cancer. Ann Oncol 27:225–232. https://doi.org/10.1093/annonc/mdv560

100. Ayers M et al (2017) IFN-gamma-related mRNA profile predicts clinical response to PD-1 blockade. J Clin Invest 127:2930–2940. https://doi.org/10.1172/JCI91190

101. Ichinokawa K et al (2019) Downregulated expression of human leukocyte antigen class I heavy chain is associated with poor prognosis in non-small-cell lung cancer. Oncol Lett 18:117–126. https://doi.org/10.3892/ol.2019.10293

102. Perea F et al (2017) The absence of HLA class I expression in non-small cell lung cancer correlates with the tumor tissue structure and the pattern of T cell infiltration. Int J Cancer 140:888–899. https://doi.org/10.1002/ijc.30489

103. Yeh CH, Bellon M, Nicot C (2018) FBXW7: a critical tumor suppressor of human cancers. Mol Cancer 17:115. https://doi.org/10.1186/s12943-018-0857-2

104. Li J et al (2019) Prognostic value of TGF-beta in lung cancer: systematic review and meta-analysis. BMC Cancer 19:691. https://doi.org/10.1186/s12885-019-5917-5

105. Ganesh K, Massague J (2018) TGF-beta inhibition and immunotherapy: checkmate. Immunity 48:626–628. https://doi.org/10.1016/j.immuni.2018.03.037

106. Mariathasan S et al (2018) TGFbeta attenuates tumour response to PD-L1 blockade by contributing to exclusion of T cells. Nature 554:544–548. https://doi.org/10.1038/nature25501

107. Botticelli A et al (2018) Can IDO activity predict primary resistance to anti-PD-1 treatment in NSCLC? J Transl Med 16:219. https://doi.org/10.1186/s12967-018-1595-3

108. Routy B et al (2018) Gut microbiome influences efficacy of PD-1-based immunotherapy against epithelial tumors. Science 359:91–97. https://doi.org/10.1126/science.aan3706

109. Sharma A et al (2019) Non-genetic intra-tumor heterogeneity is a major predictor of phenotypic heterogeneity and ongoing evolutionary dynamics in lung tumors. Cell Rep 29:2164–2174 e2165. https://doi.org/10.1016/j.celrep.2019.10.045

110. Jia Q et al (2018) Local mutational diversity drives intratumoral immune heterogeneity in non-small cell lung cancer. Nat Commun 9:5361. https://doi.org/10.1038/s41467-018-07767-w

Chapter 2
Biomarkers: Is Tumor Mutational Burden the New Prognostic Grail?

Natalie I. Vokes and Mark M. Awad

Abstract Immune checkpoint inhibitors (ICI) have improved outcomes for patients with advanced non-small cell lung cancer (NSCLC). However, only a minority of patients experience benefit, and biomarkers of response are needed to improve patient selection. Tumor mutational burden (TMB), defined as the number of somatic mutations in a tumor, has been identified as a potential predictive biomarker. Studies assessing TMB and outcome in NSCLC have demonstrated improved response rates and progression-free survival to ICIs in patients with higher TMB compared to lower TMB, and patients with high TMB have a higher likelihood of benefit to ICI compared to chemotherapy. However, TMB imperfectly stratifies responders from non-responders, and these data are heterogenous with respect to treatment context, drug, TMB assay, and TMB threshold. Importantly, many of these analyses are retrospective, and few prospective clinical trials implementing TMB as a biomarker have been completed. Additional limitations to the implementation of TMB include the need for adequate tissue to perform sequencing, and heterogeneity in TMB assays. Efforts to develop blood-based TMB assays and standardization procedures may help address these limitations. Finally, further research to understand why TMB associates with response, and how TMB interacts with other biomarkers including PD-L1 and interferon-gamma expression, may help improve its predictive power.

Keywords Tumor mutational burden · Immunotherapy · PD-1 · PD-L1 · CTLA-4 · Biomarker · Immune checkpoint inhibitor · Neoantigen

N. I. Vokes
Dana-Farber Cancer Institute, Harvard Medical School, Boston, MA, USA

Broad Institute, Cambridge, MA, USA

M. M. Awad (✉)
Dana-Farber Cancer Institute, Harvard Medical School, Boston, MA, USA
e-mail: mark_awad@dfci.harvard.edu

© Springer Nature Switzerland AG 2021
A. C. Chiang, R. S. Herbst (eds.), *Lung Cancer*, Current Cancer Research,
https://doi.org/10.1007/978-3-030-74028-3_2

1 Introduction

The treatment of non-small cell lung cancer (NSCLC) has changed dramatically over the last 15 years. The development of biomarker-driven therapies, such as agents targeting *EGFR* and *BRAF* mutations and *ALK* and *ROS1* rearrangements, helped initiate the era of 'precision oncology' and has improved outcomes in patients harboring these alterations [1–9]. However, these therapies only benefit the subset of patients harboring a targetable alteration, and the majority of cancers treated with targeted therapies will develop resistance, making further therapeutic approaches necessary.

More recently, immune checkpoint inhibitors (ICIs) targeting cytotoxic T-lymphocyte-associated protein 4 (CTLA-4), programmed cell death 1 (PD-1), and its ligand PD-L1, have improved outcomes in patients with advanced NSCLC in both the upfront and relapsed settings [10–14]. Particularly notable have been the prolonged, durable responses that occur in a subset of patients which can persist for years, even off therapy, representing an unprecedented outcome in the treatment of solid tumors. Unfortunately, however, response rates to ICIs in patients with NSCLC are as low as 20% in the relapsed setting [10–12], and only 16–38% experience prolonged overall survival (OS) lasting three years or longer [15–17]. This discrepancy between the magnitude of potential benefit and its limited scope has generated considerable interest in applying the framework of precision medicine to immunotherapy, with the hope of identifying biomarkers that can improve patient selection and provide a rational framework for subsequent clinical trial design.

Initial biomarker analyses focused on markers of immune activity [18–21]. In that context PD-L1 expression by immunohistochemistry was found to correlate with response [12, 22] was the first FDA-approved biomarker in NSCLC. However, PD-L1 expression has proven an imperfect response predictor. The predictive utility of PD-L1 has varied across trials, and even among patients with PD-L1 expression ≥50%, response rates to pembrolizumab are only 30–45% [12, 13], suggesting that additional features modulate differential response to ICIs.

Concurrent with these immune-focused analyses, ongoing large-scale cancer sequencing efforts had identified genomic differences across cancers, including differences in the number of mutations within and across tumor types (Fig. 2.1) [23, 24]. These analyses, coupled with the observation that ICIs were active in highly mutated cancers such as melanoma and NSCLC, led to the hypothesis that these cancer-specific or somatic alterations could mediate the tumor-immune interaction by giving rise to novel epitopes (termed neo-antigens) [25–27]. These findings raised the possibility that number of somatic mutations in a tumor, or tumor mutational burden (TMB), might associate with better outcomes to immune checkpoint inhibitors.

Multiple studies have now confirmed this association, though the application to clinical practice remains under investigation. In this chapter, we present the evidence linking TMB and ICI outcomes, and further discuss TMB as a predictive biomarker, barriers to clinical application, and remaining questions about TMB and its association with ICI response.

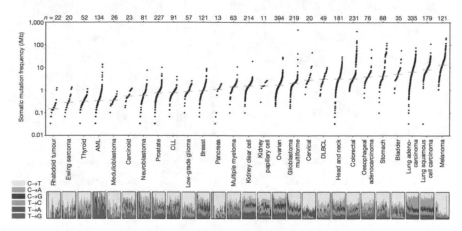

Fig. 2.1 Somatic mutation frequencies observed in exomes from 3083 tumor-normal pairs. Each point corresponds to a tumor-normal pair. The y-axis indicates the number of somatic mutations in each sample, the x-axis indicates the tumor type. Tumor types are ordered by median number of somatic mutations. Tumor types in which immune checkpoint inhibitors are active include melanoma, non-small cell lung cancer, bladder cancer, gastroesophageal cancer, and head and neck cancer, which tend to have higher numbers of somatic mutations. (Reproduced from Lawrence et al. [23])

2   Definition of TMB and TMB Assessment Methods

Most fundamentally, TMB describes the number of somatic mutations in a tumor. Because TMB is thought to associate with response to ICIs by the formation of neoantigens, TMB typically is defined as the number of protein-altering or nonsynonymous mutations. The earliest studies assessed TMB by performing whole exome sequencing (WES) on tumor/normal pairs and summing the number of somatic nonsynonymous mutations. However, the utility of whole exome sequencing in routine clinical practice is limited due to time and expense [28, 29], and, increasingly, targeted next-generation sequencing (NGS) panels have been used to calculate TMB. To enable these comparisons, TMB is now commonly expressed as number of mutations per megabase (Mb) sequenced, thereby adjusting for assay differences in how much of the genome is assessed (typically ~30 Mb in WES, 0.5–1.5 Mb in targeted panels).

Several initial *in silico* analyses validated TMB calculation via targeted panel by demonstrating high correlation between TMB obtained directly from WES, and TMB inferred from the subset of genes contained within the targeted panels ($r^2 > 0.9$) [28, 30–32]. Importantly, these *in silico* analyses demonstrated that the strength of the correlation depended on the size of the gene panel and the number of mutations detected; smaller gene panels and low TMB tumors were associated with higher deviation in the predicted TMB from the actual TMB [31, 30], suggesting that a minimum panel length of 0.8 Mb or higher is necessary for accurate quantification (Fig. 2.2). Additional work directly sequencing the same tumor samples by

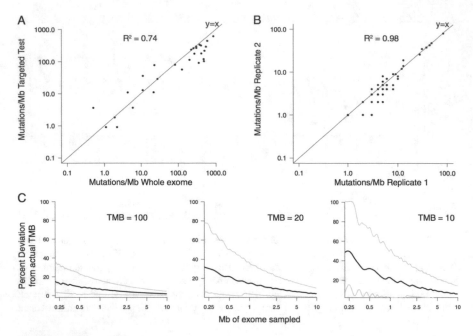

Fig. 2.2 Accuracy and precision of targeted panel sequencing compared to whole exome sequencing (WES) for inferring tumor mutational burden (TMB). (**a**) Comparison of TMB measured by WES vs targeted panel in n = 29 samples which were assessed by both assays. The line y = x is plotted in red. (**b**) TMB measured by targeted panel in 60 pairs of replicates. (**c**) Results of simulations of percentage deviation from actual TMB when sampling different numbers of megabases (Mb) sequenced. Median observed deviation is shown in black. 10% and 90% confidence intervals are shown in grey. Left: results of simulations with TMB equal to 100 mutations/Mb; center: results of simulations with TMB equal to 20 mutations/Mb; right: results of simulations with TMB equal to 10 mutations/Mb. (Reproduced from Chalmers et al. [31])

both WES and targeted NGS panel confirmed the positive correlation between WES and panel-derived TMB, though the association was weaker ($r^2 > 0.7$) [31, 33, 29], likely reflecting additional platform variation not captured by *in silico* analyses.

Additionally, though most studies have focused on TMB assessed from tumor tissue (tTMB), there is growing interest in assessing TMB from circulating tumor DNA (bTMB for blood TMB). Though a number of different blood-based assays with different performance characteristics are under development, initial studies have generally demonstrated a positive concordance between bTMB and tTMB with sufficiently large panels [34–39]. Additionally, analyses of patients treated on the POPLAR/OAK trials [36] and the MYSTIC trial [40] with both tTMB and bTMB demonstrated a positive correlation between bTMB and tTMB (Spearman's rho = 0.64, POPLAR and OAK; Spearman's rho = 0.6, MYSTIC).

Notably, despite the conceptual simplicity of TMB and the overall positive correlation between different TMB assessment methods, there is substantial methodologic heterogeneity across these different assays, and it is not fully understood how TMB quantification differs across assays.

3   TMB and Association with Response to ICIs

3.1   *Pembrolizumab*

The first study to demonstrate an association between TMB and ICI outcome in NSCLC analyzed WES data from 34 stage IV relapsed/refractory NSCLC patients treated with pembrolizumab through Keynote-001 [41]. These data and the studies below are summarized in Table 2.1. In their discovery cohort of 16 patients, the median number of nonsynonymous mutations in patients with durable clinical benefit (DCB, defined as complete or partial response [CR/PR] or stable disease [SD] lasting longer than 6 months) was 302 compared to 148 mutations in those with no durable benefit (NDB, defined as progressive disease [PD] or SD occurring within 6 months of starting immunotherapy) (p = 0.02). The rate of DCB in patients with a TMB above the median of 209 mutations was 73% compared to 13% in those with a TMB below the median (Fisher's p = 0.04), and the overall response rate (ORR) and progression free survival (PFS) were also improved [ORR 63% vs 0%, p = 0.03; HR for PFS = 0.19 (95% CI 0.05–0.70)]. Results were similar in an independent validation set of 18 patients. A receiver operator curve (ROC) analysis of the discovery cohort identified a cut-off of ≥178 nonsynonymous mutations, with a sensitivity of 100% and specificity of 67%, with similar performance in the validation cohort, though notably the total n of 34 was small.

Further study of TMB in association with pembrolizumab in NSCLC is limited, largely due to positive data from early PD-L1-selected trials for pembrolizumab monotherapy (PD-L1 ≥ 1% in the Keynote-010 2nd-line setting [12], PD-L1 ≥ 50% in the Keynote-024 1st-line setting [13]), and without biomarker selection in combination with chemotherapy [42], leading to NSCLC-specific FDA approvals without further biomarker development. However, as of June, 2020, pembrolizumab was approved across histologies in the second-line setting for patients with TMB > 10 as determined by the FoundationOneCDX assay, based on the results of the KEYNOTE-158 trial [43].

3.2   *Nivolumab*

Conversely, nivolumab did not demonstrate an OS benefit over chemotherapy in the phase III CheckMate-026 trial enrolling untreated advanced NSCLC patients with PD-L1 expression ≥1% [44]. In the primary efficacy analysis of patients with PD-L1 expression ≥5%, nivolumab showed no PFS benefit over chemotherapy [44], nor was a benefit observed in a subgroup analyses of NSCLCs with PD-L1 ≥ 50%. However, in an exploratory subgroup analysis of 312 patients whose tumors had undergone WES, patients with TMB in the upper tertile (>242 mutations) were found to benefit from nivolumab over chemotherapy [ORR 47% vs

Table 2.1 Sequencing assay, clinical outcome, and proposed tumor mutational burden cut-offs employed across clinical trials and analyses

Clinical trial (reference)	Outcome	Assay	Gene variants	Therapy	NSCLC patients	Sample type	TMB cut-off (rationale)	Outcome association
KEY-NOTE-001 [41]	DCB	WES	Nonsynonymous mutations	Pembrolizumab (any line)	34	Tumor	178 mutations (ROC analysis)	TMB ≥ 178 vs TMB < 178: DCB rate 75% vs 14% AUC 0.87 for TMB and DCB (discovery cohort, n = 16)
CheckMate 026 [44]	PFS, ORR, OS	WES	Missense mutations	Nivolumab vs chemotherapy (relapsed/refractory)	312	Tumor	Low <100; medium 100 to 242; high TMB ≥243 (tertiles)	TMB ≥ 243, nivolumab vs chemotherapy: ORR: 47% vs 28% Median PFS 9.7 vs 5.8 mos, HR 0.62 (95% CI 0.38–1.00) *No OS difference* TMB < 243, nivolumab vs chemotherapy: ORR: 21% vs 35% *Median PFS 4.1 vs 6.9 mos, HR 1.82 (95% CI, 1.30–2.55)* *No OS difference*
CheckMate 012 [51]	ORR, DCB, PFS	WES	Nonsynonymous mutations	Nivolumab plus ipilimumab	75	Tumor	158 mutations (50th percentile)	TMB >158 vs ≤158: ORR: 51 vs 13%, p = 0.0005 DCB: 65 vs 34%, p = 0.011 PFS: HR 0.41 (95% CI 0.23–0.73), p = 0.0024
FIR/BIRCH [46]	PFS, OS, ORR	Foundation Medicine F1 assay	Not specified	Atezolizumab, PD-L1 ≥ 5%	102 1L, 371 2L+	Tumor	1L: - ≥9 mut/Mb (50th percentile), - 13.5 mut/Mb (75th percentile); 2L+ - ≥9.9 mut/Mb (50th percentile), - ≥17.1 mut/Mb (75th percentile)	1L, TMB ≥ vs <9; TMB ≥ vs <13.5: *OS: HR 0.79 (0.39–1.58); HR 0.45 (0.17–1.16) (NS)* PFS: HR 0.58 (0.36–0.94); HR 0.53 (0.3–0.97) ORR: 28% vs 13%; 25% vs 20% 2L+, TMB ≥ vs <9.9; TMB ≥ vs <17.1 *OS: HR 0.87 (0.65–1.16), 0.7 (0.49–1.00)* PFS: HR 0.64 (0.5–0.8), 0.5 (0.38–0.67) ORR: 25%/14%, 29%/16%

| POPLAR [46] | PFS, OS, ORR | Foundation Medicine F1 assay | 92 | Atezolizumab (2L+) vs docetaxel, PD-L1 unselected | Not specified | Tumor | 9.9 mut/Mb (50th percentile), 15.8 mut/Mb (75th percentile) | Atezolizumab vs docetaxel, all pts; TMB ≥ 9.9; TMB ≥ 17.1 *OS: HR 0.65 (0.38–1.12); HR 0.48 (0.23–1.04); 0.5 (0.15–1.67)* *PFS: HR 0.98 (0.63–1.53); 0.49 (0.25–0.93); 0.49 (0.19–1.3)* ORR: 13% vs 15%; 20% vs 4%; 20% vs 8% |
| CheckMate 568 [52] | ORR | FoundationOne CDx | 98 | Nivolumab + Ipilimumab | Number of somatic mutations (inc synonymous mutations, excluding driver events) per Mb of genome examined | Tumor | 10 mut/Mb (cut-off performance) | TMB ≥ vs <10: ORR 44% vs 12% AUC 0.73 for TMB and ORR |

(continued)

Table 2.1 (continued)

Clinical trial (reference)	Outcome	Assay	NSCLC patients	Therapy	Gene variants	Sample type	TMB cut-off (rationale)	Outcome association
CheckMate 227 [45]	PFS (1ary), OS (2ary)	FoundationOne CDx	299 (139 vs 160)	Nivolumab + Ipilimumab vs chemotherapy	All somatic mutations (including synonymous mutations, excluding driver events) per Mb of genome examined	Tumor	10 mut/Mb (from CheckMate 568)	TMB ≥ 10: nivolumab + ipilimumab vs chemotherapy 1-year PFS: 42.6% vs 13.2%, HR 0.58 (95% CI 0.41–0.81, p < 0.001). TMB < 10: nivolumab + ipilimumab vs chemotherapy 1-year PFS: 25% vs 17%, HR 1.07 (95% CI 0.84–1.35) (NS) OS reported not significant
			150 (71 vs 79)	Nivolumab vs chemotherapy			13 mut/Mb (rationale not specified)	TMB ≥ 13: nivolumab vs chemotherapy *Median PFS 4.2 vs 5.6 mo, HR 0.95 (97.5% CI, 0.61 to 1.48, p = 0.78)* TMB ≥ 10: nivolumab vs chemotherapy *Median PFS 7.1 vs 4.2 mo, HR 0.75 (95% CI, 0.53 to 1.07)*
POPLAR/OAK [36]	PFS, OS OS, PFS	Foundation Medicine F1 assay	794 (211 + 583)	Atezolizumab (2L/3L) vs docetaxel	All somatic mutations (including synonymous mutations, excluding driver events) per Mb of genome examined	Blood	≥16 mutations (bTMB assay analytic performance)	POPLAR, TMB ≥ 16: atezolizumab vs chemotherapy: PFS HR 0.57 (95% CI, 0.33–0.99), OS HR 0.56 (95% CI, 0.31–0.99) OAK, TMB ≥ 16: atezolizumab vs chemotherapy PFS HR 0.65 (0.47–0.92), OS HR 0.64 (0.44–0.92)

Study	Endpoints	Assay	N	Comparison	TMB definition	Source	TMB cutoff	Results
MYSTIC	OS, PFS	Foundation Medicine F1 assay	460	Durvaumab vs Durvalumab + Tremelimumab vs chemotherapy	All somatic mutations (including synonymous mutations, excluding driver events) per Mb of genome examined	Tumor	≥10 mut/Mb (CheckMate 227)	TMB ≥ 10: durvalumab vs durvalumab + tremilimumab vs chemotherapy: Median OS 18.6 vs 16.6 vs 11.9 mos, *HR 0.7 (95% CI, 0.47–1.06) and HR 0.72 (95% CI, 0.48–1.09)* TMB < 10: durvalumab vs durvalumab + tremilimumab vs chemotherapy: Median OS 10.1 vs 8.4 vs 13.8 mos, HR 1.26 (95% CI, 0.9–1.77), HRR 1.39 (95% CI, 1.00–1.92)
		GuardantOMNI	809	Durvaumab vs Durvalumab + Tremelimumab vs chemotherapy	SNVs + indels	Blood	≥20 mut/Mb (OS HR analysis)	bTMB ≥ 20: durvalumab vs durvalumab + tremilimumab vs chemotherapy: Median OS 12.6 vs 21.9 vs 10 mos, *HR 0.72 (95% CI, 0.5–1.05), HR 0.49 (95% CI, 0.32–0.74)* bTMB < 20: durvalumab vs durvalumab + tremilimumab vs chemotherapy: Median OS 11.0 vs 8.5 vs 11.6 mos, *HR 0.93 (95% CI, 0.74–1.16), HR 1.16 (95% CI, 0.93–1.45)*
Commercial use [29]	ORR, DCB, PFS	MSK–IMPACT	240	Multiple	Nonsynonymous mutations per Mb of genome examined	Tumor	≥ 7.4 mutations/ Mb (50th percentile)	TMB ≥ 7.4 vs <7.4: DCB: 38.6% vs 25.1%, p = 0.009
Commercial use [54]	OS, time on therapy, clinical benefit rate (CBR)	FoundationOne	1290	Mixed			≥20 mut/Mb (from Goodman et al. [62])	TMB ≥ 20 vs <20: Median OS: 16.8 vs 8.5 mo, p < 0.001 (HR not provided) Duration on therapy: 7.8 mo vs 3.3 mo, p < 0.001 CBR: 80.7% vs 56.7%, p < 0.001

DCB durable clinical benefit, *PFS* progression-free survival, *ORR* overall response rate, *OS* overall survival, *TMB* tumor mutational burden

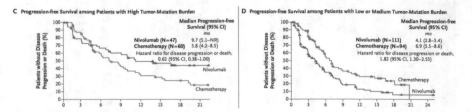

Fig. 2.3 Exploratory subgroup analysis of progression-free survival (PFS) in patients stratified by tumor mutational burden (TMB). Left: PFS of patients with TMB > 242 mutations treated with nivolumab vs chemotherapy. Right: PFS of patients with TMB ≤ 242 mutations treated with nivolumab vs chemotherapy. (Reproduced from Carbone et al. [44])

28%, median PFS 9.7 vs 5.8 months, HR 0.62 (95% CI 0.38–1.00)], while those with TMB ≤ 242 mutations had better outcomes with chemotherapy (Fig. 2.3). There was no difference in overall survival, though many chemotherapy-treated patients went on to receive subsequent treatment with a PD-1 inhibitor.

The CheckMate-227 study explored the role of TMB in predicting benefit to first-line nivolumab either alone or in combination with the CTLA-4 inhibitor ipilimumab compared to platinum doublet chemotherapy in patients with previously-untreated advanced NSCLC [45]. Assessment of PFS in patients with TMB ≥ 10 mutations/Mb, as assessed by FoundationOneCDx panel rather than WES, was included in the protocol as a coprimary endpoint, though this was added to the protocol after randomization. The hazard ratio (HR) for progression or death for nivolumab-treated patients with TMB ≥ 10 mutations/Mb was 0.75, though this was not significant (95% CI, 0.53–1.07), nor was there a significant PFS difference between nivolumab vs chemotherapy-treated patients with PD-L1 ≥ 1% and TMB ≥ 13 mutations/Mb.

It is unknown, at this point, whether the lack of benefit in nivolumab-treated patients with higher TMB reflects a differential association between TMB and outcome to nivolumab compared to other drugs; an overall lack of benefit to nivolumab; or differences in patient population or study design that contribute to the overall lack of benefit seen with single-agent nivolumab. This uncertainty reflects larger uncertainties about why nivolumab has not demonstrated benefit in first-line NSCLC patients that requires further investigation.

3.3   Atezolizumab

The association between efficacy of the PD-L1 inhibitor atezolizumab and tissue TMB was assessed retrospectively in patients treated on three phase II trials [46]: POPLAR [47], which compared atezolizumab to docetaxel in PD-L1-unselected second- or third-line patients; and BIRCH [48]/FIR [49], which were single-arm studies of first or second-line atezolizumab patients with PD-L1 expression ≥5%. TMB was assessed by the Foundation Medicine F1 panel. In the 102 first-line patients treated on BIRCH/FIR, patients whose TMB was ≥9 mutations/Mb (study median) had improved PFS and ORR compared to those with TMB < 9 mutations/ Mb; OS was not significantly different. Results were similar in 371 patients treated second-line or later, with improved PFS and ORR in patients with TMB ≥ 9.9 mutations/Mb (median) compared to those with TMBB < 9.9 mutations/Mb. In patients from the POPLAR trial with TMB ≥ 9.9 mutations/Mb, atezolizumab offered PFS and ORR benefit compared to docetaxel. Similar results were obtained upon analysis of blood TMB in 794 patients from the POPLAR and OAK trials using the Foundation Medicine F1 bait set and a bTMB threshold of 16 (Table 2.1).

3.4 Durvalumab, Durvalumab Plus Tremelimumab

The MYSTIC trial assessed the efficacy of the PD-L1 inhibitor durvalumab alone or in combination with the CTLA-4 inhibitor tremelimumab *vs* chemotherapy in patients with untreated, advanced NSCLC [50]. Patients were stratified by PD-L1 expression (<25% vs ≥25%) and histology (squamous vs adenocarcinoma), with primary endpoints of OS and PFS in the PD-L1 high population. The initial analysis did not meet its primary endpoints of improved OS in ICI-treated patients compared to chemotherapy in the PD-L1 high group, with HR for OS of 0.76 (97.54% CI, 0.564–1.019, p = 0.036) for durvalumab monotherapy, and HR 0.85 (98.77% CI 0.611–1.173, p = 0.202) for the combination. In an exploratory subgroup analysis, patients with a tissue TMB ≥ 10 as assessed by Foundation Medicine F1 assay had a median OS of 18.6 months on durvalumab, 16.6 months on durvalumab plus tremelimumab, and 11.9 months on chemotherapy; hazard ratios for durvalumab and durvalumab plus tremelimumab vs chemotherapy were 0.70 and 0.72 respectively, though these did not reach statistical significance. There was no benefit to ICI over chemotherapy in patients with tTMB < 10. Similarly, in patients with a blood TMB ≥ 20 as assessed by the GuardantOMNI assay, median OS was 12.6 months in patients treated with durvalumab; 21.9 months in durvalumab plus tremelimumab; and 10 months on chemotherapy [HR 0.72 (95% CI 0.5–1.05) for durvalumab vs chemotherapy; HR 0.49 (95% CI 0.32–0.74) for durvalumab plus tremelimumab vs chemotherapy]. There was no difference in OS across treatment arms in patients with bTMB < 20.

3.5 Nivolumab Plus Ipilimumab

The potential utility of TMB as a biomarker in dual-checkpoint blockade-treated patients was demonstrated in a retrospective analysis of 75 whole-exome sequenced tumors from NSCLC patients treated on CheckMate-012 with ipilimumab plus nivolumab. TMB was higher in patients with CR/PR compared with SD/PD (median 273 vs 114 mutations, p = 0.0004) and with DCB vs NDB (210 vs 113, p = 0.0071) [51]. ORR, DCB rate, and PFS were all improved in patients with TMB ≥ 158 mutations (median) (ORR 51% vs 13% p = 0.0005; DCB 65% vs 34% p = 0.011, PFS HR = 0.41, p = 0.0024). ROC analysis of TMB as a predictor of outcome was associated with an AUC of 0.68 for DCB and 0.75 for ORR.

CheckMate-568 was performed to confirm this association and identify a TMB threshold for further prospective studies [52]. This open-label, phase II trial evaluated the efficacy and safety of nivolumab plus low-dose ipilimumab for untreated stage IIIB/IV NSCLC. Efficacy on the basis of TMB as assessed by the FoundationOne CDx panel was added as a secondary endpoint after completion of enrollment. 98 patients were evaluable for TMB, and 95 patients were evaluable for both PD-L1 expression and TMB. Both PD-L1 and TMB were found to be informative classifiers for ORR (AUC 0.70 for PD-L1, AUC 0.73 for TMB). ORR plateaued at TMB $\geq$ 10 mutations/Mb (ORR 44% vs 12% in TMB < 10 mutations/Mb) without additional ORR benefit in patients with TMB $\geq$ 15, leading the investigators to select 10 mutations/Mb as a cut-off, though notably they did not appear to use their ROC analysis to generate this threshold. TMB $\geq$ 10 was associated with higher ORR independent of PD-L1 expression $\geq$1% or <1%.

This threshold of 10 mutations/Mb was then applied to CheckMate-227, an open-label phase III trial investigating multiple hypotheses regarding the efficacy of first-line nivolumab-based regimens in biomarker selected NSCLC populations [45]. The protocol was amended to add a coprimary endpoint evaluating PFS with nivolumab plus ipilimumab compared to chemotherapy among patients with TMB $\geq$ 10 mut/Mb as determined by the FoundationOne CDx assay. Among the 444 patients with TMB $\geq$ 10 mut/Mb, 138 were treated with ipilimumab plus nivolumab and 160 were treated with chemotherapy. PFS and ORR were significantly improved in the ipilimumab plus nivolumab treated patients compared to the chemotherapy-treated patients, with ORR 45.3% vs 26.9% for nivolumab plus ipilimumab vs chemotherapy. HR for progression or death was 0.58 (95% CI 0.41–0.81, p < 0.001). Neither PFS nor ORR favored ICI therapy in patients with TMB < 10. Notably, although CheckMate 227 met its primary endpoint, an interim exploratory analysis showed no improvement in OS for nivolumab plus ipilimumab vs chemotherapy, whether comparing among the TMB-high patients (HR 0.77; 95% CI, 0.56–1.06) or among the TMB-low patients (HR, 0.78; 95% CI, 0.61–1.00) [53]. Ipilimumab plus nivolumab have since been approved in the first-line setting in NSCLC patients with PD-L1 > 1%, independent of TMB, based positive PFS and OS results from CheckMate-227 [https://www.nejm.org/doi/10.1056/ NEJMoa1910231?url_ver=Z39.88-2003&rfr_id=ori:rid:crossref.org&rfr_dat=cr_ pub%20%200pubmed;   https://www.fda.gov/drugs/resources-information-approved-drugs/fda-approves-nivolumab-plus-ipilimumab-first-line-mnsclc-pd-l1-tumor-expression-1]

3.6   Real-World Analyses

Several retrospective analyses using real-world datasets have identified a similar association between higher TMB and improved outcomes to ICIs. In their analysis of 240 patients treated with ICIs, Rizvi et al. [29] demonstrated higher TMB in patients with DCB or CR/PR vs NDB or PD, respectively. Odds ratio of DCB and likelihood of progression free survival increased with increasing TMB percentile cut-offs. AUC of the ROC analysis for DCB at varying TMB cut-points was 0.601. A similar retrospective analysis of patients in the Foundation Medicine/Flatiron database demonstrated improved OS in ICI-treated patients with TMB $\geq$ 20 mutations/Mb compared to those with TMB < 20 [54] (16.8 vs 8.5 months, p < 0.001). Duration of therapy (7.8 vs 3.3 mo, p < 0.001) and rate of CR/PR or SD (80.7% vs 56.7%, p < 0.001) were also improved. However, in contrast to CheckMate-026 [44] and CheckMate-568 [52] where this association was independent of PD-L1 expression (Fig. 2.3), PD-L1 negative patients in this study with TMB $\geq$ 20 did not do better than PD-L1 negative patients with TMB < 20.

4   Efficacy of TMB as a Predictive Biomarker

Taken together, these studies comprise a growing evidence base associating higher TMB with increased likelihood of benefit to ICI therapy (studies summarized in Table 2.1). Notably, the association seems to hold across line of therapy and specific drug. Moreover, similar findings in other cancer subtypes, including melanoma, bladder cancer, and head and neck cancer, support the inference that this association describes a generalized (though not universal) feature of ICI response [55–61].

However, there are important differences underlying the seeming consistency of the overall association across these studies. First, there is heterogeneity in which outcomes and comparator groups are analyzed; some studies compare TMB high vs TMB low ICI-treated patients, while others compare outcomes in TMB high patients treated with ICI vs chemotherapy. If TMB is to be used clinically to select patients who will benefit from ICI over chemotherapy, only the latter analysis provides direct evidence for this approach. Additionally, many of these analyses did not demonstrate an OS benefit, and there are additional inconsistencies across studies as to the outcome measure used, as well as the magnitude and statistical significance of the findings. It is not yet known whether these discrepancies arise from differential efficacy of these drugs, different patient populations, different stratification by PD-L1 thresholds or line of therapy, or differential sensitivity of TMB as a biomarker in these contexts. The interplay between TMB and these factors requires further study, and there is a need for prospective clinical trials that incorporate TMB into the study design, rather than post-hoc analysis of largely negative clinical trials.

Another important distinction between studies is in how TMB thresholds were identified and applied (Table 2.1). While most studies used a percentile-based threshold to stratify their cohort into TMB high vs low sub-groups, the actual selected thresholds range from the median (most common) to the 90th percentile [31, 54, 56, 62]. Most analyses do not justify how these thresholds were selected, nor do they discuss how the response association changes with differential threshold application. This variability makes it unclear whether these different threshold values reflect sequencing assay and TMB algorithm differences; selection bias for thresholds that demonstrated a significant difference; variation in the distribution of TMB values across cohorts; or meaningful context-specific differences in how TMB should be used to stratify patients into responders vs non-responders. For example, it may be the case that the TMB threshold predictive of ICI benefit will differ in the second-line setting compared to the first-line setting, just as it is likely that the TMB values from the FoundationOne CDx assay differ from WES (more on this below).

More broadly speaking, the studies that have more thoroughly scrutinized how different thresholds affect the response association differed in whether the association between TMB and response is linear, with increasing benefit at higher and higher values, or whether there is an inflection point beyond which benefit plateaus. In their analysis of CheckMate-568 [52], the authors found no improvement with a threshold of 15 compared to 10 mutations/Mb, whereas the blood TMB analyses of POPLAR/OAK [36] and MYSTIC [40] found decreasing HRs with increasing thresholds, leading them to propose higher thresholds of 16 and 20 mutations/Mb respectively. More formal quantification of TMB as a response discriminator through receiver operator curve analyses (ROC) [29, 41, 51, 52] is broadly consistent with the interpretation that the association between TMB and outcome does not have a clear cut-point. Indeed, most ROC analyses have demonstrated an AUC of 0.6–0.75, indicating only weak discrimination between responders and non-responders, without a clear inflection point (Fig. 2.4). This suggests that any clinical application of TMB thresholds are likely to come with trade-offs in sensitivity and specificity, and corroborates the simple observation that there are responders across the TMB spectrum. Any threshold that gets selected, therefore, must be defined within a goal-specific clinical context that considers the relative efficacy of the alternative therapy, and, as above, must be evaluated in a prospective clinical trial.

Fig. 2.4 Receiver operator characteristic (ROC) curve of sensitivity vs 1-specificity of durable clinical benefit (DCB) at varying tumor mutational burden (TMB) and PD-L1 values. Area under the curve (AUC) for TMB = 0.601, AUC for PD-L1 = 0.646. (Reproduced from Rizvi et al. [29])

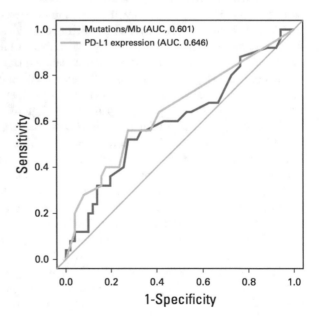

5 Pragmatic Limitations

5.1 TMB Standardization

There are additional pragmatic limitations to the implementation of TMB as a clinical biomarker. One such limitation is the considerable heterogeneity across studies in TMB assay and threshold used. Sequencing assays may report different mutations due to differences in gene panel size and composition, mutation calling pipeline, germline filtration strategy, quality control metrics, variant allele frequency thresholds, and mutation reporting practices, among others. Furthermore, different studies have employed different TMB calculation algorithms; some have included all nonsynonymous mutations, some all missense mutations, and some have employed commercial tests with their own proprietary algorithms (e.g. Foundation Medicine's TMB algorithm counts all somatic mutations, including silent mutations, but subtracts putative driver mutations). It is not yet fully known how this variation affect the values generated by one test compared to another, and this heterogeneity makes it difficult to understand whether the heterogeneity in TMB thresholds reflect assay differences or true clinical differences. It also limits the clinical application of TMB, as it is not known how to compare a patient's TMB value, which may be obtained through one assay, with a published threshold obtained via another assay.

For the time being, it is likely that any identified threshold will need to be assay-specific, and researchers and clinicians need to be aware that values from one test may not be equivalent to those from another. However, harmonization algorithms have been proposed [63], and ongoing collaborative efforts from the Quality Assurance Initiative Pathology (QuIP) and the Friends of Cancer Research consortium will help identify sources variation and standardize TMB across assays.

5.2 Feasibility of Assessing TMB in Routine Clinical Practice

While the increasing number of genetically targeted therapies in NSCLC have made NGS panel-based assessment of tumors increasingly common, the feasibility of routine assessment of TMB remains unknown. Indeed, data from clinical trials to date suggest that the need for adequate tissue may be a significant limitation; in CheckMate-227, only 1004 of 1649 available samples (60.9%) were evaluable for TMB [45]. Similarly, only 120 of 288 (42%) patients treated on CheckMate-568 [52] had sufficient tissue available after PD-L1 testing, and 460 of 1118 (41%) patients randomized in the MYSTIC trial were evaluable for tissue TMB [40].

Admittedly, TMB assessment was incorporated into these trials only after initial enrollment, and it is possible that an upfront requirement would have led to more adequate tumor tissue sampling with higher sequencing success rates. However, it is also the case that tissue availability was a precondition for enrollment in these trials, and it might be that patients treated outside a clinical trial are even less likely to have adequate tissue; by one estimate, 30% of patients do not have adequate tissue available at diagnosis for standard biomarker testing, let alone the quantities necessary for NGS [64].

One potential strategy that circumvents the need for substantial amounts of tumor tissue is the use of blood TMB. In the MYSTIC trial, for example, 809 patients were evaluable for bTMB compared to 352 for tTMB [40], demonstrating the increased availability of blood over tissue. However, as above, additional work to fully understand the differences between blood and tissue TMB assays will be necessary. While comparisons of blood and tissue TMB in POPLAR/OAK and MYSTIC trials demonstrated an overall positive correlation [36, 40], there were a range of tTMB values associated with each bTMB value, and vice versa, suggesting imperfect mapping from one test to the other. Additionally, analyses by Gandara et al. suggested that these differences were less likely due to technical variation between assays, and more likely arising from tumor characteristics such as the quantity of tumor DNA in the blood (tumor shed) and differences in mutations across metastatic sites (intratumoral heterogeneity), affecting which mutations are detected in the blood and in the tissue, respectively [36]. Notably, because these features depend on tumor and patient characteristics, it may not be straightforward to translate the values of bTMB to tTMB. Additionally, tumor shed and intratumoral heterogeneity themselves may associate with outcome [59, 65–67]. Therefore, more work to understand determinants of differential bTMB and tTMB values will be necessary to better define the set of patients in whom bTMB is sufficiently reliable. These considerations suggest that independent validation of bTMB as a biomarker will also need to be evaluated. Ongoing prospective clinical trials, including the B-F1RST trial evaluating the efficacy of first-line atezolizumab in patients with bTMB $\geq$ 16 vs <16 mutations/Mb, and the B-FAST trial comparing PFS with atezolizumab vs chemotherapy in patients with bTMB above a specified threshold [68], will be instrumental in assessing the clinical utility of bTMB.

6 Biology Underlying the Response Association

In addition to these pragmatic considerations, it is not yet known why TMB actually associates with outcome. The dominant hypothesis has been that TMB is a surrogate for neoantigen load [69], which in turn associates with more immunogenic tumors. However, there is no evidence to actually confirm this interpretation. Neoantigen load, as predicted by in silico algorithms, is very tightly correlated with TMB (R^2 > 0.9 across multiple studies) [30, 41, 51, 59, 70] (Fig. 2.5), and associates no more closely with response than TMB [51, 59, 58], suggesting that neoantigen prediction adds little information over and above TMB itself. Additionally, it is striking that most TMB algorithms, including those that count silent mutations (which do not generate neoantigens) [59], demonstrate the same response association, further suggesting that TMB may be capturing a biological feature other than neoantigen load.

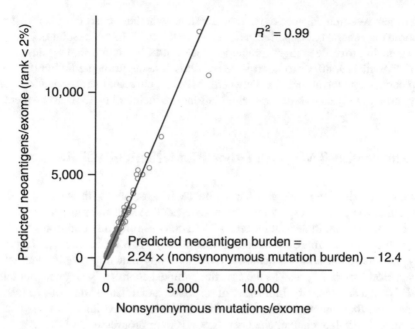

Fig. 2.5 Relationship between predicted neoantigen burden (y-axis) and nonsynonymous mutational burden (x-axis). Linear regression excludes one outlier (n = 249). (Reproduced from Miao et al. [59])

One possible explanation for these findings is that it is not the absolute number of neoantigens that matters but some feature of a subset of neoantigens that associates with response, which are themselves more probable in the setting of more mutations. Consistent with this hypothesis, in both mouse models of sarcoma [71, 72] and in ICI-responsive patients, researchers identified a much smaller number of neoantigen-specific T cells than the predicted number of neo-epitopes [27, 67, 73]. One possible distinguishing feature of response-eliciting neoantigens is clonality. Clonal neoantigens (present in all cancer cells) were found to improve the association between TMB and ICI response in NSCLC and melanoma, whereas subclonal neoantigens predominated in non-responders [67]. In another study, a higher proportion of subclonal mutations was present in patients with PD compared to CR/PR, though notably this observation did not account for all high TMB non-responders [59].

Another, not mutually exclusive possibility, is that the antigenicity of the neoantigen also plays a role. Studies have quantified the foreignness of neoantigens by comparing the neoantigen peptide sequences with those of immune epitopes that were experimentally validated as targets of adaptive immune responses [74, 75]. Quantification of neoantigens that had highest homology to known pathogenic alterations such as those from viruses was used to identify tumors with more immunogenic neoantigens, which were then found to correlate with longer survival after ICI therapy [74]. Similarly, virus-associated cancers, and tumors with aberrant expression of germline endogenous retroviruses, associate with response to checkpoint blockade [70, 76–78].

Further research is necessary to understand whether these or other features underlie the general but imperfect association between TMB and response. Ongoing efforts to improve neoantigen prediction techniques by incorporating mass spectrometry data [79, 80] or to improve MHC class II neoepitope prediction [81] may help corroborate the association between TMB, response, and neoantigen load, and may further allow us to refine which mutations are included in TMB assessment.

7   Integrating TMB with Other Biomarkers of ICI Response

The data described here suggest that, while TMB associates with outcome, it does not perfectly segregate responders from non-responders. Further prospective studies will be instrumental in defining whether TMB can meaningfully contribute to clinical practice, and an improved understanding of why TMB associates with response may help us refine how we quantify TMB in a way that improves its predictive power. However, it may also be the case that, unlike genomically targeted therapies, TMB is not a deterministic biomarker of response, and it instead describes a feature of response that interacts with other tumor intrinsic and extrinsic features that in aggregate determine whether a patient responds to or progresses on ICIs.

Evidence for this latter possibility comes from studies of TMB in association with markers of an inflamed tumor microenvironment (TME) such as PD-L1 expression. In one study, response rates were highest in patients with both high TMB (TMB $\geq$ 7.4 mutations/Mb) and high PD-L1 (PD-L1 $\geq$ 1%) (ORR 50% in PD-L1 high/TMB high; 35.3% in PD-L1 high/TMB low; 29.4% in TMB high/PD-L1 low; 18% in TMB low/PD-L1 low) [29]. Similar results were demonstrated in Checkmate-026, where patients with PD-L1 expression $\geq$50% and TMB in the upper tertile had a 75% response rate compared to 32% in patients with TMB high/PD-L1 low; 34% with PD-L1 high/TMB low; or 16% in with both low [44]. Another marker of an inflamed TME, an interferon-gamma gene expression profile (GEP) as assessed by nanostring, was also shown to associate with highest response rates when combined with TMB (Fig. 2.6) [61]. Interestingly, despite the assumption that TMB should associate with more antigenic tumors and therefore a more inflamed TME, TMB has been found to be independent of PD-L1 expression and the interferon-gamma GEP [29, 44, 52, 61, 82].

8   Conclusion

TMB has been found to associate with response to immune checkpoint inhibitors across multiple treatment contexts, leading to growing interest in developing TMB as a clinical biomarker. However, further work is necessary to define the optimal clinical context and thresholds for TMB application, and to better understand whether and in what context TMB associates with improved overall survival rather

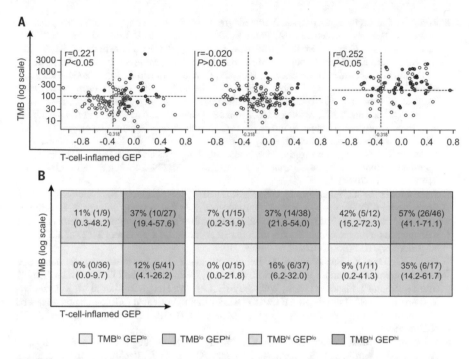

Fig. 2.6 Joint relationship of tumor mutational burden (TMB) or T cell-inflamed gene expression profile (GEP) with anti-PD-1 response across multiple patient cohorts. (a) Relationships of both TMB and T cell-inflamed GEP signatures with best overall response (BOR). A responder is defined as having complete response (CR) or partial response (PR) (filled circles), and a non-responder as having no CR/PR (open circles). Dashed horizontal lines represent the Youden Index-associated cut-offs for TMB in each cohort as derived from receiver operator characteristic (ROC) analyses. Dashed vertical lines represented a discovery cut-off for the T-cell inflamed GEP. (b) CR/PR rates per TMB cut-off status and T cell-inflamed GEP cut-off status as designated in (a). Cohorts from left to right: pan-cancer cohort (n = 119) from Keynote-028 and Keynote-012); head and neck squamous cell carcinoma cohort (n = 107) from Keynote-012 B1 and Keynote-012 B2; melanoma cohort (n = 89) from Keynote-001 and Keynote-006. (Reproduced from Cristescu et al. [61])

than simply response and progression free survival. Efforts to standardize TMB assessment and to validate blood-based TMB assays are also necessary if this biomarker is to be widely used. Finally, additional research to better understand why TMB associates with response and to develop models that integrate TMB with other continuously-scored biomarkers such as PD-L1 or interferon-gamma expression may be instrumental in improving the predictive power of this potential biomarker.

References

1. Mok TS, Wu YL, Thongprasert S, Yang CH, Chu DT, Saijo N, Sunpaweravong P, Han B, Margono B, Ichinose Y, Nishiwaki Y, Ohe Y, Yang JJ, Chewaskulyong B, Jiang H, Duffield EL, Watkins CL, Armour AA, Fukuoka M (2009) Gefitinib or carboplatin-paclitaxel in pulmonary adenocarcinoma. N Engl J Med 361(10):947–957. https://doi.org/10.1056/NEJMoa0810699

2. Rosell R, Carcereny E, Gervais R, Vergnenegre A, Massuti B, Felip E, Palmero R, Garcia-Gomez R, Pallares C, Sanchez JM, Porta R, Cobo M, Garrido P, Longo F, Moran T, Insa A, De Marinis F, Corre R, Bover I, Illiano A, Dansin E, de Castro J, Milella M, Reguart N, Altavilla G, Jimenez U, Provencio M, Moreno MA, Terrasa J, Munoz-Langa J, Valdivia J, Isla D, Domine M, Molinier O, Mazieres J, Baize N, Garcia-Campelo R, Robinet G, Rodriguez-Abreu D, Lopez-Vivanco G, Gebbia V, Ferrera-Delgado L, Bombaron P, Bernabe R, Bearz A, Artal A, Cortesi E, Rolfo C, Sanchez-Ronco M, Drozdowskyj A, Queralt C, de Aguirre I, Ramirez JL, Sanchez JJ, Molina MA, Taron M, Paz-Ares L, Spanish Lung Cancer Group in collaboration with Groupe Francais de P-C, Associazione Italiana Oncologia T (2012) Erlotinib versus standard chemotherapy as first-line treatment for European patients with advanced EGFR mutation-positive non-small-cell lung cancer (EURTAC): a multicentre, open-label, randomised phase 3 trial. Lancet Oncol 13(3):239–246. https://doi.org/10.1016/S1470-2045(11)70393-X
3. Sequist LV, Yang JC, Yamamoto N, O'Byrne K, Hirsh V, Mok T, Geater SL, Orlov S, Tsai CM, Boyer M, Su WC, Bennouna J, Kato T, Gorbunova V, Lee KH, Shah R, Massey D, Zazulina V, Shahidi M, Schuler M (2013) Phase III study of afatinib or cisplatin plus pemetrexed in patients with metastatic lung adenocarcinoma with EGFR mutations. J Clin Oncol 31(27):3327–3334. https://doi.org/10.1200/JCO.2012.44.2806
4. Soria JC, Ohe Y, Vansteenkiste J, Reungwetwattana T, Chewaskulyong B, Lee KH, Dechaphunkul A, Imamura F, Nogami N, Kurata T, Okamoto I, Zhou C, Cho BC, Cheng Y, Cho EK, Voon PJ, Planchard D, Su WC, Gray JE, Lee SM, Hodge R, Marotti M, Rukazenkov Y, Ramalingam SS, Investigators F (2018) Osimertinib in untreated EGFR-mutated advanced non-small-cell lung cancer. N Engl J Med 378(2):113–125. https://doi.org/10.1056/NEJMoa1713137
5. Solomon BJ, Mok T, Kim DW, Wu YL, Nakagawa K, Mekhail T, Felip E, Cappuzzo F, Paolini J, Usari T, Iyer S, Reisman A, Wilner KD, Tursi J, Blackhall F, Investigators P (2014) First-line crizotinib versus chemotherapy in ALK-positive lung cancer. N Engl J Med 371(23):2167–2177. https://doi.org/10.1056/NEJMoa1408440
6. Soria JC, Tan DSW, Chiari R, Wu YL, Paz-Ares L, Wolf J, Geater SL, Orlov S, Cortinovis D, Yu CJ, Hochmair M, Cortot AB, Tsai CM, Moro-Sibilot D, Campelo RG, McCulloch T, Sen P, Dugan M, Pantano S, Branle F, Massacesi C, de Castro G Jr (2017) First-line ceritinib versus platinum-based chemotherapy in advanced ALK-rearranged non-small-cell lung cancer (ASCEND-4): a randomised, open-label, phase 3 study. Lancet 389(10072):917–929. https://doi.org/10.1016/S0140-6736(17)30123-X
7. Shaw AT, Ou SH, Bang YJ, Camidge DR, Solomon BJ, Salgia R, Riely GJ, Varella-Garcia M, Shapiro GI, Costa DB, Doebele RC, Le LP, Zheng Z, Tan W, Stephenson P, Shreeve SM, Tye LM, Christensen JG, Wilner KD, Clark JW, Iafrate AJ (2014) Crizotinib in ROS1-rearranged non-small-cell lung cancer. N Engl J Med 371(21):1963–1971. https://doi.org/10.1056/NEJMoa1406766
8. Planchard D, Besse B, Groen HJM, Souquet PJ, Quoix E, Baik CS, Barlesi F, Kim TM, Mazieres J, Novello S, Rigas JR, Upalawanna A, D'Amelio AM Jr, Zhang P, Mookerjee B, Johnson BE (2016) Dabrafenib plus trametinib in patients with previously treated BRAF(V600E)-mutant metastatic non-small cell lung cancer: an open-label, multicentre phase 2 trial. Lancet Oncol 17(7):984–993. https://doi.org/10.1016/S1470-2045(16)30146-2
9. Planchard D, Smit EF, Groen HJM, Mazieres J, Besse B, Helland A, Giannone V, D'Amelio AM Jr, Zhang P, Mookerjee B, Johnson BE (2017) Dabrafenib plus trametinib in patients with previously untreated BRAF(V600E)-mutant metastatic non-small-cell lung cancer: an open-label, phase 2 trial. Lancet Oncol 18(10):1307–1316. https://doi.org/10.1016/S1470-2045(17)30679-4
10. Brahmer J, Reckamp KL, Baas P, Crino L, Eberhardt WE, Poddubskaya E, Antonia S, Pluzanski A, Vokes EE, Holgado E, Waterhouse D, Ready N, Gainor J, Aren Frontera O, Havel L, Steins M, Garassino MC, Aerts JG, Domine M, Paz-Ares L, Reck M, Baudelet C, Harbison CT, Lestini B, Spigel DR (2015) Nivolumab versus docetaxel in advanced squamous-cell non-small-cell lung cancer. N Engl J Med 373(2):123–135. https://doi.org/10.1056/NEJMoa1504627

11. Borghaei H, Paz-Ares L, Horn L, Spigel DR, Steins M, Ready NE, Chow LQ, Vokes EE, Felip E, Holgado E, Barlesi F, Kohlhaufl M, Arrieta O, Burgio MA, Fayette J, Lena H, Poddubskaya E, Gerber DE, Gettinger SN, Rudin CM, Rizvi N, Crino L, Blumenschein GR Jr, Antonia SJ, Dorange C, Harbison CT, Graf Finckenstein F, Brahmer JR (2015) Nivolumab versus docetaxel in advanced nonsquamous non-small-cell lung cancer. N Engl J Med 373(17):1627–1639. https://doi.org/10.1056/NEJMoa1507643

12. Herbst RS, Baas P, Kim DW, Felip E, Perez-Gracia JL, Han JY, Molina J, Kim JH, Arvis CD, Ahn MJ, Majem M, Fidler MJ, de Castro G, Garrido M, Lubiniecki GM, Shentu Y, Im E, Dolled-Filhart M, Garon EB (2016) Pembrolizumab versus docetaxel for previously treated, PD-L1-positive, advanced non-small-cell lung cancer (KEYNOTE-010): a randomised controlled trial. Lancet 387(10027):1540–1550. https://doi.org/10.1016/S0140-6736(15)01281-7

13. Reck M, Rodriguez-Abreu D, Robinson AG, Hui R, Csoszi T, Fulop A, Gottfried M, Peled N, Tafreshi A, Cuffe S, O'Brien M, Rao S, Hotta K, Leiby MA, Lubiniecki GM, Shentu Y, Rangwala R, Brahmer JR, Investigators K (2016) Pembrolizumab versus chemotherapy for PD-L1-positive non-small-cell lung cancer. N Engl J Med 375(19):1823–1833. https://doi.org/10.1056/NEJMoa1606774

14. Rittmeyer A, Barlesi F, Waterkamp D, Park K, Ciardiello F, von Pawel J, Gadgeel SM, Hida T, Kowalski DM, Dols MC, Cortinovis DL, Leach J, Polikoff J, Barrios C, Kabbinavar F, Frontera OA, De Marinis F, Turna H, Lee JS, Ballinger M, Kowanetz M, He P, Chen DS, Sandler A, Gandara DR, Group OAKS (2017) Atezolizumab versus docetaxel in patients with previously treated non-small-cell lung cancer (OAK): a phase 3, open-label, multicentre randomised controlled trial. Lancet 389(10066):255–265. https://doi.org/10.1016/S0140-6736(16)32517-X

15. Nadal E, Massuti B, Domine M, Garcia-Campelo R, Cobo M, Felip E (2019) Immunotherapy with checkpoint inhibitors in non-small cell lung cancer: insights from long-term survivors. Cancer Immunol Immunother 68(3):341–352. https://doi.org/10.1007/s00262-019-02310-2

16. Garon EB, Hellmann MD, Rizvi NA, Carcereny E, Leighl NB, Ahn MJ, Eder JP, Balmanoukian AS, Aggarwal C, Horn L, Patnaik A, Gubens M, Ramalingam SS, Felip E, Goldman JW, Scalzo C, Jensen E, Kush DA, Hui R (2019) Five-year overall survival for patients with advanced nonsmall-cell lung cancer treated with Pembrolizumab: results from the phase I KEYNOTE-001 study. J Clin Oncol:JCO1900934. https://doi.org/10.1200/JCO.19.00934

17. Gettinger S, Horn L, Jackman D, Spigel D, Antonia S, Hellmann M, Powderly J, Heist R, Sequist LV, Smith DC, Leming P, Geese WJ, Yoon D, Li A, Brahmer J (2018) Five-year follow-up of Nivolumab in previously treated advanced non-small-cell lung Cancer: results from the CA209-003 study. J Clin Oncol 36(17):1675–1684. https://doi.org/10.1200/JCO.2017.77.0412

18. Ku GY, Yuan J, Page DB, Schroeder SE, Panageas KS, Carvajal RD, Chapman PB, Schwartz GK, Allison JP, Wolchok JD (2010) Single-institution experience with ipilimumab in advanced melanoma patients in the compassionate use setting: lymphocyte count after 2 doses correlates with survival. Cancer 116(7):1767–1775. https://doi.org/10.1002/cncr.24951

19. Gajewski TF, Louahed J, Brichard VG (2010) Gene signature in melanoma associated with clinical activity: a potential clue to unlock cancer immunotherapy. Cancer J 16(4):399–403. https://doi.org/10.1097/PPO.0b013e3181eacbd8

20. Ji RR, Chasalow SD, Wang L, Hamid O, Schmidt H, Cogswell J, Alaparthy S, Berman D, Jure-Kunkel M, Siemers NO, Jackson JR, Shahabi V (2012) An immune-active tumor microenvironment favors clinical response to ipilimumab. Cancer Immunol Immunother 61(7):1019–1031. https://doi.org/10.1007/s00262-011-1172-6

21. Lee SJ, Jang BC, Lee SW, Yang YI, Suh SI, Park YM, Oh S, Shin JG, Yao S, Chen L, Choi IH (2006) Interferon regulatory factor-1 is prerequisite to the constitutive expression and IFN-gamma-induced upregulation of B7-H1 (CD274). FEBS Lett 580(3):755–762. https://doi.org/10.1016/j.febslet.2005.12.093

22. Garon EB, Rizvi NA, Hui R, Leighl N, Balmanoukian AS, Eder JP, Patnaik A, Aggarwal C, Gubens M, Horn L, Carcereny E, Ahn MJ, Felip E, Lee JS, Hellmann MD, Hamid O, Goldman JW, Soria JC, Dolled-Filhart M, Rutledge RZ, Zhang J, Lunceford JK, Rangwala R, Lubiniecki GM, Roach C, Emancipator K, Gandhi L, Investigators K (2015) Pembrolizumab for the treatment of non-small-cell lung cancer. N Engl J Med 372(21):2018–2028. https://doi.org/10.1056/NEJMoa1501824

23. Lawrence MS, Stojanov P, Polak P, Kryukov GV, Cibulskis K, Sivachenko A, Carter SL, Stewart C, Mermel CH, Roberts SA, Kiezun A, Hammerman PS, McKenna A, Drier Y, Zou L, Ramos AH, Pugh TJ, Stransky N, Helman E, Kim J, Sougnez C, Ambrogio L, Nickerson E, Shefler E, Cortes ML, Auclair D, Saksena G, Voet D, Noble M, DiCara D, Lin P, Lichtenstein L, Heiman DI, Fennell T, Imielinski M, Hernandez B, Hodis E, Baca S, Dulak AM, Lohr J, Landau DA, Wu CJ, Melendez-Zajgla J, Hidalgo-Miranda A, Koren A, McCarroll SA, Mora J, Crompton B, Onofrio R, Parkin M, Winckler W, Ardlie K, Gabriel SB, Roberts CWM, Biegel JA, Stegmaier K, Bass AJ, Garraway LA, Meyerson M, Golub TR, Gordenin DA, Sunyaev S, Lander ES, Getz G (2013) Mutational heterogeneity in cancer and the search for new cancer-associated genes. Nature 499(7457):214–218. https://doi.org/10.1038/nature12213

24. Alexandrov LB, Nik-Zainal S, Wedge DC, Aparicio SA, Behjati S, Biankin AV, Bignell GR, Bolli N, Borg A, Borresen-Dale AL, Boyault S, Burkhardt B, Butler AP, Caldas C, Davies HR, Desmedt C, Eils R, Eyfjord JE, Foekens JA, Greaves M, Hosoda F, Hutter B, Ilicic T, Imbeaud S, Imielinski M, Jager N, Jones DT, Jones D, Knappskog S, Kool M, Lakhani SR, Lopez-Otin C, Martin S, Munshi NC, Nakamura H, Northcott PA, Pajic M, Papaemmanuil E, Paradiso A, Pearson JV, Puente XS, Raine K, Ramakrishna M, Richardson AL, Richter J, Rosenstiel P, Schlesner M, Schumacher TN, Span PN, Teague JW, Totoki Y, Tutt AN, Valdes-Mas R, van Buuren MM, van 't Veer L, Vincent-Salomon A, Waddell N, Yates LR, Australian Pancreatic Cancer Genome I, Consortium IBC, Consortium IM-S, PedBrain I, Zucman-Rossi J, Futreal PA, McDermott U, Lichter P, Meyerson M, Grimmond SM, Siebert R, Campo E, Shibata T, Pfister SM, Campbell PJ, Stratton MR (2013) Signatures of mutational processes in human cancer. Nature 500(7463):415–421. https://doi.org/10.1038/nature12477

25. Segal NH, Parsons DW, Peggs KS, Velculescu V, Kinzler KW, Vogelstein B, Allison JP (2008) Epitope landscape in breast and colorectal cancer. Cancer Res 68(3):889–892. https://doi.org/10.1158/0008-5472.CAN-07-3095

26. Matsushita H, Vesely MD, Koboldt DC, Rickert CG, Uppaluri R, Magrini VJ, Arthur CD, White JM, Chen YS, Shea LK, Hundal J, Wendl MC, Demeter R, Wylie T, Allison JP, Smyth MJ, Old LJ, Mardis ER, Schreiber RD (2012) Cancer exome analysis reveals a T-cell-dependent mechanism of cancer immunoediting. Nature 482(7385):400–404. https://doi.org/10.1038/nature10755

27. van Rooij N, van Buuren MM, Philips D, Velds A, Toebes M, Heemskerk B, van Dijk LJ, Behjati S, Hilkmann H, El Atmioui D, Nieuwland M, Stratton MR, Kerkhoven RM, Kesmir C, Haanen JB, Kvistborg P, Schumacher TN (2013) Tumor exome analysis reveals neoantigen-specific T-cell reactivity in an ipilimumab-responsive melanoma. J Clin Oncol 31(32):e439–e442. https://doi.org/10.1200/JCO.2012.47.7521

28. Johnson DB, Frampton GM, Rioth MJ, Yusko E, Xu Y, Guo X, Ennis RC, Fabrizio D, Chalmers ZR, Greenbowe J, Ali SM, Balasubramanian S, Sun JX, He Y, Frederick DT, Puzanov I, Balko JM, Cates JM, Ross JS, Sanders C, Robins H, Shyr Y, Miller VA, Stephens PJ, Sullivan RJ, Sosman JA, Lovly CM (2016) Targeted next generation sequencing identifies markers of response to PD-1 blockade. Cancer Immunol Res 4(11):959–967. https://doi.org/10.1158/2326-6066.CIR-16-0143

29. Rizvi H, Sanchez-Vega F, La K, Chatila W, Jonsson P, Halpenny D, Plodkowski A, Long N, Sauter JL, Rekhtman N, Hollmann T, Schalper KA, Gainor JF, Shen R, Ni A, Arbour KC, Merghoub T, Wolchok J, Snyder A, Chaft JE, Kris MG, Rudin CM, Socci ND, Berger MF, Taylor BS, Zehir A, Solit DB, Arcila ME, Ladanyi M, Riely GJ, Schultz N, Hellmann MD (2018) Molecular determinants of response to anti-programmed cell death (PD)-1 and anti-programmed death-ligand 1 (PD-L1) blockade in patients with non-small-cell lung cancer profiled with targeted next-generation sequencing. J Clin Oncol 36(7):633–641. https://doi.org/10.1200/JCO.2017.75.3384

30. Garofalo A, Sholl L, Reardon B, Taylor-Weiner A, Amin-Mansour A, Miao D, Liu D, Oliver N, MacConaill L, Ducar M, Rojas-Rudilla V, Giannakis M, Ghazani A, Gray S, Janne P, Garber J, Joffe S, Lindeman N, Wagle N, Garraway LA, Van Allen EM (2016) The impact of tumor profiling approaches and genomic data strategies for cancer precision medicine. Genome Med 8(1):79. https://doi.org/10.1186/s13073-016-0333-9

31. Chalmers ZR, Connelly CF, Fabrizio D, Gay L, Ali SM, Ennis R, Schrock A, Campbell B, Shlien A, Chmielecki J, Huang F, He Y, Sun J, Tabori U, Kennedy M, Lieber DS, Roels S, White J, Otto GA, Ross JS, Garraway L, Miller VA, Stephens PJ, Frampton GM (2017) Analysis of 100,000 human cancer genomes reveals the landscape of tumor mutational burden. Genome Med 9(1):34. https://doi.org/10.1186/s13073-017-0424-2

32. Campesato LF, Barroso-Sousa R, Jimenez L, Correa BR, Sabbaga J, Hoff PM, Reis LF, Galante PA, Camargo AA (2015) Comprehensive cancer-gene panels can be used to estimate mutational load and predict clinical benefit to PD-1 blockade in clinical practice. Oncotarget 6(33):34221–34227. https://doi.org/10.18632/oncotarget.5950

33. Zehir A, Benayed R, Shah RH, Syed A, Middha S, Kim HR, Srinivasan P, Gao J, Chakravarty D, Devlin SM, Hellmann MD, Barron DA, Schram AM, Hameed M, Dogan S, Ross DS, Hechtman JF, DeLair DF, Yao J, Mandelker DL, Cheng DT, Chandramohan R, Mohanty AS, Ptashkin RN, Jayakumaran G, Prasad M, Syed MH, Rema AB, Liu ZY, Nafa K, Borsu L, Sadowska J, Casanova J, Bacares R, Kiecka IJ, Razumova A, Son JB, Stewart L, Baldi T, Mullaney KA, Al-Ahmadie H, Vakiani E, Abeshouse AA, Penson AV, Jonsson P, Camacho N, Chang MT, Won HH, Gross BE, Kundra R, Heins ZJ, Chen HW, Phillips S, Zhang H, Wang J, Ochoa A, Wills J, Eubank M, Thomas SB, Gardos SM, Reales DN, Galle J, Durany R, Cambria R, Abida W, Cercek A, Feldman DR, Gounder MM, Hakimi AA, Harding JJ, Iyer G, Janjigian YY, Jordan EJ, Kelly CM, Lowery MA, Morris LGT, Omuro AM, Raj N, Razavi P, Shoushtari AN, Shukla N, Soumerai TE, Varghese AM, Yaeger R, Coleman J, Bochner B, Riely GJ, Saltz LB, Scher HI, Sabbatini PJ, Robson ME, Klimstra DS, Taylor BS, Baselga J, Schultz N, Hyman DM, Arcila ME, Solit DB, Ladanyi M, Berger MF (2017) Mutational landscape of metastatic cancer revealed from prospective clinical sequencing of 10,000 patients. Nat Med 23(6):703–713. https://doi.org/10.1038/nm.4333

34. Adalsteinsson VA, Ha G, Freeman SS, Choudhury AD, Stover DG, Parsons HA, Gydush G, Reed SC, Rotem D, Rhoades J, Loginov D, Livitz D, Rosebrock D, Leshchiner I, Kim J, Stewart C, Rosenberg M, Francis JM, Zhang CZ, Cohen O, Oh C, Ding H, Polak P, Lloyd M, Mahmud S, Helvie K, Merrill MS, Santiago RA, O'Connor EP, Jeong SH, Leeson R, Barry RM, Kramkowski JF, Zhang Z, Polacek L, Lohr JG, Schleicher M, Lipscomb E, Saltzman A, Oliver NM, Marini L, Waks AG, Harshman LC, Tolaney SM, Van Allen EM, Winer EP, Lin NU, Nakabayashi M, Taplin ME, Johannessen CM, Garraway LA, Golub TR, Boehm JS, Wagle N, Getz G, Love JC, Meyerson M (2017) Scalable whole-exome sequencing of cell-free DNA reveals high concordance with metastatic tumors. Nat Commun 8(1):1324. https://doi.org/10.1038/s41467-017-00965-y

35. Koeppel F, Blanchard S, Jovelet C, Genin B, Marcaillou C, Martin E, Rouleau E, Solary E, Soria JC, Andre F, Lacroix L (2017) Whole exome sequencing for determination of tumor mutation load in liquid biopsy from advanced cancer patients. PLoS One 12(11):e0188174. https://doi.org/10.1371/journal.pone.0188174

36. Gandara DR, Paul SM, Kowanetz M, Schleifman E, Zou W, Li Y, Rittmeyer A, Fehrenbacher L, Otto G, Malboeuf C, Lieber DS, Lipson D, Silterra J, Amler L, Riehl T, Cummings CA, Hegde PS, Sandler A, Ballinger M, Fabrizio D, Mok T, Shames DS (2018) Blood-based tumor mutational burden as a predictor of clinical benefit in non-small-cell lung cancer patients treated with atezolizumab. Nat Med 24(9):1441–1448. https://doi.org/10.1038/s41591-018-0134-3

37. Chaudhuri AA, Chabon JJ, Lovejoy AF, Newman AM, Stehr H, Azad TD, Khodadoust MS, Esfahani MS, Liu CL, Zhou L, Scherer F, Kurtz DM, Say C, Carter JN, Merriott DJ, Dudley JC, Binkley MS, Modlin L, Padda SK, Gensheimer MF, West RB, Shrager JB, Neal JW, Wakelee HA, Loo BW Jr, Alizadeh AA, Diehn M (2017) Early detection of molecular residual disease in localized lung cancer by circulating tumor DNA profiling. Cancer Discov 7(12):1394–1403. https://doi.org/10.1158/2159-8290.CD-17-0716

38. Muller JN, Falk M, Talwar J, Neemann N, Mariotti E, Bertrand M, Zacherle T, Lakis S, Menon R, Gloeckner C, Tiemann M, Heukamp LC, Thomas RK, Griesinger F, Heuckmann JM (2017) Concordance between comprehensive cancer genome profiling in plasma and tumor specimens. J Thorac Oncol 12(10):1503–1511. https://doi.org/10.1016/j.jtho.2017.07.014

39. Davis AA, Chae YK, Agte S, Pan A, Simon NI, Taxter TJ, Behdad A, Carneiro BA, Cristofanilli M, Giles FJ (2017) Comparison of tumor mutational burden (TMB) across tumor tissue and circulating tumor DNA (ctDNA). J Clin Oncol 35(15_suppl):e23028–e23028. https://doi.org/10.1200/JCO.2017.35.15_suppl.e23028

40. Peters S (2019) Tumor mutational burden (TMB) as a biomarker of survival in metastatic non-small cell lung cancer (mNSCLC): Blood and tissue TMB analysis from MYSTIC, a Phase III study of first-line durvalumab±tremelimumab vs chemotherapy. In: American Association for Cancer Research Annual Meeting

41. Rizvi NA, Hellmann MD, Snyder A, Kvistborg P, Makarov V, Havel JJ, Lee W, Yuan J, Wong P, Ho TS, Miller ML, Rekhtman N, Moreira AL, Ibrahim F, Bruggeman C, Gasmi B, Zappasodi R, Maeda Y, Sander C, Garon EB, Merghoub T, Wolchok JD, Schumacher TN, Chan TA (2015) Cancer immunology. Mutational landscape determines sensitivity to PD-1 blockade in non-small cell lung cancer. Science 348(6230):124–128. https://doi.org/10.1126/science.aaa1348

42. Gandhi L, Rodriguez-Abreu D, Gadgeel S, Esteban E, Felip E, De Angelis F, Domine M, Clingan P, Hochmair MJ, Powell SF, Cheng SY, Bischoff HG, Peled N, Grossi F, Jennens RR, Reck M, Hui R, Garon EB, Boyer M, Rubio-Viqueira B, Novello S, Kurata T, Gray JE, Vida J, Wei Z, Yang J, Raftopoulos H, Pietanza MC, Garassino MC, Investigators K (2018) Pembrolizumab plus chemotherapy in metastatic non-small-cell lung cancer. N Engl J Med 378(22):2078–2092. https://doi.org/10.1056/NEJMoa1801005

43. Marabelle A, Fakih M, Lopez J, Shah M, Shapira-Frommer R, Nakagawa K, Chung HC, Kindler HL, Lopez-Martin JA, Miller WH Jr, Italiano A, Kao S, Piha-Paul SA, Delord JP, McWilliams RR, Fabrizio DA, Aurora-Garg D, Xu L, Jin F, Norwood K, Bang YJ, (2020) Association of tumour mutational burden with outcomes in patients with advanced solid tumours treated with pembrolizumab: prospective biomarker analysis of the multicohort, open-label, phase 2 KEYNOTE-158 study. Lancet Oncol. Oct;21(10):1353–1365. https://doi.org/10.1016/S1470-2045(20)30445-9. Epub 2020 Sep 10. PMID: 32919526. https://www.fda.gov/drugs/drug-approvals-and-databases/fda-approves-pembrolizumab-adults-and-children-tmb-h-solid-tumors

44. Carbone DP, Reck M, Paz-Ares L, Creelan B, Horn L, Steins M, Felip E, van den Heuvel MM, Ciuleanu TE, Badin F, Ready N, Hiltermann TJN, Nair S, Juergens R, Peters S, Minenza E, Wrangle JM, Rodriguez-Abreu D, Borghaei H, Blumenschein GR Jr, Villaruz LC, Havel L, Krejci J, Corral Jaime J, Chang H, Geese WJ, Bhagavatheeswaran P, Chen AC, Socinski MA, CheckMate I (2017) First-line Nivolumab in stage IV or recurrent non-small-cell lung cancer. N Engl J Med 376(25):2415–2426. https://doi.org/10.1056/NEJMoa1613493

45. Hellmann MD, Ciuleanu TE, Pluzanski A, Lee JS, Otterson GA, Audigier-Valette C, Minenza E, Linardou H, Burgers S, Salman P, Borghaei H, Ramalingam SS, Brahmer J, Reck M, O'Byrne KJ, Geese WJ, Green G, Chang H, Szustakowski J, Bhagavatheeswaran P, Healey D, Fu Y, Nathan F, Paz-Ares L (2018) Nivolumab plus Ipilimumab in lung cancer with a high tumor mutational burden. N Engl J Med 378(22):2093–2104. https://doi.org/10.1056/NEJMoa1801946

46. Kowanetz M, Zou W, Shames D, Cummings C, Rizvi N, Spira A, Frampton G, Leveque V, Flynn S, Mocci S, Shankar G, Funke R, Ballinger M, Waterkamp D, Chen D, Sandler A, Hampton G, Amler L, Hegde P, Hellmann M (2017) OA20.01 tumor mutation burden (TMB) is associated with improved efficacy of Atezolizumab in 1L and 2L+ NSCLC patients. J Thorac Oncol 12(1, Supplement):S321–S322. https://doi.org/10.1016/j.jtho.2016.11.343

47. Fehrenbacher L, Spira A, Ballinger M, Kowanetz M, Vansteenkiste J, Mazieres J, Park K, Smith D, Artal-Cortes A, Lewanski C, Braiteh F, Waterkamp D, He P, Zou W, Chen DS, Yi J, Sandler A, Rittmeyer A, Group PS (2016) Atezolizumab versus docetaxel for patients with previously treated non-small-cell lung cancer (POPLAR): a multicentre, open-label, phase 2 randomised controlled trial. Lancet 387(10030):1837–1846. https://doi.org/10.1016/S0140-6736(16)00587-0

48. Peters S, Gettinger S, Johnson ML, Janne PA, Garassino MC, Christoph D, Toh CK, Rizvi NA, Chaft JE, Carcereny Costa E, Patel JD, Chow LQM, Koczywas M, Ho C, Fruh M, van den

Heuvel M, Rothenstein J, Reck M, Paz-Ares L, Shepherd FA, Kurata T, Li Z, Qiu J, Kowanetz M, Mocci S, Shankar G, Sandler A, Felip E (2017) Phase II trial of Atezolizumab as first-line or subsequent therapy for patients with programmed death-ligand 1-selected advanced non-small-cell lung cancer (BIRCH). J Clin Oncol 35(24):2781–2789. https://doi.org/10.1200/JCO.2016.71.9476

49. Spigel DR, Chaft JE, Gettinger S, Chao BH, Dirix L, Schmid P, Chow LQM, Hicks RJ, Leon L, Fredrickson J, Kowanetz M, Sandler A, Funke R, Rizvi NA (2018) FIR: efficacy, safety, and biomarker analysis of a phase II open-label study of Atezolizumab in PD-L1-selected patients with NSCLC. J Thorac Oncol 13(11):1733–1742. https://doi.org/10.1016/j.jtho.2018.05.004

50. Rizvi NA, Chul Cho B, Reinmuth N, Lee KH, Ahn M-J, Luft A, van den Heuvel M, Cobo M, Smolin A, Vicente D, Moiseyenko V, Antonia SJ, Le Moulec S, Robinet G, Natale R, Nakagawa K, Zhao L, Stockman PK, Chand V, Peters S (2018) LBA6Durvalumab with or without tremelimumab vs platinum-based chemotherapy as first-line treatment for metastatic non-small cell lung cancer: MYSTIC. Ann Oncol 29(suppl_10). https://doi.org/10.1093/annonc/mdy511.005

51. Hellmann MD, Nathanson T, Rizvi H, Creelan BC, Sanchez-Vega F, Ahuja A, Ni A, Novik JB, Mangarin LMB, Abu-Akeel M, Liu C, Sauter JL, Rekhtman N, Chang E, Callahan MK, Chaft JE, Voss MH, Tenet M, Li XM, Covello K, Renninger A, Vitazka P, Geese WJ, Borghaei H, Rudin CM, Antonia SJ, Swanton C, Hammerbacher J, Merghoub T, McGranahan N, Snyder A, Wolchok JD (2018) Genomic features of response to combination immunotherapy in patients with advanced non-small-cell lung cancer. Cancer Cell 33(5):843–852. e844. https://doi.org/10.1016/j.ccell.2018.03.018

52. Ready N, Hellmann MD, Awad MM, Otterson GA, Gutierrez M, Gainor JF, Borghaei H, Jolivet J, Horn L, Mates M, Brahmer J, Rabinowitz I, Reddy PS, Chesney J, Orcutt J, Spigel DR, Reck M, O'Byrne KJ, Paz-Ares L, Hu W, Zerba K, Li X, Lestini B, Geese WJ, Szustakowski JD, Green G, Chang H, Ramalingam SS (2019) First-line Nivolumab plus Ipilimumab in advanced non-small-cell lung cancer (CheckMate 568): outcomes by programmed death ligand 1 and tumor mutational burden as biomarkers. J Clin Oncol:JCO1801042. https://doi.org/10.1200/JCO.18.01042

53. Squibb B-M (2018, Oct 19) Bristol-Myers Squibb provides update on the ongoing regulatory review of Opdivo Plus low-dose Yervoy in first-line lung cancer patients with tumor mutational burden ≥10 mut/Mb. https://bit.ly/2ySdgOC. Accessed 20 May 2019

54. Singal G, Miller PG, Agarwala V, Li G, Kaushik G, Backenroth D, Gossai A, Frampton GM, Torres AZ, Lehnert EM, Bourque D, O'Connell C, Bowser B, Caron T, Baydur E, Seidl-Rathkopf K, Ivanov I, Alpha-Cobb G, Guria A, He J, Frank S, Nunnally AC, Bailey M, Jaskiw A, Feuchtbaum D, Nussbaum N, Abernethy AP, Miller VA (2019) Association of patient characteristics and tumor genomics with clinical outcomes among patients with non-small cell lung cancer using a clinicogenomic database. JAMA 321(14):1391–1399. https://doi.org/10.1001/jama.2019.3241

55. Yarchoan M, Hopkins A, Jaffee EM (2017) Tumor mutational burden and response rate to PD-1 inhibition. N Engl J Med 377(25):2500–2501. https://doi.org/10.1056/NEJMc1713444

56. Samstein RM, Lee CH, Shoushtari AN, Hellmann MD, Shen R, Janjigian YY, Barron DA, Zehir A, Jordan EJ, Omuro A, Kaley TJ, Kendall SM, Motzer RJ, Hakimi AA, Voss MH, Russo P, Rosenberg J, Iyer G, Bochner BH, Bajorin DF, Al-Ahmadie HA, Chaft JE, Rudin CM, Riely GJ, Baxi S, Ho AL, Wong RJ, Pfister DG, Wolchok JD, Barker CA, Gutin PH, Brennan CW, Tabar V, Mellinghoff IK, DeAngelis LM, Ariyan CE, Lee N, Tap WD, Gounder MM, D'Angelo SP, Saltz L, Stadler ZK, Scher HI, Baselga J, Razavi P, Klebanoff CA, Yaeger R, Segal NH, Ku GY, DeMatteo RP, Ladanyi M, Rizvi NA, Berger MF, Riaz N, Solit DB, Chan TA, Morris LGT (2019) Tumor mutational load predicts survival after immunotherapy across multiple cancer types. Nat Genet 51(2):202–206. https://doi.org/10.1038/s41588-018-0312-8

57. Snyder A, Makarov V, Merghoub T, Yuan J, Zaretsky JM, Desrichard A, Walsh LA, Postow MA, Wong P, Ho TS, Hollmann TJ, Bruggeman C, Kannan K, Li Y, Elipenahli C, Liu C, Harbison CT, Wang L, Ribas A, Wolchok JD, Chan TA (2014) Genetic basis for clinical

response to CTLA-4 blockade in melanoma. N Engl J Med 371(23):2189–2199. https://doi.org/10.1056/NEJMoa1406498

58. Van Allen EM, Miao D, Schilling B, Shukla SA, Blank C, Zimmer L, Sucker A, Hillen U, Foppen MHG, Goldinger SM, Utikal J, Hassel JC, Weide B, Kaehler KC, Loquai C, Mohr P, Gutzmer R, Dummer R, Gabriel S, Wu CJ, Schadendorf D, Garraway LA (2015) Genomic correlates of response to CTLA-4 blockade in metastatic melanoma. Science 350(6257):207–211. https://doi.org/10.1126/science.aad0095

59. Miao D, Margolis CA, Vokes NI, Liu D, Taylor-Weiner A, Wankowicz SM, Adeegbe D, Keliher D, Schilling B, Tracy A, Manos M, Chau NG, Hanna GJ, Polak P, Rodig SJ, Signoretti S, Sholl LM, Engelman JA, Getz G, Janne PA, Haddad RI, Choueiri TK, Barbie DA, Haq R, Awad MM, Schadendorf D, Hodi FS, Bellmunt J, Wong KK, Hammerman P, Van Allen EM (2018) Genomic correlates of response to immune checkpoint blockade in microsatellite-stable solid tumors. Nat Genet 50(9):1271–1281. https://doi.org/10.1038/s41588-018-0200-2

60. Rosenberg JE, Hoffman-Censits J, Powles T, van der Heijden MS, Balar AV, Necchi A, Dawson N, O'Donnell PH, Balmanoukian A, Loriot Y, Srinivas S, Retz MM, Grivas P, Joseph RW, Galsky MD, Fleming MT, Petrylak DP, Perez-Gracia JL, Burris HA, Castellano D, Canil C, Bellmunt J, Bajorin D, Nickles D, Bourgon R, Frampton GM, Cui N, Mariathasan S, Abidoye O, Fine GD, Dreicer R (2016) Atezolizumab in patients with locally advanced and metastatic urothelial carcinoma who have progressed following treatment with platinum-based chemotherapy: a single-arm, multicentre, phase 2 trial. Lancet 387(10031):1909–1920. https://doi.org/10.1016/S0140-6736(16)00561-4

61. Cristescu R, Mogg R, Ayers M, Albright A, Murphy E, Yearley J, Sher X, Liu XQ, Lu H, Nebozhyn M, Zhang C, Lunceford JK, Joe A, Cheng J, Webber AL, Ibrahim N, Plimack ER, Ott PA, Seiwert TY, Ribas A, McClanahan TK, Tomassini JE, Loboda A, Kaufman D (2018) Pan-tumor genomic biomarkers for PD-1 checkpoint blockade-based immunotherapy. Science 362(6411). https://doi.org/10.1126/science.aar3593

62. Goodman AM, Kato S, Bazhenova L, Patel SP, Frampton GM, Miller V, Stephens PJ, Daniels GA, Kurzrock R (2017) Tumor mutational burden as an independent predictor of response to immunotherapy in diverse cancers. Mol Cancer Ther 16(11):2598–2608. https://doi.org/10.1158/1535-7163.MCT-17-0386

63. Vokes NI, Liu D, Ricciuti B, Jimenez-Aguilar E, Rizvi H, Dietlein F, He MX, Margolis CA, Elmarakeby HA, Girshman J, Adeni A, Sanchez-Vega F, Schultz N, Dahlberg S, Zehir A, Jänne PA, Nishino M, Umeton R, Sholl LM, Van Allen EM, Hellmann MD, Awad MM. (2019) Harmonization of Tumor Mutational Burden Quantification and Association With Response to Immune Checkpoint Blockade in Non-Small-Cell Lung Cancer. JCO Precis Oncol.; 3:PO.19.00171. https://doi.org/10.1200/PO.19.00171. Epub 2019 Nov 12. PMID: 31832578

64. Lim C, Tsao MS, Le LW, Shepherd FA, Feld R, Burkes RL, Liu G, Kamel-Reid S, Hwang D, Tanguay J, da Cunha SG, Leighl NB (2015) Biomarker testing and time to treatment decision in patients with advanced nonsmall-cell lung cancer. Ann Oncol 26(7):1415–1421. https://doi.org/10.1093/annonc/mdv208

65. Sacher AG, Paweletz C, Dahlberg SE, Alden RS, O'Connell A, Feeney N, Mach SL, Janne PA, Oxnard GR (2016) Prospective validation of rapid plasma genotyping for the detection of EGFR and KRAS mutations in advanced lung Cancer. JAMA Oncol 2(8):1014–1022. https://doi.org/10.1001/jamaoncol.2016.0173

66. Sacher AG, Komatsubara KM, Oxnard GR (2017) Application of plasma genotyping technologies in non-small cell lung cancer: a practical review. J Thorac Oncol 12(9):1344–1356. https://doi.org/10.1016/j.jtho.2017.05.022

67. McGranahan N, Furness AJ, Rosenthal R, Ramskov S, Lyngaa R, Saini SK, Jamal-Hanjani M, Wilson GA, Birkbak NJ, Hiley CT, Watkins TB, Shafi S, Murugaesu N, Mitter R, Akarca AU, Linares J, Marafioti T, Henry JY, Van Allen EM, Miao D, Schilling B, Schadendorf D, Garraway LA, Makarov V, Rizvi NA, Snyder A, Hellmann MD, Merghoub T, Wolchok JD, Shukla SA, Wu CJ, Peggs KS, Chan TA, Hadrup SR, Quezada SA, Swanton C (2016) Clonal

neoantigens elicit T cell immunoreactivity and sensitivity to immune checkpoint blockade. Science 351(6280):1463–1469. https://doi.org/10.1126/science.aaf1490

68. Mok TSK, Gadgeel S, Kim ES, Velcheti V, Hu S, Riehl T, Schleifman E, Paul SM, Mocci S, Shames DS, Phan S, Yun C, Mathisen M, Kowanetz M, Sweere U, Socinski MA (2017) 1383TiPBlood first line ready screening trial (B-F1RST) and blood first assay screening trial (BFAST) enable clinical development of novel blood-based biomarker assays for tumor mutational burden (TMB) and somatic mutations in 1L advanced or metastatic NSCLC. Ann Oncol 28(suppl_5). https://doi.org/10.1093/annonc/mdx380.084

69. Schumacher TN, Schreiber RD (2015) Neoantigens in cancer immunotherapy. Science 348(6230):69–74. https://doi.org/10.1126/science.aaa4971

70. Rooney MS, Shukla SA, Wu CJ, Getz G, Hacohen N (2015) Molecular and genetic properties of tumors associated with local immune cytolytic activity. Cell 160(1–2):48–61. https://doi.org/10.1016/j.cell.2014.12.033

71. Gubin MM, Zhang X, Schuster H, Caron E, Ward JP, Noguchi T, Ivanova Y, Hundal J, Arthur CD, Krebber WJ, Mulder GE, Toebes M, Vesely MD, Lam SS, Korman AJ, Allison JP, Freeman GJ, Sharpe AH, Pearce EL, Schumacher TN, Aebersold R, Rammensee HG, Melief CJ, Mardis ER, Gillanders WE, Artyomov MN, Schreiber RD (2014) Checkpoint blockade cancer immunotherapy targets tumour-specific mutant antigens. Nature 515(7528):577–581. https://doi.org/10.1038/nature13988

72. Fehlings M, Simoni Y, Penny HL, Becht E, Loh CY, Gubin MM, Ward JP, Wong SC, Schreiber RD, Newell EW (2017) Checkpoint blockade immunotherapy reshapes the high-dimensional phenotypic heterogeneity of murine intratumoural neoantigen-specific CD8(+) T cells. Nat Commun 8(1):562. https://doi.org/10.1038/s41467-017-00627-z

73. Le DT, Durham JN, Smith KN, Wang H, Bartlett BR, Aulakh LK, Lu S, Kemberling H, Wilt C, Luber BS, Wong F, Azad NS, Rucki AA, Laheru D, Donehower R, Zaheer A, Fisher GA, Crocenzi TS, Lee JJ, Greten TF, Duffy AG, Ciombor KK, Eyring AD, Lam BH, Joe A, Kang SP, Holdhoff M, Danilova L, Cope L, Meyer C, Zhou S, Goldberg RM, Armstrong DK, Bever KM, Fader AN, Taube J, Housseau F, Spetzler D, Xiao N, Pardoll DM, Papadopoulos N, Kinzler KW, Eshleman JR, Vogelstein B, Anders RA, Diaz LA Jr (2017) Mismatch repair deficiency predicts response of solid tumors to PD-1 blockade. Science 357(6349):409–413. https://doi.org/10.1126/science.aan6733

74. Luksza M, Riaz N, Makarov V, Balachandran VP, Hellmann MD, Solovyov A, Rizvi NA, Merghoub T, Levine AJ, Chan TA, Wolchok JD, Greenbaum BD (2017) A neoantigen fitness model predicts tumour response to checkpoint blockade immunotherapy. Nature 551(7681):517–520. https://doi.org/10.1038/nature24473

75. Balachandran VP, Luksza M, Zhao JN, Makarov V, Moral JA, Remark R, Herbst B, Askan G, Bhanot U, Senbabaoglu Y, Wells DK, Cary CIO, Grbovic-Huezo O, Attiyeh M, Medina B, Zhang J, Loo J, Saglimbeni J, Abu-Akeel M, Zappasodi R, Riaz N, Smoragiewicz M, Kelley ZL, Basturk O, Australian Pancreatic Cancer Genome I, Garvan Institute of Medical R, Prince of Wales H, Royal North Shore H, University of G, St Vincent's H, Institute QBMR, University of Melbourne CfCR, University of Queensland IfMB, Bankstown H, Liverpool H, Royal Prince Alfred Hospital COBL, Westmead H, Fremantle H, St John of God H, Royal Adelaide H, Flinders Medical C, Envoi P, Princess Alexandria H, Austin H, Johns Hopkins Medical I, Cancer AR-NCfARo, Gonen M, Levine AJ, Allen PJ, Fearon DT, Merad M, Gnjatic S, Iacobuzio-Donahue CA, Wolchok JD, DeMatteo RP, Chan TA, Greenbaum BD, Merghoub T, Leach SD (2017) Identification of unique neoantigen qualities in long-term survivors of pancreatic cancer. Nature 551(7681):512–516. https://doi.org/10.1038/nature24462

76. Seiwert TY, Burtness B, Mehra R, Weiss J, Berger R, Eder JP, Heath K, McClanahan T, Lunceford J, Gause C, Cheng JD, Chow LQ (2016) Safety and clinical activity of pembrolizumab for treatment of recurrent or metastatic squamous cell carcinoma of the head and neck (KEYNOTE-012): an open-label, multicentre, phase 1b trial. Lancet Oncol 17(7):956–965. https://doi.org/10.1016/S1470-2045(16)30066-3

77. Nghiem PT, Bhatia S, Lipson EJ, Kudchadkar RR, Miller NJ, Annamalai L, Berry S, Chartash EK, Daud A, Fling SP, Friedlander PA, Kluger HM, Kohrt HE, Lundgren L, Margolin K, Mitchell A, Olencki T, Pardoll DM, Reddy SA, Shantha EM, Sharfman WH, Sharon E, Shemanski LR, Shinohara MM, Sunshine JC, Taube JM, Thompson JA, Townson SM, Yearley JH, Topalian SL, Cheever MA (2016) PD-1 blockade with Pembrolizumab in advanced Merkel-cell carcinoma. N Engl J Med 374(26):2542–2552. https://doi.org/10.1056/NEJMoa1603702
78. Panda A, de Cubas AA, Stein M, Riedlinger G, Kra J, Mayer T, Smith CC, Vincent BG, Serody JS, Beckermann KE, Ganesan S, Bhanot G, Rathmell WK (2018) Endogenous retrovirus expression is associated with response to immune checkpoint blockade in clear cell renal cell carcinoma. JCI Insight 3(16). https://doi.org/10.1172/jci.insight.121522
79. Yadav M, Jhunjhunwala S, Phung QT, Lupardus P, Tanguay J, Bumbaca S, Franci C, Cheung TK, Fritsche J, Weinschenk T, Modrusan Z, Mellman I, Lill JR, Delamarre L (2014) Predicting immunogenic tumour mutations by combining mass spectrometry and exome sequencing. Nature 515(7528):572–576. https://doi.org/10.1038/nature14001
80. Abelin JG, Keskin DB, Sarkizova S, Hartigan CR, Zhang W, Sidney J, Stevens J, Lane W, Zhang GL, Eisenhaure TM, Clauser KR, Hacohen N, Rooney MS, Carr SA, Wu CJ (2017) Mass spectrometry profiling of HLA-associated Peptidomes in mono-allelic cells enables more accurate epitope prediction. Immunity 46(2):315–326. https://doi.org/10.1016/j.immuni.2017.02.007
81. Graham DB, Luo C, O'Connell DJ, Lefkovith A, Brown EM, Yassour M, Varma M, Abelin JG, Conway KL, Jasso GJ, Matar CG, Carr SA, Xavier RJ (2018) Antigen discovery and specification of immunodominance hierarchies for MHCII-restricted epitopes. Nat Med 24(11):1762–1772. https://doi.org/10.1038/s41591-018-0203-7
82. Yarchoan M, Albacker LA, Hopkins AC, Montesion M, Murugesan K, Vithayathil TT, Zaidi N, Azad NS, Laheru DA, Frampton GM, Jaffee EM (2019) PD-L1 expression and tumor mutational burden are independent biomarkers in most cancers. JCI Insight 4(6). https://doi.org/10.1172/jci.insight.126908

Chapter 3
Liquid Biopsies: New Technology and Evidence

Daniel Morgensztern

Abstract Liquid biopsy refers to a broad category of minimally invasive test done on blood or other fluid specimens to detect fragments of tumor-derived DNA, extracellular vesicles (EVs) and circulating tumor cells (CTCs). The most common method for liquid biopsy in lung cancer is the circulating tumor DNA (ctDNA), which may be used for the initial genotype profiling and detection of mechanisms of acquired resistance to targeted therapy. Other potential uses for ctDNA include evaluation of therapeutic response and detection of postsurgical minimal residual disease. In contrast to ctDNA which is originated from dying cells, EVs originates from living cells and may provide a better evaluation of the cancer biology. Early studies have shown comparable sensitivity for EVs and ctDNA in the detection of targetable alterations. CTCs may be useful to evaluate the risk of tumor relapse after treatment with curative intention.

Keywords NSCLC · Liquid biopsy · ctDNA · Extracellular vesicles · Circulating tumor cells

1 Introduction

The molecular profile of cancer has traditionally been performed with the use of samples obtained from the primary tumor or a single metastatic lesion [1]. However, although tissue biopsy represents the gold standard for the diagnosis and initial genome testing, it has limitations. Needle biopsies may lead to complications, and are often associated with difficulty in obtaining adequate samples for genomic profiling as well as sampling bias due to genetic tumor heterogeneity [2]. Furthermore, although genomic features of the initial biopsy are used to guide the therapeutic strategy, the molecular profile of tumors evolve over time, particularly among patients treated with targeted drugs. Although repeated biopsies the tumor may

D. Morgensztern (✉)
Department of Medicine, Division of Medical Oncology, Washington University School of Medicine, St. Louis, MO, USA
e-mail: danielmorgensztern@wustl.edu

© Springer Nature Switzerland AG 2021
A. C. Chiang, R. S. Herbst (eds.), *Lung Cancer*, Current Cancer Research,
https://doi.org/10.1007/978-3-030-74028-3_3

provide information on the tumor evolution, the procedural risks often discourage both clinical providers and patients. An alternative to tissue profile is the use of liquid biopsy.

Liquid biopsy refers to a broad category minimally invasive test done on blood or other fluid specimens to detect fragments of tumor-derived DNA, extracellular vesicles (EVs) and circulating tumor cells (CTCs).

2   Circulating Tumor DNA

Cell-free DNA (cfDNA) represents fragmented DNA found in the non-cellular component of the blood and may originate from multiple sources including tumors, where it is termed circulating tumor DNA (ctDNA). [3] The fraction of ctDNA in the overall cfDNA is typically small and variable among cancer patients. Nevertheless, ctDNA levels in individual patients may correlate with tumor burden and treatment response, particularly due to the short half-life of approximately one hour in the circulation.

Some of the applications of ctDNA in patients with cancer include molecular profiling, evaluation of therapeutic response, evaluation of the mechanisms of acquired resistance and detection of postsurgical minimal residual disease (MRD).

Methods for ctDNA detection range from targeted allele-specific polymerase chain reaction (PCR) to next generation sequencing (NGS). The detection of this small fraction of ctDNA in the plasma depends on the release of tumor DNA into the circulation, making the ability of plasma genotyping assays to detect ctDNA directed related to tumor shed, which in turn is dependent on tumor burden and possibly metastatic sites [4]. The detection of genomic alterations in plasma ctDNA also requires isolation by methods that minimize contamination with leukocyte-derived DNA and the use of highly sensitive genotyping assays. The main challenges for all methods include a low amount plasma ctDNA in a background of abundant cfDNA from nontumor cells in addition to the unclear origin of some of the detected variants. Another factor to be considered when interpreting cfDNA is the clonal hematopoiesis of indeterminate potential (CHIP). Clonal hematopoiesis is defined as an expansion of blood cells derived from a single hematopoietic stem cell, which in addition to be a defining feature of hematologic cancers, may also be found during aging [5]. Although CHIP is not considered a hematologic disorder, it is a risk factor for evolution to one of the defined diseases. Despite the lack of uniform consensus on the specific mutations or criteria for CHIP, it is estimated to be seen in up to 15% of people older than 70 years and more than 30% of those aged 85 or older. The detection of these non-malignant mutations from hematopoietic cells may confound the interpretation of the ctDNA results. In a study evaluating 221 patients with non-small cell lung cancer (NSCLC) evaluated with cfDNA, mutations in JAK2, TP53 and KRAS G12X were detected in both cfDNA and peripheral blood cells, indicating that they are originated from clonal hematopoiesis and not the tumors [6].

3 Initial Molecular Profiling in NSCLC

NSCLC, particularly adenocarcinomas, may be associated with several actionable gene alterations, including mutations in Epidermal Growth Factor Receptor (*EGFR*), *BRAF* V600E, and rearrangements of Anaplastic Lymphoma Kinase (*ALK*) and *ROS1* genes among others. Targeted therapy in these patients is associated with prolonged benefit, with response rates and median progression-free survival (PFS) higher than standard first-line chemotherapy and with a better safety profile [7–12]. Although tissue profile remains the standard of care, some patient may have insufficient tissue material for clinical sequencing. In these patients, since identification of actionable gene alterations remains very important to guide the treatment decision, ctDNA may be particularly valuable by providing an alternative method for molecular profile while avoiding the risks from repeated biopsy. The main role for ctDNA test in patients with NSCLC is to rule in actionable alterations.

Using the Scorpion Amplified Refractory Mutation System (ARMS) technology, Kimura and colleagues detected *EGFR* exon 19 deletion or L858R mutations in the serum, with were associated with benefit from treatment with the first-generation EGFR tyrosine kinase inhibitor (TKI) gefitinib [13]. Other studies using the Scorpion-ARMS platform showed a sensitivity of 43% to 85% in the detection of *EGFR* exon 19 and L858R mutations [13–15]. Newer platforms include the highly sensitive droplet digital polymerase chain reaction (ddPCR) and beads, emulsions, amplification and magnetics (BEAMing) PCR. In the ASSESS study, the concordance of *EGFR* mutation status between matched tissue and plasma in 1288 patients with metastatic NSCLC was 89% [16]. In this study, the most commonly used testing methodologies for plasma testing were Cycleave, QUIAGEN therascreen and Roche cobas. More recently, NGS platforms such as Guardant360 and InVision have allowed more extensive panels of genomic alterations and rearrangements, with sensitivity ranging from 67% to 100% [17–20]. The Non-invasive versus Invasive Lung Evaluation (NILE) was a multicenter study where 307 patients with biopsy-proven and previously untreated advanced stage NSCLC underwent ctDNA test using the Guardant360 method with the results compared to tissue genotyping for eight alterations including *EGFR* mutation, *ALK* fusion, *ROS1* fusion, *BRAF* V600E mutation, *RET* fusion, *ERBB2* mutation, *MET* exon 14 skipping variant, *MET* amplification, and *KRAS* mutation [21]. Among the 282 patients evaluable for analysis, the turnaround time was significantly faster for ctDNA compared to tissue (9 vs 15 days, P < 0.0001). One of the eight alterations was found in 60 patients by tissue genotyping and 77 patients by ctDNA (21.3% vs 27.3%, P < 0.0001). Among the 60 patients with tissue positive tumors, 48 (80%) had positive ctDNA whereas among patients with tissue negative tumors, 29 had ctDNA positive. The addition of ctDNA increased the detection of the pre-specified alterations from 60 in tissue alone to 89 patients in total. The modeling of the results suggested that starting with tissue genotyping, 67% of patients would have the target alterations detected, with an additional 33% detected by subsequent ctDNA, whereas ctDNA first would have detected 87% of the alterations. Therefore, with shorter turnaround time, good correlation with tissue genotyping and similar detection rates, it seems reasonable to pursue a "plasma-first" approach to allow a faster initiation of targeted therapy, particularly in patients with high tumor burden and biopsy performed outside the treating facility who did not undergo reflex genotyping.

4   Detection of the Mechanism of Acquired Resistant to Targeted Therapy

Despite the initial response to targeted therapy, virtually all patients eventually developed acquired resistance. For patients treated with earlier generation EGFR TKIs, the most common mechanism of acquired resistance is a threonine to methionine substitution on exon 20, codon 790 (T790M) [22, 23] Since the third-generation EGFR inhibitor osimertinib is effective in patients harboring acquired *EGFR* T790M mutation, repeated molecular profiling became an important component in the treatment of *EGFR* mutant NSCLC [24]. Although the initial method for the detection was through repeated tissue biopsy, ctDNA has emerged as a more feasible alternative. In an exploratory analysis of the dose escalation and expansion of the phase I AURA study [24, 25], where patients where patients with *EGFR* mutant NSCLC were treated with osimertinib, plasma genotype using BEAMing was compared to central tissue genotype [26]. Plasma *EGFR* T790M was detected in 111 of the 158 patients (70%) with positive tissue test. The objective response rate (ORR) was 62% for patients with T790M positive tumors by tissue analysis and 63% in those with T790M positive by plasma genotyping, with median PFS of 9.7 months in both groups. The results from this study indicated that plasma genotype could be used as the initial step. In the case of positive T790M mutation, there would be no need for a repeated biopsy for tissue testing due to the similar outcomes among patients treated with osimertinib regardless of the method of T790M detection. In contrast, patients with negative plasma genotype would require a biopsy due to the risks of false-negative results, particularly in the absence of detectable initial sensitizing *EGFR* mutations.

The role for detection of *EGFR* T790M mutation as the mechanism of acquired resistant for EGFR TKIs is likely to be reduced with the results from the FLAURA study, where in comparison with gefitinib or erlotinib, first-line osimertinib was associated with increased median PFS and median overall survival (OS) [9, 27]. Nevertheless, similar to earlier generation EGFR TKIs, acquired resistance develops in virtually all patients treated with osimertinib. Several mechanisms of resistance have been detected in patients treated with osimertinib, including additional *EGFR* mutations (*EGFR* C797S, *EGFR* G724S), other mutations (*BRAF* V600E, *KRAS*), fusions (*RET*, *BRAF*) and amplifications (*MET*, *ERBB2*) [28]. These alterations may be detected with ctDNA and some may have therapeutic implications [29].

Similar to *EGFR* mutation, patients with *ALK* rearrangements usually achieve excellent and response to ALK inhibitors but eventually develop acquired resistance, which may be broadly classified as on-targed genetic alterations, including *ALK* mutations or amplification, and off-target mechanisms [30]. Although *ALK* resistance mutations occur less frequently after treatment with the first-generation ALK TKI crizotinib, they are present in the majority of patients treated with second-generation inhibitors including ceritinib, alectinib and brigatinib. Preclinical data also suggests that some mutations may be associated with resistance to some but not all second-generation drugs. Furthermore, ALK *G1020R* mutation, the most commonly seen mechanism of acquired resistance to second-generation ALK inhibitors, is sensitive only to the third-generation lorlatinib, which was approved based on a multi-arm phase II trial showing efficacy in patients receiving up to three prior lines of ALK inhibitors [31]. In a planned analysis of this phase II using both tissue and ctDNA through Guardant360, patients previously treated with one or more second-generation ALK TKIs were more likely to respond to lorlatinib in the presence of ALK mutations, either by tissue or ctDNA [32]. In contrast, the absence of an *ALK* mutation suggests an ALK-independent mechanism of resistance, decreasing the probability of response to ALK TKI inhibitors. These findings constitute the basis for the ALK Master Protocol, a clinical trial currently accruing patients with tumor progression after second-generation ALK TKis, that uses both plasma and tissue genotyping to define the next line of therapy.

5 Detection of Minimal Residual Disease

The rationale for using ctDNA to assess minimal residual disease is the potential to detect microscopic remnants and hidden metastases beyond the resolution of imaging studies [33]. This application may be particularly useful in patients undergoing surgical resection where changes in ctDNA levels before and after surgery may predict for tumor relapse. In the TRACERx study, tissue and ctDNA were collected from patients with early stage NSCLC treated surgically. The tissue study showed that intratumor heterogeneity was associated with increased risk for recurrence or death after surgery [34]. The ctDNA study used multiplex-PCR assay panels that were developed for each patient, targeting clonal and subclonal single-nucleotide varians (SNVs) [35]. At least two SNVs were detected preoperatively in 46 out of 96 (48%) of patients, with an additional 12 patients harboring single SNV. ctDNA was detected more frequently in squamous cell carcinomas (30 out of 31) than adenocarcinomas (11 out of 58), including in those with stage I (16 out of 17 for squamous versus 5 out of 39 in adenocarcinoma). In addition to histology, lymphovascular invasion and high Ki67 proliferation index were independent predictors for ctDNA detection. Among patients with ctDNA positive results, clonal SNVs were present in all cases whereas subclonal SNVs were detected in 27 patients (68%). Both the tumor volume by computer tomography (CT) and the pathologic tumor size were correlated with the mean clonal variant allele frequency (VAF). The longitudinal phase of the study included 24 patients with preoperative and postoperative ctDNA samples, which were followed every 3 months for the first two years followed by every 6 months thereafter. After a median follow-up of 775 days, 14 patients had confirmed tumor relapse. At least two SNVs were detected in 13 out of 14 (93%) patients with relapse and 1 out of 10 (10%) without relapse, with the median interval between ctDNA detection and relapse by CT scan of 70 days. The detection of ctDNA in patients with early stage NSCLC may be increased with the use of cancer personalizing profiling by deep sequencing (CAPP-Seq). In a study evaluating 40 patients with stage I to III lung cancer, including 37 with NSCLC and 3 with small cell lung cancer treated with curative intent, the freedom from progression at 36 months was 0% in patients with detectable ctDNA and 93% for those with undetectable ctDNA [36]. In a subsequent study using this method, ctDNA was detected in 20 out of 48 (42%) of patients with stage I, 14 out of 21 (82%) of those with stage II and 14 out of 16 (88%) of those with stage III [37]. The study also found that high pretreatment ctDNA levels were associated with lower relapse-free survival for all stages combined (hazard ratio [HR] 4.48, P = 0.0004) and for stage I (HR 9.3, P = 0.0004).

6 Small Cell Lung Cancer

SCLC accounts for approximately 13% of patients with lung cancer and is characterized by rapid doubling time and early development of distant metastases [38]. Despite the usual response to the first-line therapy, virtually all patients with metastatic disease eventually developed tumor progression, for which subsequent therapy has been associated with suboptimal outcomes [39–41]. Although a more comprehensive characterization of the mechanisms of resistance to therapy could help the development of new therapeutic modalities, obtaining repeated tissue biopsy is particularly challenging in SCLC since most of the relapses are symptomatic and require prompt treatment. Therefore, tissue data on treatment resistant SCLC is limited [42]. A retrospective study evaluating 609 samples collected from 564 patients between 2014 and 2017 analyzed ctDNA through Guardant 360 [43]. At least one non-synonymous mutation or amplification was detected in 552 samples (90.6%). When the samples were classified as being collected at diagnosis or at relapse, the allele frequencies were higher for samples collected at diagnosis whereas there were no differences in the number of nonsynonymous mutations or amplifications between groups. Alterations in the androgen receptor gene was detected with higher frequency among relapsed samples compared to those obtained at diagnosis (14% vs 2%, P < 0.05), with both mutations and amplifications occurring predominantly in women. Potentially actionable or alterations predictive to responses to specific therapies were detected in DNA repair genes (*BRCA1*, *BRCA2*, *ATM*), *ARID1A*, *BRAF*, *MET* and *ERBB2*. Another possible application for ctDNA in SCLC is as a rapid and non-invasive monitoring of the tumor burden. In a prospective study evaluating 27 patients with SCLC, ctDNA was tested for 14 genes using a custom SCLC-specific panel [44]. ctDNA was detected in 80% of patients with the most common alterations including *TP53* (70%) and *RB1* (52%). Allele frequencies and copy number alterations correlated with occult disease and recurrence that were not detected by radiographic imaging.

7 Extracellular Vesicles

EVs are lipid membrane encapsulated particles released by cells into the intercellular space or circulation in response to cell activation, injury and cellular stress [45]. They are involved in multiple physiologic functions including blood coagulation, immunity, stem cell differentiation, tissue regeneration and angiogenesis. EVs may contain mRNA transcripts of oncogenes and DNA fragments with cancer driver mutation genes. The two major classes of extracellular vesicles are the exosomes and shed microvesicles. A possible important difference between exosomes and ctDNA is that while the latter originates from dying cells, the latter originates from living cells, possibly providing a better reflection of the cancer biology. A prospective study compared plasma exosomal nucleic acids (exoNA) to ctDNA in 43 patients with advanced cancer, including 6 patients with NSCLC, who had tissue genotyping available [46]. *EGFR* exon 19 deletion, *EGFR* L858R mutation, *BRAF* V600E mutation, *KRAS* G12C and *KRAS* G12D mutations were detected in 95% of plasma exoNA samples, 92% of ctDNA by ddPCR and 97% of BEAMing ctDNA. When subdivided according to the median allele frequency (MAF), the median OS for patients with exoNA MAF above the median and below the median was 11.8 months and 5.9 months respectively, P = 0.006). The median OS was also higher in patient with lower MAF according to ddPCR (8.5 vs 5.9 months, P = 0.023) and BEAMing (7.4 vs 6.5 months, P = 0.06) although to a lesser extent. In the TIGER-X study, which evaluated the third-generation EGFR TKI rociletinib in patients with activating *EGFR* mutations a subset of patients with matched tissue and plasma pretreatment specimens were further evaluated for ctDNA by BEAMing and exoNA [47]. The sensitivities for detection of activating *EGFR* mutation and *EGFR* T790M mutations were 98% and 90% respectively for exoNA and 82% and 84% respectively for ctDNA.

8 Circulating Tumor Cells

CTCs can be found in the bloodstream of patients with cancer and are presumably originated from the primary tumor or metastatic sites and postulated to be responsible for the metastatic seeding [48].

In a study evaluating 92 patients with stage I NSCLC treated with stereotactic radiation therapy, 38 (41%) had positive CTCs prior to therapy [49]. A pretreatment cutoff of ≥5 CTCs/ml predicted for an increased risk for nodal or distant failure. In a pooled analysis of 550 patients with advanced stage NSCLC participating into the CellSearch CTC studies from 2003 to 2017, CTC was an independent prognostic indicator for both PFS and OS using cutoffs of both ≥2 CTCs and ≥5/7.5 ml [50].

9 Conclusion

Liquid biopsy has several advantages over tissue profile including faster turnaround time, safety and better evaluation of tumor heterogeneity. ctDNA has an established role in the initial genomic profile and may be particularly suitable for the detection of mechanisms of acquired resistance to targeted therapy, avoiding the risks from repeated biopsy. Neither EVs nor CTCs have been approved for clinical use in patients with NSCLC.

References

1. Siravegna G, Marsoni S, Siena S, Bardelli A (2017) Integrating liquid biopsies into the management of cancer. Nat Rev Clin Oncol 14:531–548
2. Wan JCM, Massie C, Garcia-Corbacho J et al (2017) Liquid biopsies come of age: towards implementation of circulating tumour DNA. Nat Rev Cancer 17:223–238
3. Corcoran RB, Chabner BA (2018) Application of cell-free DNA analysis to cancer treatment. N Engl J Med 379:1754–1765
4. Sacher AG, Komatsubara KM, Oxnard GR (2017) Application of plasma genotyping technologies in non-small cell lung cancer: a practical review. J Thorac Oncol 12:1344–1356
5. Steensma DP (2018) Clinical implications of clonal hematopoiesis. Mayo Clin Proc 93:1122–1130
6. Hu Y, Ulrich BC, Supplee J et al (2018) False-positive plasma genotyping due to clonal hematopoiesis. Clin Cancer Res 24:4437–4443
7. Herbst RS, Morgensztern D, Boshoff C (2018) The biology and management of non-small cell lung cancer. Nature 553:446–454
8. Mok TS, Wu YL, Thongprasert S et al (2009) Gefitinib or carboplatin-paclitaxel in pulmonary adenocarcinoma. N Engl J Med 361:947–957
9. Ramalingam SS, Vansteenkiste J, Planchard D et al (2020) Overall survival with Osimertinib in untreated, EGFR-mutated advanced NSCLC. N Engl J Med 382:41–50
10. Planchard D, Smit EF, Groen HJM et al (2017) Dabrafenib plus trametinib in patients with previously untreated BRAF(V600E)-mutant metastatic non-small-cell lung cancer: an open-label, phase 2 trial. Lancet Oncol 18:1307–1316
11. Solomon BJ, Mok T, Kim DW et al (2014) First-line crizotinib versus chemotherapy in ALK-positive lung cancer. N Engl J Med 371:2167–2177
12. Shaw AT, Ou SH, Bang YJ et al (2014) Crizotinib in ROS1-rearranged non-small-cell lung cancer. N Engl J Med 371:1963–1971
13. Kimura H, Suminoe M, Kasahara K et al (2007) Evaluation of epidermal growth factor receptor mutation status in serum DNA as a predictor of response to gefitinib (IRESSA). Br J Cancer 97:778–784
14. Goto K, Ichinose Y, Ohe Y et al (2012) Epidermal growth factor receptor mutation status in circulating free DNA in serum: from IPASS, a phase III study of gefitinib or carboplatin/paclitaxel in non-small cell lung cancer. J Thorac Oncol 7:115–121
15. Douillard JY, Ostoros G, Cobo M et al (2014) Gefitinib treatment in EGFR mutated caucasian NSCLC: circulating-free tumor DNA as a surrogate for determination of EGFR status. J Thorac Oncol 9:1345–1353
16. Reck M, Hagiwara K, Han B et al (2016) ctDNA determination of EGFR mutation status in European and Japanese patients with advanced NSCLC: the ASSESS study. J Thorac Oncol 11:1682–1689

17. Paweletz CP, Sacher AG, Raymond CK et al (2016) Bias-corrected targeted next-generation sequencing for rapid, multiplexed detection of actionable alterations in cell-free DNA from advanced lung cancer patients. Clin Cancer Res 22:915–922
18. Lanman RB, Mortimer SA, Zill OA et al (2015) Analytical and clinical validation of a digital sequencing panel for quantitative, highly accurate evaluation of cell-free circulating tumor DNA. PLoS One 10:e0140712
19. Thompson JC, Yee SS, Troxel AB et al (2016) Detection of therapeutically targetable driver and resistance mutations in lung cancer patients by next-generation sequencing of cell-free circulating tumor DNA. Clin Cancer Res 22:5772–5782
20. Gale D, Lawson ARJ, Howarth K et al (2018) Development of a highly sensitive liquid biopsy platform to detect clinically-relevant cancer mutations at low allele fractions in cell-free DNA. PLoS One 13:e0194630
21. Leighl NB, Page RD, Raymond VM et al (2019) Clinical utility of comprehensive cell-free DNA analysis to identify genomic biomarkers in patients with newly diagnosed metastatic non-small cell lung cancer. Clin Cancer Res 25:4691–4700
22. Kobayashi S, Boggon TJ, Dayaram T et al (2005) EGFR mutation and resistance of non-small-cell lung cancer to gefitinib. N Engl J Med 352:786–792
23. Sequist LV, Waltman BA, Dias-Santagata D et al (2011) Genotypic and histological evolution of lung cancers acquiring resistance to EGFR inhibitors. Sci Transl Med 3:75ra26
24. Janne PA, Yang JC, Kim DW et al (2015) AZD9291 in EGFR inhibitor-resistant non-small-cell lung cancer. N Engl J Med 372:1689–1699
25. Yang JC, Ahn MJ, Kim DW et al (2017) Osimertinib in pretreated T790M-positive advanced non-small-cell lung cancer: AURA study phase II extension component. J Clin Oncol 35:1288–1296
26. Oxnard GR, Thress KS, Alden RS et al (2016) Association between plasma genotyping and outcomes of treatment with Osimertinib (AZD9291) in advanced non-small-cell lung cancer. J Clin Oncol 34:3375–3382
27. Soria JC, Ohe Y, Vansteenkiste J et al (2017) Osimertinib in untreated EGFR-mutated advanced non-small-cell lung cancer. N Engl J Med 378:113
28. Leonetti A, Sharma S, Minari R, Perego P, Giovannetti E, Tiseo M (2019) Resistance mechanisms to osimertinib in EGFR-mutated non-small cell lung cancer. Br J Cancer 121:725–737
29. Oxnard GR, Hu Y, Mileham KF et al (2018) Assessment of resistance mechanisms and clinical implications in patients with EGFR T790M-positive lung cancer and acquired resistance to Osimertinib. JAMA Oncol 4:1527–1534
30. Gainor JF, Dardaei L, Yoda S et al (2016) Molecular mechanisms of resistance to first- and second-generation ALK inhibitors in ALK-rearranged lung cancer. Cancer Discov 6:1118–1133
31. Solomon BJ, Besse B, Bauer TM et al (2018) Lorlatinib in patients with ALK-positive non-small-cell lung cancer: results from a global phase 2 study. Lancet Oncol 19:1654–1667
32. Shaw AT, Solomon BJ, Besse B et al (2019) ALK resistance mutations and efficacy of Lorlatinib in advanced anaplastic lymphoma kinase-positive non-small-cell lung cancer. J Clin Oncol 37:1370–1379
33. Chae YK, Oh MS (2019) Detection of minimal residual disease using ctDNA in lung cancer: current evidence and future directions. J Thorac Oncol 14:16–24
34. Jamal-Hanjani M, Wilson GA, McGranahan N et al (2017) Tracking the evolution of non-small-cell lung Cancer. N Engl J Med 376:2109–2121
35. Abbosh C, Birkbak NJ, Wilson GA et al (2017) Phylogenetic ctDNA analysis depicts early stage lung cancer evolution. Nature 545:446
36. Chaudhuri AA, Chabon JJ, Lovejoy AF et al (2017) Early detection of molecular residual disease in localized lung Cancer by circulating tumor DNA profiling. Cancer Discov 7:1394–1403
37. Chabon JJ, Hamilton EG, Kurtz DM et al (2020) Integrating genomic features for non-invasive early lung cancer detection. Nature 580:245–251

38. Govindan R, Page N, Morgensztern D et al (2006) Changing epidemiology of small-cell lung cancer in the United States over the last 30 years: analysis of the surveillance, epidemiologic, and end results database. J Clin Oncol 24:4539–4544
39. von Pawel J, Schiller JH, Shepherd FA et al (1999) Topotecan versus cyclophosphamide, doxorubicin, and vincristine for the treatment of recurrent small-cell lung cancer. J Clin Oncol 17:658–667
40. von Pawel J, Jotte R, Spigel DR et al (2014) Randomized phase III trial of amrubicin versus topotecan as second-line treatment for patients with small-cell lung cancer. J Clin Oncol 32:4012–4019
41. Trigo J, Subbiah V, Besse B et al (2020) Lurbinectedin as second-line treatment for patients with small-cell lung cancer: a single-arm, open-label, phase 2 basket trial. Lancet Oncol 21:645–654
42. Wagner AH, Devarakonda S, Skidmore ZL et al (2018) Recurrent WNT pathway alterations are frequent in relapsed small cell lung cancer. Nat Commun 9:3787
43. Devarakonda S, Sankararaman S, Herzog BH et al (2019) Circulating tumor DNA profiling in small-cell lung cancer identifies potentially targetable alterations. Clin Cancer Res 25:6119–6126
44. Almodovar K, Iams WT, Meador CB et al (2018) Longitudinal cell-free DNA analysis in patients with small cell lung Cancer reveals dynamic insights into treatment efficacy and disease relapse. J Thorac Oncol 13:112–123
45. Xu R, Rai A, Chen M, Suwakulsiri W, Greening DW, Simpson RJ (2018) Extracellular vesicles in cancer - implications for future improvements in cancer care. Nat Rev Clin Oncol 15:617–638
46. Mohrmann L, Huang HJ, Hong DS et al (2018) Liquid biopsies using plasma exosomal nucleic acids and plasma cell-free DNA compared with clinical outcomes of patients with advanced cancers. Clin Cancer Res 24:181–188
47. Krug AK, Enderle D, Karlovich C et al (2018) Improved EGFR mutation detection using combined exosomal RNA and circulating tumor DNA in NSCLC patient plasma. Ann Oncol 29:700–706
48. Ignatiadis M, Lee M, Jeffrey SS (2015) Circulating tumor cells and circulating tumor DNA: challenges and opportunities on the path to clinical utility. Clin Cancer Res 21:4786–4800
49. Frick MA, Feigenberg SJ, Jean-Baptiste SR et al (2020) Circulating tumor cells are associated with recurrent disease in patients with early-stage non-small cell lung cancer treated with stereotactic body radiotherapy. Clin Cancer Res 26:2372–2380
50. Lindsay CR, Blackhall FH, Carmel A et al (2019) EPAC-lung: pooled analysis of circulating tumour cells in advanced non-small cell lung cancer. Eur J Cancer 117:60–68

Chapter 4
Osimertinib in EGFR-Mutant Non-Small Cell Lung Carcinoma: Clinical Activity and Mechanisms of Resistance

Ashita Talsania, Janie Zhang, and Frederick H. Wilson

Abstract Oncogenic mutations in the epidermal growth factor receptor (EGFR) are identified in a subset of non-small cell lung carcinomas (NSCLC). These alterations lead to constitutive EGFR activation and upregulation of pathways promoting cell survival and proliferation. The development of small molecule inhibitors of EGFR has transformed the care of patients with advanced EGFR-mutant NSCLC. We review here the clinical development and activity of the third-generation EGFR inhibitor osimertinib in the advanced and adjuvant settings. As with other targeted therapies, resistance to osimertinib is common and limits the efficacy of this agent. Here we present an overview of reported acquired resistance mechanisms and potential therapeutic strategies to overcome resistance. The heterogeneity of resistance mechanisms (including secondary EGFR mutations and diverse EGFR-independent alterations) presents a major therapeutic challenge in EGFR-mutant NSCLC.

Keywords Epidermal growth factor receptor (EGFR) · Targeted therapy · EGFR inhibitor · Osimertinib · Acquired resistance · Adjuvant therapy

Activating alterations in the epithelial growth factor receptor (EGFR) are an important therapeutic target in non-small cell lung carcinoma (NSCLC). EGFR mutations are present in ~20% of lung adenocarcinomas in Caucasians [1, 2] and ~50% of adenocarcinomas in Asians [1, 3]. EGFR mutations are enriched in light or never-smokers and are identified in about 47% of nonsmokers in North America [1, 4]. EGFR mutations are observed more commonly in women compared to men with

A. Talsania · J. Zhang · F. H. Wilson (✉)
Department of Medicine (Medical Oncology), Yale School of Medicine/Yale Cancer Center, New Haven, CT, USA
e-mail: ashita.talsania@yale.edu; janie.zhang@yale.edu; frederick.wilson@yale.edu

© Springer Nature Switzerland AG 2021   65
A. C. Chiang, R. S. Herbst (eds.), *Lung Cancer*, Current Cancer Research,
https://doi.org/10.1007/978-3-030-74028-3_4

lung adenocarcinoma in the North American population (28% vs. 19% respectively) [1].

Activating in-frame deletions in Exon 19 account for 45% of EGFR mutations. The missense L858R mutation in Exon 21 comprises 40–45% of activating mutations, and the remaining 10% of mutations involve Exons 18 and 20 [5]. Most activating EGFR alterations are sensitive to FDA-approved EGFR tyrosine kinase inhibitors (TKIs). Exon 20 insertion mutations are an exception, but inhibitors with activity against these mutations are currently in clinical development [6, 7]. Acquired resistance to EGFR TKIs is common, and 50–60% of tumors that develop resistance to 1st and 2nd generation inhibitors acquire a secondary T790M EGFR mutation [8–12]. T790M confers resistance by increasing the affinity of EGFR for ATP [11].

1   Clinical Activity of Osimertinib

Osimertinib is a third generation EGFR inhibitor which irreversibly inhibits both EGFR-activating mutations (e.g. L858R, Exon 19 deletion) and T790M [8]. Osimertinib has a manageable side effect profile and crosses the blood-brain barrier [13].

The activity of osimertinib in patients with advanced EGFR-mutant NSCLC with acquired T790M after a first or second-generation EGFR inhibitor was demonstrated in the Phase I/II AURA trial. In this study of 253 patients, osimertinib was associated with a response rate of 61% and median PFS of 9.6 months [14]. In the Phase III AURA3 trial, 419 patients who progressed on a first or second-generation EGFR TKI with T790M were randomized to receive osimertinib vs. carboplatin/cisplatin + pemetrexed. Median PFS was 10.1 months for patients treated with osimertinib vs. 4.4 months with chemotherapy. At 6 months, 69% were alive and progression free in the osimertinib group vs. 37% in the chemotherapy doublet group. At 12 months, 44% were alive and progression free in the osimertinib group vs 10% in the doublet chemotherapy group. ORR was significantly better at 71% (osimertinib) vs. 31% (chemotherapy), p < 0.001 [15].

The activity of osimertinib in the first-line treatment setting has also been demonstrated. In a phase I clinical trial, a group of 60 patients with previously untreated EGFR-mutated advanced NSCLC who received osimertinib at a dose of 80 mg or 160 mg had an overall response rate of 77% and a median PFS of 20.5 months [16]. In the phase III FLAURA study which included 556 patients with previously untreated advanced NSCLC with either EGFR L858R or Exon 19 deletion, osimertinib was compared to the first generation EGFR inhibitors gefinitib or erlotinib in the first-line setting. Median PFS was 18.9 months with osimertinib vs. 10.2 months with a first generation TKI, survival rate at 18 months was 83% with osimertinib vs

71% with the first generation TKI. This benefit was observed regardless of ethnicity (Asian vs. non-Asian), type of EGFR mutation (L858R vs. Exon 19 deletion), and presence or absence of CNS metastases. Overall response rate was 80% for osimertinib vs. 76% for standard TKIs. A median OS of 38.6 months was seen with osimertinib vs 31.8 months with the first generation TKI [17]. Based on these data, the Food and Drug Administration approved the use of osimertinib in the first-line setting for patients with advanced EGFR-mutant NSCLC in April 2018.

2   Activity in CNS and Leptomeningeal Disease

Osimertinib shows improved CNS efficacy and reduced risk of progression compared with first generation EGFR TKIs. Osimertinib was shown to have activity in a mouse model of leptomeningeal cells resistant to first-generation and second-generation EGFR-TKIs [18]. Osimertinib has activity in refractory leptomeningeal disease after early generation EGFR-TKI failure and appears to be more effective in CSF T790M-positive cases [19]. In a preplanned subgroup analysis of FLAURA with CNS progression-free survival as primary objective, osimertinib demonstrated a significant improvement in CNS PFS compared to early generation EGFR-TKIs in the first-line setting, with a 52% reduction in the risk of CNS progression [20].

3   Osimertinib in the Adjuvant Setting

The safety and efficacy of osimertinib in the adjuvant setting was evaluated in the ADAURA study. This is a double-blind, phase 3 trial in which 682 patients with resected Stage IB, II, or IIIA EGFR-mutated NSCLC were randomized to receive osimertinib or placebo for 3 years. Patients were permitted but not required to receive adjuvant chemotherapy. The primary endpoint of the study was disease-free survival. 89% of patients randomized to osimertinib were alive without NSCLC recurrence at 24 months compared to 52% of patients receiving placebo with a hazard ratio of 0.20. In addition, 98% of patients receiving osimertinib were alive without central nervous system disease at 24 months compared to 85% of patients receiving placebo with a hazard ratio of 0.18. Overall survival data is not yet mature. Based on these findings, the FDA approved osimertinib in December 2020 as adjuvant therapy for patients with Stage IB, II, and IIIA EGFR-mutant NSCLC after surgical resection with curative intent [21].

4   Resistance to Osimertinib

Tyrosine kinase inhibitors have revolutionized the treatment of patients with advanced non-small cell lung cancer harboring targetable molecular alterations. Unfortunately, acquired resistance to these therapies is common and osimertinib is no exception. With osimertinib now widely adopted as the preferred first-line treatment for advanced EGFR-mutant NSCLC in the United States, resistance is an important challenge limiting the efficacy of these therapies, as shown in Fig. 4.1.

A. Acquired Secondary EGFR Mutations

The secondary EGFR mutation C797S [22–25] is identified in 10–19% of reported cases of osimertinib resistance [26]. This mutation occurs in the ATP binding site which prevents osimertinib from covalently binding to the site. Whether the C797S mutation is in *cis* (on the same allele) or *trans* (on a different allele) with T790M may have important implications [24, 27, 28]. If T790M and C797S are in *trans*, cells are resistant to 3rd generation TKIs but sensitive to a combination of first generation and 3rd generation TKIs. If T790M and C797S are in *cis*, cells are resistant to all first/second/third generation TKIs. If C797S arises without T790M during first-line therapy with osimertinib, cells may be sensitive to first generation TKIs [28].

In cell line models, the anti-EGFR antibody cetuximab was evaluated as a strategy for overcoming résistance mediated by C797S. The L858R/T790M/C797S triple-mutant EGFR protein exists as a monomer and a dimer, whereas Ex19del/T790M/C797S exists only as a monomer. Cetuximab disrupts dimerization of EGFR which results in inhibition of EGFR phosphorylation and inhibition of cell growth. Cetuximab has no effect on the monomer. Cetuximab showed activity against L858R/T790M/C797S *in vitro*. Additional *in vivo* studies may help determine if cetuximab could have a role in overcoming resistance mediated by C797S [24].

MECHANISMS OF RESISTANCE

SECONDARY EGFR MUTATIONS	MUTATIONS IN OTHER DRIVERS
➢ Secondary EGFR mutation	➢KRAS mediated
• Exon 20 C797S	➢BRAF mediated
• Exon 19 G724S	➢MET mediated
• L792H	➢RET mediated
• G796R	➢Her 2 amplification
➢EGFR amplifications	➢AXL
	➢Transformation Epithelial mesenchymal- transition

Fig. 4.1 Reported Mechanisms of Resistance to Osimertinib

The tyrosine kinase inhibitor brigatinib has activity against both ALK and EGFR. In cell lines, it showed activity against Ex19del/T790M/C797S and to a lesser degree L858R/T790M/C797S. Effects of brigatinib were enhanced with the anti-EGFR antibodies cetuximab or panitumumab by decreasing EGFR expression on the cell surface [27].

The fourth generation TKI EAI045 is an allosteric inhibitor of EGFR that binds outside the ATP-binding site and thus is not impaired by C797S. It has been shown to promote tumor regression in mouse models in combination with cetuximab, however only for L858R/T790M/C797S triple-mutant EGFR with no efficacy in Ex19del/T790M/C797S [29].

G724S is a secondary EGFR resistance mutation that induces a conformational change in the P-loop of EGFR that reduces the binding affinity of osimertinib and seems to preferentially occur in the context of an Exon 19 deletion [26, 30]. In 19 patients with osimertinib resistance and G724S, 15 had coexisting Ex19del but none had L858R. G724S was not present in biopsies before the emergence of resistance.

Variants of Ex19del that coexist with G724S are uncommon variants (e.g. E746-A750 > V, rather than the classic E746-A750 del). The combination may lead to enhanced dimerization-dependent activation of EGFR. These tumors may respond to afatinib, as *in vitro* molecular modeling suggests binding of afatinib to Ex19del/G724S is not affected [30].

L792H and G796R have also been reported as acquired EGFR mutations that confer resistance to osimertinib. They were noted in genomic analysis of patient tumor samples after treatment with osimertinib and proven *in vitro* to mediate resistance to osimertinib when in *cis* with T790M through inhibition of covalent binding of osimertinib [31].

In a transgenic mouse model of lung adenocarcinoma driven by EGFR L858R, C797S and L718Q/V secondary EGFR mutations were identified as mediators of resistance to osimertinib. L718Q/V mutations are reported in EGFR-mutant lung adenocarcinoma post osimertinib treatment. L718Q/V mutations almost always occur in the context of an L858R driver mutation [32]. Preclinical testing in mice demonstrated activity of afatinib for L718Q mutant tumors [33].

B. EGFR Amplification

EGFR amplification [25] was reported in a lung cancer cell line with Ex19del and T790M and acquired resistance to the 3rd generation EGFR TKI rociletinib [34]. This was first described in a patient with Ex19del who developed T790M on erlotinib and subsequently developed resistance to osimertinib with emergence of two tumor clones: one with C797S and one with amplification of the EGFR Ex19del allele [35]. This clinical experience corresponds to laboratory data demonstrating that higher levels of EGFR activating mutations in cell-free DNA of patients who progressed on a first or second generation TKI correlated with poorer response to osimertinib [23].

C. Non-EGFR Dependent Mechanisms of Resistance

MET-mediated

MET amplification is reported in up to 15% of tumors with resistance to osimertinib [22, 23, 25, 36, 37]. A patient who initially had T790M with L858R developed progressive disease after 10 months of osimertinib and was found to have loss of T790M and MET amplification [36]. Preclinical data suggested EGFR TKIs plus MET TKIs are a possible treatment for *EGFR* mutation-positive lung cancers with *MET*-driven acquired resistance [37]. In the TATTON study evaluating the combination of osimertinib and the MET inhibitor savolitinib, objective partial responses were observed in 66 of 138 patients (48%) with acquired resistance to a third-generation TKI and MET amplification. This combination may be a potential treatment option for patients with *MET*-driven resistance to EGFR TKI [38].

KRAS–mediated

KRAS amplification was reported in an osimertinib resistant lung cancer cell line [34]. Effects of KRAS amplification were overcome in osimertinib resistant cells by MEK inhibition + IGF1R inhibition [34]. A KRAS G12S activating mutation is reported in a patient with EGFR-mutant NSCLC with resistance to osimertinib and loss of T790M [37].

BRAF-mediated Acquired BRAF fusions (AGK-BRAF and PJA2-BRAF) are reported in approximately 2% of patients with progression on erlotinib or osimertinib and have been shown *in vitro* to mediate EGFR TKI resistance [39]. In another cell line, a PCBP2-BRAF fusion was identified in osimertinib resistance associated with loss of T790M [22]. Combination treatment with osimertinib and a MEK inhibitor (trametinib) inhibited growth of a patient-derived cell line with EGFR Ex19del and PJA2-BRAF [39]. A cell line established from a patient with acquired resistance to osimertinib harboring PCBP2-BRAF and loss of T790M was sensitive to the MEK inhibitor trametinib but not to the RAF inhibitors dabrafenib and LXH245 [22].

RET-mediated

Tumors from two patients with acquired resistance to EGFR inhibition (including one with resistance to osimertinib) were found to have activating RET fusions. A tumor response was achieved for both patients with the addition of a RET inhibitor (BLU-667) to the EGFR inhibitor [22].

HER2 amplification

HER2 amplification has been reported as a mechanism of resistance to osimertinib. A patient with acquired resistance to osimertinib and HER2 amplification was treated with the HER2-targeting antibody trastuzumab with stable disease [36].

Epithelial-Mesenchymal Transition (EMT)

NSCLC cell lines with acquired resistance to first or third generation EGFR TKIs exhibit features of EMT including a decrease in E-cadherin expression and an increase in vimentin expression. This leads to loss of cellular polarity and increased metastatic potential [40]. AXL is a mediator of EMT and is overexpressed in several cancers [33]. High levels of AXL expression in EGFR mutated lung cancer cell lines correlated inversely with susceptibility to EGFR TKIs. AXL is activated by osimertinib in lung cancer cell lines [41]. The AXL inhibitors NPS1034 and ASP2215 sensitized resistant EGFR-mutant lung cancer cell lines to osimertinib. The combination of osimertinib and NSP1034 induced tumor regression and delayed development of resistance in a xenograft mouse model with high AXL expression. NSP1034 and osimertinib co-administration in an AXL-expressing, osimertinib resistant patient derived xenograft (PDX) model resulted in stability of tumor size [41].

Transformation to Small Cell Histology
Transformation to small cell lung carcinoma (SCLC) occurs in 3% to 10% of EGFR TKI–resistant cases regardless of the generation of TKI used [42]. Transformation to SCLC may occur at any time during the course of the disease but generally occurs 13 to 18 months after the start of TKI treatment [43, 44]. These tumors have the characteristic histologic features of small cell carcinomas including neuroendocrine differentiation, though they differ from conventional SCLCs in they occur in non-smokers or light smokers and frequently retain the original EGFR mutation. They respond to conventional chemotherapy for small cell lung cancer [45].

5 Conclusion

In conclusion, osimertinib is now the standard first line therapy for advanced EGFR mutant lung cancers in the United States. Resistance is heterogeneous, and many potential resistance mechanisms exist; some are due to secondary EGFR mutations while others are independent of EGFR. Certain resistance mechanisms (such as acquired RET fusions or MET amplification) may be actionable given the availability of inhibitors of these targets. But for others, there may not be an obvious therapeutic strategy to overcome resistance. As a result, the development of strategies to delay or prevent the emergence of resistance may be important to maximize the benefit of EGFR inhibitors in the treatment of advanced EGFR-mutant NSCLC.

References

1. Midha A, Dearden S, McCormack R (2015) EGFR mutation incidence in non-small-cell lung cancer of adenocarcinoma histology: a systematic review and global map by ethnicity (mut-MapII). Am J Cancer Res 5:2892–2911
2. Dearden S, Stevens J, Wu YL et al (2013) Mutation incidence and coincidence in non small-cell lung cancer: meta-analyses by ethnicity and histology (mutMap). Ann Oncol 24:2371–2376
3. Shi Y, Au JS, Thongprasert S et al (2014) A prospective, molecular epidemiology study of EGFR mutations in Asian patients with advanced non-small-cell lung cancer of adenocarcinoma histology (PIONEER). J Thorac Oncol 9:154–162

4. Pao W, Miller V, Zakowski M et al (2004) EGF receptor gene mutations are common in lung cancers from "never smokers" and are associated with sensitivity of tumors to gefitinib and erlotinib. Proc Natl Acad Sci U S A 101:13306–13311
5. Sharma SV, Bell DW, Settleman J et al (2007) Epidermal growth factor receptor mutations in lung cancer. Nat Rev Cancer 7:169–181
6. Janne PA, Neal JW, Camidge DR et al (2019) Antitumor activity of TAK-788 in NSCLC with EGFR exon 20 insertions. J Clin Oncol 37:9007–9007
7. Heymach J, Negrao M, Robichaux J et al (2018) OA02.06 A phase II trial of Poziotinib in EGFR and HER2 exon 20 mutant Non-Small Cell Lung Cancer (NSCLC). J Thorac Oncol 13:S323–S324
8. Cross DA, Ashton SE, Ghiorghiu S et al (2014) AZD9291, an irreversible EGFR TKI, overcomes T790M-mediated resistance to EGFR inhibitors in lung cancer. Cancer Discov 4:1046–1061
9. Oxnard GR, Arcila ME, Sima CS et al (2011) Acquired resistance to EGFR tyrosine kinase inhibitors in EGFR-mutant lung cancer: distinct natural history of patients with tumors harboring the T790M mutation. Clin Cancer Res 17:1616–1622
10. Yu HA, Arcila ME, Rekhtman N et al (2013) Analysis of tumor specimens at the time of acquired resistance to EGFR-TKI therapy in 155 patients with EGFR-mutant lung cancers. Clin Cancer Res 19:2240–2247
11. Yun CH, Mengwasser KE, Toms AV et al (2008) The T790M mutation in EGFR kinase causes drug resistance by increasing the affinity for ATP. Proc Natl Acad Sci U S A 105:2070–2075
12. Sos ML, Rode HB, Heynck S et al (2010) Chemogenomic profiling provides insights into the limited activity of irreversible EGFR inhibitors in tumor cells expressing the T790M EGFR resistance mutation. Cancer Res 70:868–874
13. Ballard P, Yates JW, Yang Z et al (2016) Preclinical comparison of Osimertinib with other EGFR-TKIs in EGFR-mutant NSCLC brain metastases models, and early evidence of clinical brain metastases activity. Clin Cancer Res 22:5130–5140
14. Janne PA, Yang JC, Kim DW et al (2015) AZD9291 in EGFR inhibitor-resistant non-small-cell lung cancer. N Engl J Med 372:1689–1699
15. Mok TS, Wu YL, Ahn MJ et al (2017) Osimertinib or platinum-Pemetrexed in EGFR T790M-positive lung cancer. N Engl J Med 376:629–640
16. Ramalingam SS, Yang JC, Lee CK et al (2018) Osimertinib as first-line treatment of EGFR mutation-positive advanced non-small-cell lung cancer. J Clin Oncol 36:841–849
17. Soria JC, Ohe Y, Vansteenkiste J et al (2018) Osimertinib in untreated EGFR-mutated advanced non-small-cell lung cancer. N Engl J Med 378:113–125
18. Nanjo S, Ebi H, Arai S et al (2016) High efficacy of third generation EGFR inhibitor AZD9291 in a leptomeningeal carcinomatosis model with EGFR-mutant lung cancer cells. Oncotarget 7:3847–3856
19. Nanjo S, Hata A, Okuda C et al (2018) Standard-dose osimertinib for refractory leptomeningeal metastases in T790M-positive EGFR-mutant non-small cell lung cancer. Br J Cancer 118:32–37
20. Reungwetwattana T, Nakagawa K, Cho BC et al (2018) CNS response to Osimertinib versus standard epidermal growth factor receptor tyrosine kinase inhibitors in patients with untreated EGFR-mutated advanced non-small-cell lung cancer. J Clin Oncol:JCO2018783118
21. Wu YL, Tsuboi M, He J et al (2020) Osimertinib in resected EGFR-mutated non-small-cell lung cancer. N Engl J Med 383:1711–1723
22. Piotrowska Z, Isozaki H, Lennerz JK et al (2018) Landscape of acquired resistance to Osimertinib in EGFR-mutant NSCLC and clinical validation of combined EGFR and RET inhibition with Osimertinib and BLU-667 for acquired RET fusion. Cancer Discov 8:1529–1539
23. Bordi P, Del Re M, Minari R et al (2019) From the beginning to resistance: study of plasma monitoring and resistance mechanisms in a cohort of patients treated with osimertinib for advanced T790M-positive NSCLC. Lung Cancer 131:78–85
24. Ercan D, Choi HG, Yun CH et al (2015) EGFR mutations and resistance to irreversible pyrimidine-based EGFR inhibitors. Clin Cancer Res 21:3913–3923

25. Schmid S, Klingbiel D, Aeppli S et al (2019) Patterns of progression on osimertinib in EGFR T790M positive NSCLC: a Swiss cohort study. Lung Cancer 130:149–155
26. Brown BP, Zhang YK, Westover D et al (2019) On-target resistance to the mutant-selective EGFR inhibitor Osimertinib can develop in an allele-specific manner dependent on the original EGFR-activating mutation. Clin Cancer Res 25:3341–3351
27. Uchibori K, Inase N, Araki M et al (2017) Brigatinib combined with anti-EGFR antibody overcomes osimertinib resistance in EGFR-mutated non-small-cell lung cancer. Nat Commun 8:14768
28. Niederst MJ, Hu H, Mulvey HE et al (2015) The allelic context of the C797S mutation acquired upon treatment with third-generation EGFR inhibitors impacts sensitivity to subsequent treatment strategies. Clin Cancer Res 21:3924–3933
29. Jia Y, Yun CH, Park E et al (2016) Overcoming EGFR(T790M) and EGFR(C797S) resistance with mutant-selective allosteric inhibitors. Nature 534:129–132
30. Oztan A, Fischer S, Schrock AB et al (2017) Emergence of EGFR G724S mutation in EGFR-mutant lung adenocarcinoma post progression on osimertinib. Lung Cancer 111:84–87
31. Zhang Q, Zhang XC, Yang JJ et al (2018) EGFR L792H and G796R: two novel mutations mediating resistance to the third-generation EGFR tyrosine kinase inhibitor Osimertinib. J Thorac Oncol 13:1415–1421
32. Ma L, Chen R, Wang F et al (2019) EGFR L718Q mutation occurs without T790M mutation in a lung adenocarcinoma patient with acquired resistance to osimertinib. Ann Transl Med 7:207
33. Starrett JH, Guernet AA, Cuomo ME et al (2020) Drug sensitivity and allele specificity of first-line Osimertinib resistance EGFR mutations. Cancer Res 80:2017–2030
34. Nakatani K, Yamaoka T, Ohba M et al (2019) KRAS and EGFR amplifications mediate resistance to Rociletinib and Osimertinib in acquired Afatinib-resistant NSCLC harboring exon 19 deletion/T790M in EGFR. Mol Cancer Ther 18:112–126
35. Knebel FH, Bettoni F, Shimada AK et al (2017) Sequential liquid biopsies reveal dynamic alterations of EGFR driver mutations and indicate EGFR amplification as a new mechanism of resistance to osimertinib in NSCLC. Lung Cancer 108:238–241
36. Planchard D, Loriot Y, Andre F et al (2015) EGFR-independent mechanisms of acquired resistance to AZD9291 in EGFR T790M-positive NSCLC patients. Ann Oncol 26:2073–2078
37. Ortiz-Cuaran S, Scheffler M, Plenker D et al (2016) Heterogeneous mechanisms of primary and acquired resistance to third-generation EGFR inhibitors. Clin Cancer Res 22:4837–4847
38. Sequist LV, Han JY, Ahn MJ et al (2020) Osimertinib plus savolitinib in patients with EGFR mutation-positive, MET-amplified, non-small-cell lung cancer after progression on EGFR tyrosine kinase inhibitors: interim results from a multicentre, open-label, phase 1b study. Lancet Oncol 21:373–386
39. Vojnic M, Kubota D, Kurzatkowski C et al (2019) Acquired BRAF rearrangements induce secondary resistance to EGFR therapy in EGFR-mutated lung cancers. J Thorac Oncol 14:802–815
40. Weng CH, Chen LY, Lin YC et al (2019) Epithelial-mesenchymal transition (EMT) beyond EGFR mutations per se is a common mechanism for acquired resistance to EGFR TKI. Oncogene 38:455–468
41. Taniguchi H, Yamada T, Wang R et al (2019) AXL confers intrinsic resistance to osimertinib and advances the emergence of tolerant cells. Nat Commun 10:259
42. Sequist LV, Waltman BA, Dias-Santagata D et al (2011) Genotypic and histological evolution of lung cancers acquiring resistance to EGFR inhibitors. Sci Transl Med 3:75ra26
43. Marcoux N, Gettinger SN, O'Kane G et al (2019) EGFR-mutant adenocarcinomas that transform to small-cell lung Cancer and other neuroendocrine carcinomas: clinical outcomes. J Clin Oncol 37:278–285
44. Ferrer L, Giaj Levra M, Brevet M et al (2019) A brief report of transformation from NSCLC to SCLC: molecular and therapeutic characteristics. J Thorac Oncol 14:130–134
45. Antony J, Huang RY (2017) AXL-driven EMT state as a targetable conduit in cancer. Cancer Res 77:3725–3732

Chapter 5
Immune Therapy: What Can We Learn From Acquired Resistance?

Michael J. Grant, Katerina Politi, and Scott Gettinger

Abstract Programmed death-1 (PD-1) pathway inhibitors have revolutionized the treatment of locally advanced and advanced non-small cell lung cancer (NSCLC). Response to these agents can be durable, but most patients will go on to develop resistance after initial tumor regression or prolonged disease stability. In patients with 'acquired oligo-resistance,' in whom progression is limited to two or less disease sites, local therapy may be an effective management strategy. For those experiencing systemic progression, immunotherapy based combinations are currently under investigation. Translational work has uncovered neoantigen loss and antigen processing/presentation defects as mediators of resistance to PD-1 axis inhibitors NSCLC. In other tumor types, defects in IFN- γ signaling, upregulation of alternative immune checkpoint pathways, and various tumor genomic or epigenetic changes have been implicated. In this review, we propose clinical criteria, highlight emerging management strategies, and discuss mechanistic insights into acquired resistance to PD-1 axis inhibitors in NSCLC.

Keywords Immunotherapy · Immune Checkpoint Inhibitor · Programmed Death- 1 (PD-1) Axis Inhibitor · Cytotoxic T-lymphocyte Antigen-4 (CTLA-4) Inhibitor · Lung Cancer · Acquired Resistance · Oligo-resistance · Neoantigen loss · Beta-2 microglobulin · Nivolumab · Pembrolizumab · Atezolizumab · Durvalumab · Ipilimumab

M. J. Grant · S. Gettinger (✉)
Department of Medicine (Medical Oncology), Yale School of Medicine/Yale Cancer Center, New Haven, CT, USA
e-mail: Scott.gettinger@yale.edu

K. Politi
Department of Pathology, Yale School of Medicine/Yale Cancer Center, New Haven, CT, USA
e-mail: Scott.gettinger@yale.edu

© Springer Nature Switzerland AG 2021
A. C. Chiang, R. S. Herbst (eds.), *Lung Cancer*, Current Cancer Research,
https://doi.org/10.1007/978-3-030-74028-3_5

1   Introduction

The therapeutic landscape for stage III unresectable and stage IV non-small cell lung cancer (NSCLC) has been transformed since 2015 with the advent of immunotherapy approvals [1–4]. Immune checkpoint inhibitors (ICI) targeting the programmed death 1 (PD-1) axis, alone and in combination with chemotherapy and/or ipilimumab, another checkpoint inhibitor, provide long-term survival benefits over classic standard regimens for patients with both squamous and nonsquamous NSCLC [5–13]. However, resistance to PD-1 axis inhibitors is undoubtedly the next hurdle for further augmentation of overall survival in advanced NSCLC. Resistance, in this context, can be classified as *primary* in patients who are treated with and do not have an initial response to checkpoint inhibitor therapy, and *acquired* in patients who initially derive clinical benefit from treatment and subsequently experience progression of disease.

Long-term follow up of responders to PD-1 axis inhibitors provides some insight into the burden of acquired resistance to PD-1 axis inhibitors and demonstrates that although responses can be durable, in most cases the initial response to immunotherapy is lost (Table 5.1). In this chapter, we will focus on acquired resistance, specifically to PD-1 axis inhibitors. After defining this concept, we will dissect the existing literature to better characterize patterns of acquired resistance in NSCLC. We aim to highlight effective management strategies for subsets of this heterogeneous population and introduce a treatment algorithm for tackling acquired resistance in the context of different clinical situations. We will review lessons learned from attempts to understand mechanisms driving acquired resistance to immunotherapy in NSCLC and other malignancies. Finally, we will discuss concepts and strategies for future study.

2   Defining Acquired Resistance

Whereas primary resistance to ICIs refers to patients with disease that fails to regress or stabilize upon initial challenge with these agents, acquired resistance is more challenging to define. At the cellular level, acquired resistance manifests as a shift from a state of tumor elimination or tumor-immune equilibrium to a state of tumor-immune-escape. Drivers of immune-escape fall into one of two categories—either acquired alterations in anti-tumor immune cell function or tumor-intrinsic changes that prevent immune-mediated destruction/control. At the clinical level, we classify acquired resistance to PD-1 axis inhibitors in NSCLC patients according to the initial response to therapy. **"Acquired resistance after initial response" describes a scenario in which a patient achieves a partial or complete response to PD-1 axis inhibitor followed by subsequent progression at ≥1 site while on therapy or within 12 weeks of therapy cessation** (Table 5.2). **Alternatively, "acquired resistance after initial prolonged stability" describes a scenario in which a patient experiences disease stability on PD-1 axis inhibitor for ≥24 weeks followed by subsequent progression at ≥1 site while on therapy or within 12 weeks of therapy cessation.**

Table 5.1 Long-term response data for patients with advanced NSCLC achieving objective response to PD-1 axis inhibitors on various clinical trials

PD-1 Axis Inhibitor	Trial	Population	Response Criteria Used	ORR (n/N)	Minimum followup (mos.)	% Ongoing response at 24 months	Median Duration of response (months)	Long-term Survival (all patients)	References
Nivolumab (PD-1)	CA209-003	Previously treated advanced NSCLC	RECIST v1.1	17.1% (22/129)	75.2	41	19.1	5-year OS: 15.6% 6-year OS: 14.7%	[14–16]
	Checkmate 017/ 057 (Pooled Analysis)	Previously treated advanced NSCLC	RECIST v1.1	ORR 19.6% (84/427) ORR at 6 months: 16.4% (70/427)	51.6	47 (post-6-month landmark)	19.9	5-year OS for pooled 017/057: 13.6%	[15, 22]
Pembrolizumab (PD-1)	KEYNOTE-001	PD-L1 expressing (≥1%) advanced NSCLC (treatment naïve and previously treated cohorts)	irRC	Treatment naive: 41.6% (42/101) Previously treated: 22.9% (103/449)	52 52	NR NR	Treatment naïve: 16.8 Previously treated: 38.9	5-year OS: 23.3% 5-year OS: 15.5%	[18]
	KEYNOTE-010	Previously treated PD-L1 expressing advanced NSCLC	RECIST v1.1	18% (64/344)	35.2	NR	NR	3-year OS: 23%	[20]
	KEYNOTE-024	Treatment-naive PD-L1 high (≥50%) advanced NSCLC	RECIST v1.1	45% (69/154)	55.1	NR	29.1	5-year OS: 32%	[5, 19, 21]
	KEYNOTE-042	Treatment-naive PD-L1 expressing(≥1%) (advanced NSCLC)	RECIST v1.1	27% (174/637)	NR (median 12.8)	48	20.2	2-year OS: 39%	[9]

(continued)

Table 5.1 (continued)

PD-1 Axis Inhibitor	Trial	Population	Response Criteria Used	ORR (n/N)	Minimum followup (mos.)	% Ongoing response at 24 months	Median Duration of response (months)	Long-term Survival (all patients)	References
Atezolizumab (PD-L1)	OAK	Previously treated advanced NSCLC	RECIST v1.1	13.7 (84/613)	21	50	24	2-year OS: 31%	[17]
	IMPower 110	Treatment-naive PD-L1 expressing(≥1%) (advanced NSCLC)	RECIST v1.1	TC3 or IC3: 38.3%	0, (median 15.7)	NR	Not evaluable	1-year OS: 64.9%	[13, 49]
				TC2/3 or IC2/3: 30.7%	0, (median 15.2)	NR	Not Evaluable	1-year OS: 60.7%	

Abbreviations: *RECISTv1.1* Response Evaluation Criteria in Solid Tumors version 1.1, *irRC* immune-related response criteria, *OS* overall survival. *NR* not reported. *CM* Checkmate. *TC3 or IC3* ≥50% expression of PD-L1 on tumor cells (TC3) or ≥10% expression on tumor-infiltrating immune cells (IC3), *TC2/3 or IC2/3* ≥5% expression of PD-L1 on tumor cells (TC2/3) or ≥5% expression on tumor-infiltrating immune cells (IC2/3)

Table 5.2 Definitions pertaining to acquired resistance to PD-1 axis inhibitors in advanced NSCLC

Term	Clinical Scenario
Acquired Resistance after initial response	The patient achieves a partial or complete response to PD-1 axis inhibitor followed by subsequent progression at ≥1 site while on therapy or within 12 weeks of therapy cessation
Acquired resistance after initial prolonged stability	The patient has stable disease on PD-1 axis inhibitor for ≥24 weeks followed by subsequent progression at ≥1 site while on therapy or within 12 weeks of therapy cessation
Off-therapy Progression	The patient has initial partial response, complete response, or stable disease ≥24 weeks on PD-1 axis inhibitor, followed by progression at ≥1 site more than 12 weeks after cessation of PD-1 axis inhibitor[a]
Acquired Oligoresistance	Acquired resistance that occurs at ≤2 sites of disease
Acquired Resistance with systemic progression	Acquired resistance that occurs at >2 sites of disease

[a]Does not exclude late onset acquired resistance

2.1 Classification Based on Initial Response

Generally, patients with substantial tumor shrinkage, meeting RECIST criteria for a partial or complete response, derive initial clinical benefit from ICIs [23–25]. This is less clear for patients with prolonged stable disease (≥6 months) as the best initial response. Data from a pooled long-term 6-month landmark analysis from CHECKMATE 017 and 057 clinical trials substantiates the notion that prolonged stable disease with PD-1 axis inhibitors may be clinically meaningful, relative to stability with cytotoxic chemotherapy [15, 26]. These two trials randomized patients with pre-treated, immunotherapy naïve advanced NSCLC to the PD-1 axis inhibitor nivolumab or standard salvage chemotherapy with docetaxel. Response assessment at 6 months demonstrated stable disease for 24% of patients treated with nivolumab compared to 39% of patients treated with docetaxel. The 4-year overall survival (OS) and progression free survival (PFS) for the patients with stable disease at 6 months was 19% and 14% for nivolumab vs. 2% and 0% for docetaxel.

Although patients with advanced NSCLC experiencing prolonged stable disease (SD) on PD-1 axis inhibitors have favorable long-term outcomes compared to patients with SD on chemotherapy, how do outcomes compare to patients with RECIST objective response to PD-1 axis inhibitors? Pooled analysis of CHECKMATE 017 and 057 demonstrated that objective response (complete or partial response) vs. stable disease at 6 months was associated with a hazard ratio (HR) for progression of 0.42 (95% CI 0.27–0.65) with 4-year PFS of 38% vs 14% respectively. The 4-year survival rate was also significantly improved for patients with partial response (PR) or complete response (CR) at 6 months (58%) compared to patients with SD at 6 months (19%) with non-overlapping 95% confidence intervals. Still, prolonged SD was clearly a favorable outcome compared to progressive disease for nivolumab-treated patients on these trials, with a HR for death over the course of follow-up of 0.52 (95% CI 0.37–0.71). It is likely that patients with

SD $\geq$ 6 months on immunotherapy comprise a heterogeneous group, with some patients achieving minor responses, some patients with indolent disease experiencing slow progression, and potentially some patients with immunotherapy-mediated growth stabilization or slowing [23]. Though we include patients with prolonged stable disease in our acquired resistance definitions, we distinguish them from patients achieving initial response of CR/PR (initial responders). This distinction not only has prognostic implications, but it will also allow us to study differences in outcomes among these groups and potentially develop tools to more accurately identify patients with true acquired resistance in the future. Stratification by prior RECIST response versus prolonged stability may also be useful in clinical trials enrolling patients with acquired resistance to PD-1 axis inhibitors.

2.2   Acquired Resistance Versus Off-Therapy Progression

For our definition of off-therapy progression, the 12-week cutoff after cessation of PD-1 axis inhibitor therapy was chosen based on the high affinity binding properties of PD-1 axis inhibitors. Because these antibodies bind PD-1 with high affinity, serum drug concentration does not reflect receptor occupancy. Preclinical data from the phase I trial of Nivolumab in refractory solid tumors demonstrated that receptor occupancy remained high and only began to decline at a mean duration of 85 days after the first infusion [27]. Therefore, it is unlikely that the direct PD-1 antagonistic effects of these high affinity antibodies wane significantly before 12 weeks. After initial response or prolonged stability, progression that occurs within 12 weeks of stopping therapy is likely related to ICI resistance and not inadequate PD-1 blockade in the immune microenvironment. Moreover, this 12-week cutoff delineating acquired resistance from off-treatment progression is consistent with the Society for Immunotherapy in Cancer (SITC) Immunotherapy Resistance Task Force guidelines for defining tumor resistance to PD-1 pathway blockade [24].

Clinically the distinction between acquired resistance and off-therapy recurrence is supported, albeit with limited data, by analysis from the KEYNOTE-010 clinical trial randomizing patients with advanced pre-treated PD ligand 1 (L1) positive NSCLC to pembrolizumab vs docetaxel. Fourteen patients who had initial clinical benefit and completed 2 years of therapy with pembrolizumab were rechallenged on progression [20]. Of the 7 patients who progressed within 12 weeks of completing pembrolizumab, only one had an objective response to re-challenge. Of the 7 patients who had disease progression more than 12 weeks after completing pembrolizumab, 5 achieved second response to re-challenge (overall response rate (ORR) 71%) and all patients had disease control after 6 months of retreatment (2 patients had stable disease for 6+ months). Though we cannot draw firm conclusions or select strict cutoffs based on these limited data, the findings allude to the importance of thoughtfully distinguishing acquired resistance from off-treatment progression.

3   Clinical Observations in Patients with Advanced NSCLC and Acquired Resistance to PD-1 Axis Inhibitors

Acquired resistance to immunotherapy is a heterogeneous phenomenon, but retrospective analyses have helped to identify common patterns of occurrence. In a single-center series, 26 patients with advanced NSCLC developed disease progression after deriving initial clinical benefit from PD-1 axis inhibitors. Progression occurred within a year of starting anti-PD-1 therapy in most patients (median time to acquired resistance 313 days) [28]. Only three patients (12%) experienced progression more than 2 years after initiation of therapy. Most patients (77%, n = 20/26) were receiving a PD-1 axis inhibitor at the time of progression. Six patients (23%) were off therapy at the time of progression, most having discontinued after the development of immune-related toxicity. In these patients, time from last dose of PD-1 axis inhibitor to progression of disease was less than three months for one patient (40 days) and less than four months for two others (102, 110 days). All 23 patients who had a biopsy at the time of recurrence retained the NSCLC histologic subtype present at initial diagnosis. Recurrences had a predilection for nodal sites and most frequently occurred as oligoprogression- 54% of patients experienced acquired resistance at one site of disease, while 89% of patients had recurrence at ≤2 sites of disease. In a similar series of 57 patients with NSCLC and initial clinical benefit from PD-1 axis inhibitors, 33 patients (58%) subsequently experienced progression of disease [29]. All 33 patients were receiving PD-1 axis inhibitor at the time of progression. The median progression-free survival from the time of first CT scan was 4.4 months. Like the above series, most (67%) patients developed progression at one site of disease. Twenty patients (60%) had progression at pre-existing sites of disease rather than development of new lesions. It is important to note that this study's definition of acquired resistance differed from ours in that initial benefit was defined as 'alive with stable disease, partial response, or complete response by RECIST criteria at first CT scan.' Our definition would not include patients with stable disease at first CT scan unless these patients remained with stable disease at 24 weeks.

4   Concepts in the Management of Acquired Resistance to PD-1 Axis Inhibitors in Advanced NSCLC

To date, the management of patients with acquired resistance to immunotherapy is largely empiric. There are several strategies that have been described, yet existing literature on the topic is limited to small single-center case series [28, 29]. As we learn more about the specific mechanisms that lead to acquired resistance, we may be able to tailor systemic treatment approaches to individuals or patient subsets. In Fig. 5.1, we propose a management algorithm for patients with progression after initial benefit from PD-1 axis inhibitors.

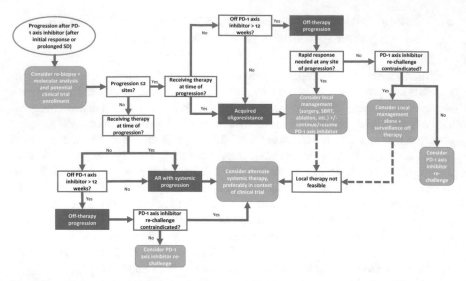

Fig. 5.1 PD-1 Axis Inhibitor acquired resistance in NSCLC management algorithm. Abbreviations: CNS Central Nervous System, SBRT Stereotactic Body Radiation Therapy, AR Acquired Resistance

4.1 Local Therapy

In cases of acquired resistance limited to one to two sites, so-called 'oligoresistant disease', one management strategy has been to treat with local therapy to progressing sites without changing or starting a new systemic therapy. This approach is standardly used in patients with driver-mutated NSCLC responding to tyrosine kinase inhibitors who experience one site of progressive disease [30–34]. In the 26-patient series previously discussed, 15 patients with acquired oligo-resistance underwent local therapy without initiation of alternative systemic therapy; two-year post-resistance survival rate was 92%. In contrast, in the 33 patient series, local therapy was rarely used to treat oligoprogressive disease [29]. Two patients out of twenty-two (9%) received local ablative radiotherapy to single sites of disease progression, and both experienced 9-month progression-free intervals that were sustained at the time of manuscript publication without further systemic therapy.

The allure of local therapy in these patients extends beyond local disease control. There may be additional immune-priming effects of different types of local therapy (e.g. radiation, ablative therapy) that enhance the systemic response to PD-1 axis inhibition through various mechanisms. These mechanisms include increased antigen release and presentation, modification of the tumor microenvironment, and enhanced immune trafficking to sites of disease [35–38]. The abscopal effect describes a phenomenon by which local therapy can induce a systemic response at distant sites of disease. This effect is thought to be enhanced by PD-1 axis inhibition, although the biologic rationale and preclinical data are presently stronger than the clinical data supporting this notion [39–42]. It is suspected that the timing of immunotherapy administration as well as the timing, dose, anatomical sites, and number of sites of radiotherapy may be important for optimizing synergy between local radio-therapy and PD-1 axis inhibition. The combination of immunotherapy and radiation is currently under investigation in several clinical trials for advanced NSCLC [43, 44].

Though it is rare, isolated central nervous system (CNS) acquired resistance can occur in patients receiving PD-1 axis inhibitors. Of note, PD-1 axis inhibitors do have activity in the brain, as demonstrated in a trial of pembrolizumab, which reported that response of brain metastases paralleled response outside the brain in patients with advanced NSCLC with asymptomatic untreated brain metastases [45]. In the 26-patient cohort previously discussed, 2/26 patients had isolated CNS pro-gression with de novo brain metastases developing well into their course of anti-PD-1 therapy [28]. Lesion-targeted stereotactic radiosurgery (SRS) is often employed for patients with NSCLC and CNS metastases. When combined with immunotherapy, SRS appears well tolerated initially with more rapid responses; however, may lead to increased risk of subsequent radiation necrosis, a tissue inflammatory response to irreversible injury that develops at sites exposed to high doses of radiation [46–48] Radiation necrosis typically occurs between 12 weeks and 2 years after SRS and it can be difficult to distinguish, both radiographically and clinically, from progression of disease. SRS with concurrent PD-1 axis inhibitor may also result in earlier onset of radiation necrosis.

4.2 Resume/Re-Challenge with PD-1 Axis Inhibitor Therapy

PD-1 axis inhibitor re-challenge has been considered in patients who experience progression of disease 12 or more weeks after discontinuation of initial therapy. Ultimately, the decision to retreat with PD-1 axis inhibitors hinges on the safety of re-challenge and the probability of inducing a meaningful response to retreatment. The literature on this topic is scant but properly designed prospective studies could potentially provide more insight into predictors of benefit from PD-1 axis inhibitor re-challenge.

In certain cases, patients responding to a PD-1 axis inhibitor may discontinue therapy after completion of a predefined treatment course. The pivotal trials leading to U.S. Federal Drug Administration approval of first-line monotherapy with pem-brolizumab and atezolizumab for advanced PD-L1 expressing NSCLC had pre-specified PD-1 axis inhibitor treatment durations of 24 months and 58 months respectively [5, 9, 11, 49]. Similarly, the registrational trials evaluating nivolumab combined with ipilimumab treated for up to 2 years [11, 12]. In contrast, trials exploring currently approved combination chemotherapy with either pembroli-zumab or atezolizumab did not specify a maximum duration for PD-1 axis inhibitor maintenance therapy [6, 8].

Outcomes to PD-1 axis inhibitor re-treatment have been reported for select patients enrolled on several clinical trials (Table 5.3). In a prior section, we dis-cussed re-challenge data from KEYNOTE-010 in the context of distinguishing acquired resistance and off-therapy progression [20]. In an updated analysis of the first line KEYNOTE-024 trial at the 2019 World Conference on Lung Cancer

Table 5.3 Reported experience with PD-1 axis inhibitor re-challenge in patients enrolled in major clinical trials for advanced NSCLC

Trial	PD-1 axis inhibitor	Patient population	Reported patients rechallenged	Response to initial PD-1 axis inhibitor course; course length	Reason for discontinuation	Interval of rechallenge	Intervening systemic therapy	Response to rechallenge; long-term outcomes	References
KEYNOTE-001	Pembrolizumab	Pretreated and treatment naïve Advanced PD-L1-expressing NSCLC	1	PR; 44 months	Presumed maximal benefit	11 weeks	None	PR; DOR 6.5 months	[18]
KEYNOTE-010	Pembrolizumab	Pretreated advanced PD-L1-expressing NSCLC	14	NR; 24 months (median)	Completed trial therapy	28 weeks (median); 8–52 weeks (range)	None	5 PR (36%), 6 SD (43%); patients with PR/SD, rechallenge PFS range 6.5–21+ months with 9 patients remaining progression-free at time of analysis (min follow-up 8 mos.)	[20]
KEYNOTE-024	Pembrolizumab	Treatment-naïve PD-L1 high (≥50%) advanced NSCLC	10	7 PR, 3 SD; 24 months	Completed trial therapy	56 weeks (median); 24–80 weeks (range)	None	3 PR (30%), 4 SD (40%); NR (short follow-up)	[52]

CA209-003	Nivolumab	Pretreated advanced NSCLC	2	Patient 1: PR, 24 months	Completed trial therapy	104 weeks	None	PR; DOR 11 months	[16]
				Patient 2: PR, 24 months	Completed trial therapy	> 260 weeks	None	PR; DOR 2+ months (ongoing)	
CHECKMATE 153	Nivolumab	Pretreated advanced NSCLC	39	NR, 12 months	Completed trial therapy	~20 weeks (median)	None	NR; 36% of retreatment patients alive at minimum follow-up of 13.5 months	[50]
NCT01693562	Durvalumab	Advanced solid tumors	21 (NSCLC)	NR, 12 months	Completed trial therapy	NR	None	3 PR (14%), 8 SD (38%); DOR 13.4 (7.2 to 25.1+)	[51]

Abbreviations: NR not reported, DOR duration of response

(WCLC), 10 patients with high (≥50%) PD-L1-expressing advanced NSCLC who completed 2 years of first-line pembrolizumab were re-treated at the time of subsequent progression [52]. Of note, 7/10 patients had an initial partial response to the first course of pembrolizumab, and the remaining three patients had a best response of stable disease. For these patients, the median interval between progression and re-challenge was 56 weeks (range 24–80 weeks). Upon retreatment, 3 patients achieved a partial response (30%), all of whom had initial partial response to the first pembrolizumab course. Four additional patients had stable disease upon re-challenge. The durability of these responses could not be assessed due to short follow-up at the time of reporting.

Two NSCLC patients that survived to 5 years in the first trial with a NSCLC cohort evaluating nivolumab were re-treated with a PD-1 inhibitor after disease progression [16]. The first patient had an early response to nivolumab, completed 2 years of treatment, then experienced disease progression 16 months after cessation of therapy. This patient had a partial response to re-challenge with nivolumab lasting 11 months. The second patient also had initial response to therapy but then progressed 5 years after completing 2 years of therapy. On re-challenge with an experimental PD-1 inhibitor, the disease responded again (2+ month duration of response at last follow-up prior to publication).

Patients with premature therapy discontinuation due to immune-related toxicity may also be considered for re-challenge at the time of disease progression. A subset of these patients may have long-term disease control from their abbreviated course of ICI, but it is not uncommon for others to experience progression during the subsequent treatment-free interval. Certainly, for these patients, the risks and benefits of re-challenge and possible recrudescence of immune toxicity need to be considered. The severity and reversibility of the initial immune toxicity should be scrutinized prior to re-challenge but current data show that 58–67% of patients will not experience re-emergence of the same immune-related adverse event (irAE) [53, 54]. In a retrospective analysis, 40 patients with NSCLC, colorectal cancer, or metastatic melanoma treated with PD-1 axis inhibitor therapy who experienced ≥ grade 2 irAEs were eventually re-challenged with a PD-1 axis inhibitor [54]. Fifty-five percent (n = 22) experienced a second irAE of any kind, while 42% (n = 17) experienced recrudescence of their initial irAE. Twenty percent of patients with pneumonitis had recurrence (n = 1/5), while 60% of patients with hepatitis or colitis had recurrence (n = 3/5 for both). There were no re-treatment related deaths. In another report, four patients experienced progressive disease after nivolumab was held for some irAE [55]. All patients benefitted from nivolumab treatment prior to toxicity (1 CR, 2 PR, 1 SD) and upon re-challenge (2 PR, 2 SD) with PFS after retreatment ranging from 110 days to 244 days. Upon retreatment, none of these patients experienced grade ≥3 or treatment-limiting irAEs.

Currently, we lack evidence to guide patient selection for re-challenge. One retrospective study looked at 10,452 patients treated with nivolumab for advanced NSCLC, of which 1517 patients were re-treated with a PD-1 axis inhibitor after some immunotherapy-free interval [56]. In these re-treated patients, outcomes were significantly better in patients who had received a longer duration of initial nivolumab therapy. This was true for patients with no intervening therapy as well as for patients with intervening chemotherapy. Though further study is needed, it may be that longer duration of initial treatment with a PD-1 inhibitor enriches for patients who previously experienced clinical benefit from these agents. A patient would be more likely to receive a longer initial course of PD-1 axis inhibitor if he or she experienced radiographic/clinical response or disease control. Alternatively, the longer duration of exposure to PD-1 axis inhibitor therapy may foster development of an immune memory response that can be re-stimulated during later line PD-1 axis inhibition. The PD-1 axis inhibitor re-treated cohort in this study had a median OS > 12 months from the time of re-treatment, which compares favorably to that of later-line chemotherapy [57]. Other series have proposed that response to re-challenge may correlate with tumor PD-L1 expression or development of irAEs [55, 58]. However, caution must be exercised before drawing conclusions from this limited data and at this time these are observations that can serve only to generate hypotheses for future prospective studies.

In a patient that progresses after completing a PD-1 axis inhibitor course, we consider re-treatment if the patient was deriving clinical benefit at the time of therapy cessation, and if progression occurred more than 12 weeks after cessation. We also consider re-treatment in patients that progress after discontinuation due to irAEs. In this setting, the risks of irAE recrudescence need to be considered and discussed with the patient.

4.3 PD-1 Axis Inhibitor Combinations

Acquired resistance to PD-1 axis inhibitors may occur from selection of resistant clones present at the time of treatment initiation, or from de novo genetic, epigenetic, or other expression-level changes that give rise to resistant clones. Combination strategies with PD-1 axis inhibitors hinge on the idea that the introduction of another agent can either expand the anti-tumor immune response against immune-evasive clonal populations or enhance an existing immune response that has been stifled. In part, the rationale to continue PD-1 axis inhibition with other therapies relates to the possibility of ongoing disease control at some disease sites despite radiographic progression. Additionally, other therapies may induce PD-L1 expression therefore dampening the efficacy of these treatments without concurrent PD-1 axis inhibition. Further, PD-1 axis inhibitors are generally well-tolerated, and experience with combination approaches have also demonstrated favorable toxicity profiles.

4.3.1 PD-1 Axis Inhibitors + CTLA-4 Inhibitors

Currently, combined PD-1 axis/ CTLA-4 inhibition with nivolumab and ipilimumab is approved for use in advanced PD-1 axis inhibitor naïve melanoma, renal cell carcinoma, non-small cell lung cancer, hepatocellular carcinoma, microsatellite instability-high or mismatch repair deficient metastatic colorectal cancer, and mesothelioma. It is unknown if the combination can rescue patients with either primary or acquired resistance to PD-1 axis inhibitor therapy.

The biologic rationale for combining PD-1 axis inhibitors with anti-CTLA-4 agents to subvert resistant disease is based on the differential roles of the PD-1 and CTLA-4 pathways. Broadly, CTLA-4 plays a larger role in the priming phase of the adaptive immune response whereas the PD-1 pathway predominates in peripheral tissues during the effector phase [59, 60]. It is important to note that this priming vs. effector checkpoint categorization is not absolute, e.g. CTLA-4 is expressed by tumor-associated T-regulatory (Treg) cells which may mediate peripheral immune evasion [61].

Trials are currently accruing which seek to determine the efficacy of combination PD-1 axis inhibitors and anti-CTLA-4 agents in PD-1 axis inhibitor acquired resistance populations (NCT03262779, NCT02000947). Early data from one trial evaluating Durvalumab (anti-PD-L1) and Tremelimumab (anti-CTLA-4) in IO-pretreated advanced NSCLC, was presented at the American Association of Clinical Oncology (ASCO) Annual Meeting 2018 [62]. Efficacy data were similar for IO-relapsed (prior response or stability to PD-1 axis inhibitor therapy) and IO-refractory patients. Of the 40 patients in the IO-relapsed cohort, only two patients experienced objective response (5%) and 9 (22.5%) achieved disease control at 24 weeks. With a median follow-up of 18 months, the 12-month OS for IO-relapsed patients was 37.5% (n = 15/40).

4.3.2 Novel Combination Strategies for PD-1 Axis Inhibitor Relapsed/ Refractory NSCLC

Several PD-1 axis inhibitor-based novel combination regimens have been evaluated in trials enrolling patients with immunotherapy (IO)- relapsed and refractory disease (Table 5.4). The phrase "IO-refractory" is often used to describe patients with primary resistance to PD-1 axis inhibitor-containing regimens. Similarly, "IO-relapsed" disease generally describes patients that have progressed after a period of response or disease control to PD-1 axis inhibitors. Of note, not all patients enrolled in these trials will fulfill criteria for acquired resistance in accordance with our definitions. Although a subset of patients with IO-relapsed disease have acquired resistance, others may have experienced progression more than 12 weeks after cessation of PD-1 axis inhibitor therapy, and therefore should be classified as having off-therapy progression. Moreover, some patients have had intervening systemic treatment with non-immunotherapy regimens immediately prior to trial enrollment. Only a handful of trials have specified enrollment criteria for NSCLC patients with

PD-1 axis inhibitor acquired resistance (Table 5.5). Therefore, it is difficult to gauge efficacy of these regimens for patients meeting our acquired resistance criteria. Here we highlight several novel combination regimens in IO-relapsed/refractory populations with promising biological rationale and some evidence for early efficacy.

PD-1 Axis Inhibitor + Interleukin Receptor Agonist

ALT-803 is an IL-15 superagonist mutant complexed to a dimeric IL-15RαSushi-Fc fusion protein shown to enhance CD8+ T-cell and NK cell efficacy [78]. This agent has exhibited more potent activity than recombinant IL-15 with a favorable toxicity profile [79–81]. Like IL-15, ALT-803 increases PD-L1 expression on immune cells, supporting combination with a PD-1 axis inhibitor. Considering ALT-803 is a potent driver of NK cell expansion, it may have particular value in reinvigorating the anti-tumor immune response in PD-1 axis inhibitor-resistant tumors that have lost or downregulated major histocompatibility complex (MHC) I. Of note, this agent has previously demonstrated safety but did not demonstrate efficacy as monotherapy in a phase I trial in patients with advanced solid tumors [81].

ALT-803 combined with nivolumab was evaluated in a phase 1b trial enrolling 11 patients with advanced NSCLC who experienced progression of disease on or after treatment with PD-1 axis inhibitors [63]. Three of these 11 patients experienced a partial response to ALT8-803/ nivolumab, with stable disease in another 7 patients (91% disease control rate). Five patients had disease control lasting more than 5 months, including one with primary refractory disease to prior PD-1 axis inhibitor therapy. All three responses occurred in patients with prior response or prolonged stability on nivolumab, including two patients who had ALT-803 added to uninterrupted nivolumab. Based on this experience, another trial evaluating the combination of ALT-803 and PD-1 axis inhibition is currently enrolling patients with acquired resistance to PD-1 axis inhibitor therapy (NCT03228667) (Table 5.5).

NKTR-214 is a human recombinant IL-2 attached to multiple releasable polyethylene glycol (PEG) chains [65]. PEGylation is used to alter the pharmacokinetics of IL-2 and bias receptor selectivity to limit binding to IL2Rα subunit and favor the dimeric IL2Rβγ. Since IL2Rα (CD25) is constitutively expressed on Treg cells, this limited binding to IL2Rα allows NKTR-214 to increase the proliferation, activation, and effector function of CD8+ T-cells and NK cells without expanding inhibitory Treg cells in the tumor microenvironment. The proposed mechanism of synergy with PD-1 axis inhibitor therapy is through the molecule's promotion of PD-1 expression on effector T-cells and its effects on increased proliferation of tumor infiltrating lymphocytes in the tumor microenvironment [65, 82]. NKTR-214 combined with nivolumab was studied in a phase 1/2 trial in patients with advanced solid tumors. Three patients with advanced NSCLC who had progression after PD-1 axis inhibitor-containing regimens experienced disease control with the combination of NKTR-214 and nivolumab [64]. One patient with lung adenocarcinoma who initially responded to combination anti-CTLA-4/ anti-PD-1 in the second line setting had progression of disease 10 months after initial response. This patient

Table 5.4 PD-1 axis inhibitor combination regimens with potential efficacy in PD-1 axis inhibitor relapsed/refractory patients

Trial	Combination	PD-1 axis inhibitor partner mechanism	Clinical Trial Phase	# patients (NSCLC PD-1 R/R)	Intervening systemic therapy between anti-PD-1 and trial (Yes/No)	ORR (# PR)	DCR (#SD+PR)	Interval between PD-1 axis inhibitor and trial	Details for select patients	References
NCT02000947	Durva/Treme	Anti-CTLA-4	Ib	40 Relapsed	No	5% (2)	28% (11)	NR	Two PR.	[62]
NCT02523469	Nivo/ALT-803	IL-15 superagonist	Ib	11 R/R	No	27% (3)	91% (10)	Could not be >3 mos.	DCR among patients with prior benefit from anti-PD-1 monotherapy was 100% (n = 6). 2PR in AR patients with addition of ALT-803 to uninterrupted nivolumab. 1PR on study treatment in a relapsed patient whose best response to 9-5 months of previous nivolumab therapy was SD.	[63]

NCT02983045	Nivo/ NKTR-214	IL-2 agonist	Ib/II	NR	NR (see details for select patients)	NR (2)	NR (3)	NR (see details for select patients)	[64, 65]
								Three patients with anti-PD-1-relapsed disease experienced disease control. 2PR, 1 SD. Patient 1 best response to prior Anti-Pd-1/Anti-CTLA-4 was PR subsequently off all therapy for 9 mos. Confirmed PR w. NKRT-214/Nivo. Patient 2 also with PR to Pt-Db/Anti-PD-1/ Anti-CTLA-4 and maintenance anti-PD-1, unknown interval between this combination and trial. PR to NKTR-214/ Nivo; Patient 3 with PR to prior anti-PD-1, unknown interval between anti-PD-1 and trial. SD on NKTR-214/Nivo.	

Table 5.4 (continued)

Trial	Combination	PD-1 axis inhibitor partner mechanism	Clinical Trial Phase	# patients (NSCLC PD-1 R/R)	Intervening systemic therapy between anti-PD-1 and trial (Yes/No)	ORR (# PR)	DCR (#SD+PR)	Interval between PD-1 axis inhibitor and trial	Details for select patients	References
NCT02437136	Pembro/ Entinostat	HDAC inhibitor	Ib/II	72 R/R	NR	10% (7)	60% (43)	Median 67 days	Median DOR 5 months; 4 patients remained on combination at reporting, longest response over 18 months.	[66, 67]
NCT02638090	Pembro/ Vorinostat	HDAC inhibitor	Ib/II	24 R/R	NR	12.5% (3)	58% (14)	NR	Median time to progression on prior PD-1 axis inhibitor treatment was 10 months (range 7–52 months) for relapsed patients and 2 months (range 1–3 months) for refractory patients. Responses: confirmed PR lasting 12 months; 2 unconfirmed PR (1 relapsed, 1 refractory); DCR for relapsed disease 54% (n = 6/11). One relapsed patient with stable disease for over 16 months.	[68]

NCT02805660	Durva/ Mocetinostat	HDAC inhibitor	Ib/II	29 R/R	No	16% (6)	NR	NR	Six PR; 4 confirmed and 2 unconfirmed (uPR). 2PRs in prior clinical benefit group (24 patients); 2PRs and 2uPRs in no prior clinical benefit cohort (13 patients); 11/37 pts demonstrated tumor reductions; longest treatment duration exceeding 55 weeks	[69]
NCT02655822	Atezo/ CPI-444	Adenosine A2AR antagonist	Ib	7 R/R	NR	28.5% (2)	71% (5)	NR	Two PR in patients with prior anti-PD-1 axis exposure, one lasting > 6 months, both ongoing at the time of data reporting.	[70, 71]

(continued)

Table 5.4 (continued)

Trial	Combination	PD-1 axis inhibitor partner mechanism	Clinical Trial Phase	# patients (NSCLC PD-1 R/R)	Intervening systemic therapy between anti-PD-1 and trial (Yes/No)	ORR (# PR)	DCR (#SD+PR)	Interval between PD-1 axis inhibitor and trial	Details for select patients	References
NCT02954991	Nivo/ Sitravatinib	Spectrum selective receptor TKI	II	56 R/R	NR	20% (11)	75% (42)	NR	Median DOR was 9.2 months, PFS 6.8 months, OS 15.1 months; 2 PRs with clinical benefit lasting over a year on trial; 3 PR (2 confirmed, 1 unconfirmed) with ongoing disease control lasting over 24 weeks	[72]
NCT02817633	TSR-042/ TSR-022	Anti-TIM-3	II	20 R/R[a]	NR	15% (3)	55% (11)	NR	One patient with nivolumab-refractory disease experienced lasting PR.	[73]
NCT03268057	Avelu/ Pepinemab	Anti-SEMA4D	Ib/II	29 R/R	NR	7% (2)	59% (17)	NR	Two PR (63% and 52% tumor reduction) in patients with progression after prior pembrolizumab; 5 SD patients with durable clinical benefit of ≥23 weeks.	[74]
NCT02439450	Nivo/ Viagenpumatucel-L	Cellular Vaccine	Ib	20 R/R	30% (6/20) had intervening non-ICI therapy	15% (3)	55% (11)	NR	Progression-free survival (PFS) was 2.7 months (95% CI, 1.8–4.0 months) with a median follow-up of	[75]

NCT02043665	Pembro/ CVA21	Oncolytic virus	Ib	7 R/R	No	28% (2)	57% (4)	NR	Two PR observed in PD-1 axis inhibitor pre-treated patients. Both responders continuing at data cut-off, 240 and 120 days since commencement; two SD; 3 non-evaluable (1 early non-treatment-related death, 3 awaiting first scan).	[76]
NCT02517398	M7824	Bifunctional fusion protein targeting PD-L1 and TGF-β	I	83 R/R	NR	2.5% (2)	23% (19)	NR	Population was heavily pretreated (74.7% received ≥3 prior therapies); 2 confirmed partial responses (ongoing at 4.5 and 7.5 months) and 17 patients with stable disease (15 ongoing at 3 months)	[77]

Abbreviations: *HDAC* Histone Deacetylase, *Durva* Durvalumab, *Treme* Tremelimumab, *Nivo* Nivolumab, *Pembro* Pembrolizumab, *Atezo* Atezolizumab, *Avelu* Avelumab, *TKI* tyrosine kinase inhibitor, *PR* partial response, *SD* stable disease, *DCR* Disease control rate, *DOR* Duration of response, *ORR* Objective response rate, *R/R* Relapsed/Refractory, *Pt-Db* Platinum Doublet Chemotherapy

[a]includes only patients treated with 300 mg dose TSR-022

Table 5.5 Trials specifying enrollment criteria for NSCLC patients with PD-1 axis inhibitor acquired resistance

Regimen for AR Patients	Trial	Phase	AR-specific Enrollment Criteria
ALT-803 (IL-15 superagonist) + one of several PD-1/PD-L1 inhibitors	NCT03228667	Ib/II	"Cohort 1: RECIST v1.1 progression on or after single-agent checkpoint inhibitor therapy after initial response (ie, confirmed CR or PR by RECIST V1.1) while taking ICI. Cohort 2: NSCLC, tumor PD-L1 expression (TPS $\geq$ 50%), relapsed on first-line PD-1 agent monotherapy after initial CR or PR. Cohort 3: NSCLC, initial CR or PR but subsequent relapse on maintenance PD-1 agent after first-line ICI + chemotherapy Cohort 4: Progression on PD-1/PD-L1 checkpoint inhibitor therapy after experiencing stable disease (SD) for at least 6 months during previous treatment with PD-1/PD-L1 checkpoint inhibitor therapy"[a]
Ipilimumab + Nivolumab	NCT03262779	II	"Acquired resistance cohort must have had stable disease for at least 24 weeks, partial response, or complete response as the best clinical response to anti-PD-1-axis monotherapy, with subsequent progression of disease"[b]
RO7121661 (PD-1/ TIM-3 Bispecific Antibody)	NCT03708328	I	"NSCLC participants must have experienced initial clinical benefit from ICI therapy for at least 4 months in which there was at least one interval scan prior to 4 months demonstrating no progression of disease"[c]
Liquid tumor infiltrating lymphocytes + PD-1 inhibitor	NCT04268108	I	Group 1, arm 1:" Secondary resistance to anti-PD-1 therapy"[d]

[a]https://clinicaltrials.gov/ct2/show/NCT03228667
[b]https://clinicaltrials.gov/ct2/show/NCT03262779
[c]https://clinicaltrials.gov/ct2/show/NCT03708328
[d]https://clinicaltrials.gov/ct2/show/NCT04268108

achieved a confirmed PR on NKTR-214 plus nivolumab in the third line setting. Another patient with squamous NSCLC was treated with combination chemotherapy (platinum doublet) plus immunotherapy (anti-CTLA-4 + anti-PD-1) as first-line therapy with partial response and ongoing disease control with anti-PD-1 maintenance for 1.5 years. On progression, this patient started trial therapy with NKTR-214 plus nivolumab and had a confirmed partial response. Lastly, one patient with KRAS mutant NSCLC with sarcomatoid features who experienced a partial response to second line anti-PD-1 therapy developed progression after 11 months on anti-PD-1 maintenance. This patient was treated with NKTR-214 plus nivolumab as third-line therapy and had prolonged stable disease with 23% decrease in tumor target lesions.

PD-1 Axis Inhibitor + Histone Deacetylase Inhibitors (HDACi)

Epigenetic modifiers have been shown in preclinical studies to increase antigen presentation on tumor cells and thwart the immunosuppressive activity of myeloid derived suppressor cells and Tregs [83–85]. HDACis tip the scale in the tumor microenvironment in favor of more anti-tumor immune effector activity, sensitizing tumors to PD-1 checkpoint blockade.

At both the 2018 WCLC and the 2019 American Association for Cancer Research (AACR) meetings, preliminary efficacy data was presented for ENCORE-601, a Phase II clinical trial investigating entinostat (Class I HDAC inhibitor) plus pembrolizumab in PD-1 axis inhibitor pretreated patients with NSCLC [66, 67]. Of 72 treated patients evaluable for efficacy, 7 (10%) achieved response, with an additional 50% (n = 35/72) achieving stable disease. Prior response, duration of response, or intervening therapy between initial course of PD-1 axis inhibitor and this combination were not reported. This study also showed that *MYC* target gene sets were enriched in responders as compared to non-responders, and the authors proposed a possible mechanism for overcoming acquired resistance involving entinostat-mediated MYC downregulation. This genetic signature represents a potential targetable biomarker, and we await further data on this combination in NSCLC with PD-1 axis inhibitor acquired resistance.

In a phase Ib/II study, 24 patients with ICI pretreated NSCLC were treated with pembrolizumab plus the oral HDAC inhibitor, vorinostat [68]. In this trial, ICI refractory patients were those who experienced disease progression within 3 months of prior ICI and ICI-relapsed patients were those who had achieved stable disease or better for at least 3 months of prior ICI treatment. Of these 24 patients, three (12.5%) achieved a PR (one confirmed), while 11 (46%) experienced SD, resulting in a disease control rate (DCR) of 58%. One patient with ICI-refractory NSCLC had a confirmed PR lasting 12 months. Among the 11 ICI-relapsed patients, the median time to progression on prior ICI therapy was 10 months (range 7–52 months). No further information was provided regarding systemic therapy between prior ICI and trial enrollment, or response to initial ICI therapy. The DCR for patients with ICI-relapsed disease was 54% (n = 6/11). One patient with ICI relapsed disease had stable disease for 16 months on the combination.

PD-1 Axis Inhibitor + Adenosine A2A Receptor Antagonists

Adenosine A2A Receptor (A2AR) signaling in immune cells induces immunosuppressive signals such that when this receptor is antagonized *in vitro*, T-cell signaling, IL2 production, and IFN-γ production are restored [71]. Moreover, preclinical studies demonstrate increased expression of A2AR and CD73, which plays a key role in generating extracellular adenosine, after exposure to PD-1 axis inhibitors, suggesting that A2A receptor signaling may contribute to therapeutic resistance to immunotherapy [86, 87]. The oral A2AR antagonist, CPI-444, in combination with PD-1 axis inhibition has demonstrated anti-tumor activity in IO-responsive colon cancer mouse models that incompletely respond to PD-1 axis inhibitor monotherapy [71]. Early data was presented at both the ASCO and AACR annual meetings in 2017 from the phase I/Ib trial of CPI-444 alone and in combination with Atezolizumab (anti-PD-L1) in advanced solid tumors [70, 88]. Two patients with NSCLC and prior PD-1 axis inhibitor exposure achieved partial responses when treated with CPI-444 plus Atezolizumab, one lasting over 6 months and both ongoing at the time of data reporting. The DCR for the combination in PD-1 axis inhibitor relapsed or refractory patients was 71% (n = 5/7) with a DCR of 25% (n = 2/8) for CPI-444 alone. A more recent presentation at the SITC 24th Annual Meeting in 2019 showed that induction of an adenosine gene expression signature correlated with tumor regression in the renal cell carcinoma cohort [89].

PD-1 Axis Inhibitor + Sitravatinib

MTRX-500, or Sitravatinib, is a "spectrum-selective tyrosine kinase inhibitor" which targets receptors including TAM (Tyro3/Axl/MERTK) receptors, split family receptors (VEGFR2 and KIT), RET, and MET among others. It is thought to modulate immune-functioning in the tumor microenvironment via depletion of Type 2 tumor associated macrophages, Tregs, myeloid derived suppressor cells (MDSCs), as well as by increasing the antigen presenting capacity of tumor microenvironment dendritic cells [72, 90, 91]. Sitravatinib was evaluated in combination with nivolumab in a phase II trial enrolling patients with NSCLC who experienced disease progression following treatment with an ICI; this included patients that were PD-1 axis inhibitor relapsed or refractory [72, 90]. As of August 2018, 56 patients from this ongoing trial were evaluable, with a DCR of 75% (n = 42/56) and a confirmed ORR of 16% (n = 9/56) with 2 unconfirmed partial responses awaiting second scan for confirmation at the time of reporting. Median duration of response (DOR) was 9.2 months, PFS 6.8 months and OS 15.1 months.

PD-1 Axis Inhibitor + Anti-TIM-3

T cell immunoglobulin and mucin-domain containing-3 (TIM-3) is a known immune checkpoint often co-expressed with PD-1, which mediates T-cell exhaustion and induces immune-suppression in the tumor microenvironment through downstream effects in myeloid cells [73]. Preclinical studies have shown combination anti-TIM-3/ anti-PD-1 to have more potent anti-tumor activity than anti-PD-1 therapy alone [92]. Early results from the Phase I AMBER trial, combining TSR-022 (anti-TIM-3) with TSR-042 (anti-PD-1), demonstrated clinical activity in patients with progression on prior anti-PD-1 therapy [73]. As of the 2018 SITC Annual Meeting, thirty-nine patients with anti-PD-1 relapsed or refractory NSCLC had been treated with this combination. Among the 20 evaluable patients treated with the 300 mg dose of TSR-022, 3 had confirmed partial responses and 8 had stable disease (DCR 55%, ORR 15%). One patient with advanced NSCLC refractory to prior nivolumab had a lasting PR after 6 cycles of TSR-022 300 mg + TSR-042 500 mg given every 3 weeks (1 cycle).

Retinoic Acid Receptor-Related Orphan Receptor γ (RORγ) +/− PD-1 Axis
Inhibitor

LYC-55716 (cintirorgon), an oral small molecule activator of the transcription factor Retinoic Acid Receptor-Related Orphan Receptor γ (RORγ) has been shown in
preclinical models to increase anti-tumor T-cell activation and decrease tumor
immune suppression [93, 94]. This agent has shown promise as monotherapy and in
combination with PD-1 axis inhibitor therapy in various syngeneic tumor models
including a breast tumor model which is known to be resistant to PD-1 axis inhibition and CTLA-4 inhibition [95, 96]. In the LYC-55716 early phase monotherapy
experience, two NSCLC patients were treated in separate dose cohorts [94]. One
NSCLC patient was enrolled after progression on pembrolizumab monotherapy
(4 cycles) followed by progression on carboplatin/pemetrexed (3 cycles). He began
LYC55716 monotherapy on trial and experienced a partial response, remaining on
trial for 10 months with ongoing clinical benefit. LYC-55716 plus pembrolizumab
has been evaluated in phase Ib investigation in advanced solid tumors
(NCT03396497). In one early reported case, a patient with metastatic PD-L1 high
NSCLC with c-MET amplification had previously been treated with combination
chemotherapy and pembrolizumab followed by pembrolizumab monotherapy maintenance for 15 cycles before experiencing progressive disease [97]. The patient was
also treated with a MET antibody-drug conjugate, achieving a partial response prior
to progression on that agent as well. After 4 cycles of LYC-55716 plus pembrolizumab, the patient achieved a partial response.

4.4   Chemotherapy Sensitization

Retrospective analyses have suggested that exposure to PD-1 axis inhibitors may
sensitize patients to subsequent chemotherapy, resulting in higher than expected
response rates with more durability [28, 98, 99]. In patients receiving docetaxel and
ramucirumab immediately after nivolumab failure, the response rate and disease
control rate were 60% (n = 12/20) and 90% (n = 18/20) respectively [98]. The
median PFS and OS for docetaxel plus ramucirumab after nivolumab failure were
5.6 and 11.4 months in this cohort. These outcomes are notable considering that
IO-naïve, platinum-doublet relapsed/refractory patients treated with docetaxel plus
ramucirumab on the phase 3 REVEL trial had an ORR of just 23% [100]. PFS and
OS for the REVEL docetaxel plus ramucirumab arm was 4.2 and 10.5 months.
Furthermore, the patients in REVEL received docetaxel plus ramucirumab in the
second-line setting, while patients in the IO-pretreated cohort received this combination in the third-, fourth-, or fifth- line settings [98, 100]. A similar analysis
showed a comparable ORR for gemcitabine-based salvage regimens after exposure
to PD-1 axis inhibitors [101]. In a retrospective review of 28 patients receiving
single-agent chemotherapy after second-line PD-1 axis inhibitor exposure, the ORR
and DCR were 39% and 71% respectively [99]. Remarkably, all patients had
received platinum-based chemotherapy regimens as first-line therapy and the

upfront ORR was 37%. Historically, for patients progressing on first-line platinum doublets chemotherapy, single-agent chemotherapy was associated with a response rate of 7.1–9.1% and a median progression-free survival (PFS) of 2.6–2.9 months [102–105]. Median PFS for the 28 patients receiving single-agent chemo following IO was 4.7 months [99]. Of note, it is unknown if the observations in the retrospective series described above were influenced by prior response to immunotherapy, as this information was not provided. In the previously discussed 26-patient AR cohort, of the seven patients receiving first- or later-line salvage chemotherapy after PD-1 axis inhibitor AR, six patients achieved objective response [28].

5   Mechanisms Mediating Acquired Resistance to PD-1 Axis Inhibitors in NSCLC

5.1   Acquired Neoantigen Loss

Somatic mutations are prominent in the DNA of tumor cells and accumulate during the process of tumorigenesis. Nonsynonymous mutations lead to amino acid changes that cause tumor-specific amino acid variations which, when presented by human leukocyte antigen (HLA) molecules on the surface of tumor cells, can be recognized by T-cells as "non-self" peptide sequences. When expressed and presented, these "mutation-associated neoantigens" generate anti-tumor immune responses and their relative abundance has been shown to be associated with favorable response to immune checkpoint inhibition in NSCLC [106]. Acquired compromise of effective neoantigen processing and presentation represents one mechanism of resistance to PD-1 axis inhibitors.

In four patients with advanced NSCLC and acquired resistance to either PD-1 axis inhibitor alone or in combination with a CTLA-4 inhibitor, investigators performed whole-exome sequencing on pretreatment and post-progression tumor specimens [107]. Neoantigen prediction software was used to predict peptide sequences that would be processed and presented by patient-specific MHC Class I proteins. This analysis demonstrated overall genome-wide gain of mutations and predicted neoantigens in each patient, however, there were a higher fraction of mutations not encoding for neoantigens among gained versus eliminated mutations. No acquired alterations or copy number changes were identified potentially explaining resistance, including genomic alterations in *CD274* (encoding PD-L1), *HLA, beta-2 microglobulin (B2M)* or other antigen presentation associated genes. Loss of 6 to 18 putative neoantigens were observed in the resistance tumor specimens from the four patients. Lost high affinity neoantigens had higher predicted MHC binding that those retained or gained in resistant tumors. Mutations in several of the lost neoantigens were found in positions thought to be important in TCR binding and anchor or auxiliary anchor residues, affecting MHC binding of these neoantigens. Loss of neoantigens occurred through either deletion of chromosomal regions containing truncal alterations or elimination of tumor subclones. To show these peptides were not only *candidates* for immune recognition but were *involved in* a specific patient's anti-tumor response, investigators carried out functional T-cell assays to directly measure the ability of peptides to generate an immune response. This approach utilized next-generation sequencing of TCR-Vβ regions to measure T-cell clonality. *In vitro*, TCR-Vβ clonality was measured before and after stimulation with synthesized mutation-associated neoantigen peptides. Then DNA from patients' individual tumor samples was sequenced to confirm these clonal populations were present in respective tumor microenvironments. Three of the four patients went on to have peripheral T-cells challenged with autologous mononuclear cells loaded with the eliminated neoantigen, retained neoantigen, and gained neoantigen peptides to re-elicit T-cell expansion and compare respective T-cell responses. Results demonstrated that specific T-cell expansion occurred in response to lost neoantigen peptide challenge, confirming evidence of prior immune response to lost antigens. Retained/gained neoantigen peptides were rare to elicit T-cell expansion; in one of three patients, only a subset of retained/gained neoantigen peptides elicited a neoantigen-specific clonal T-cell expansion. For 2 patients with available peripheral blood samples obtained at various clinical timepoints throughout treatment response and progression, eliminated-neoantigen-specific T-cell clonal populations increased at time points associated with tumor response and fell to pretreatment levels on progression.

5.2 Acquired Antigen Processing and Presentation Defects

In another attempt to characterize mechanisms of acquired resistance to immunotherapy in NSCLC, 14 patients with acquired resistance to either PD-1 axis inhibitor monotherapy (n = 10), PD-1 axis inhibitor + CTLA-4 inhibitor (n = 3), or PD-1 axis inhibitor + erlotinib (EGFR TKI) after progression on erlotinib alone (n = 1) were studied [108]. Eight patients had paired pre- and post- progression tumor specimens which were subjected to whole exome sequencing. The number of neoantigens in the ICI-resistant specimens ranged from 71% to 278% that of pretreatment specimens and both mutational load and neoantigens were higher in post-progression samples in 6/8 cases.

To investigate acquired defects in HLA Class I antigen presentation, 72 genes known to be involved in antigen processing and presentation were interrogated for mutations and copy number variations. In one patient with stage IV lung squamous cell carcinoma who developed acquired resistance to anti-PD-1/anti-CTLA-4 combination therapy, copy-number variation analysis showed acquired homozygous loss of *B2M* at the time of ICI resistance. The patient's first biopsy at initial diagnosis of NSCLC (pre-chemotherapy) had both copies of *B2M* although one allele harbored a subclonal (non-reference allele frequency of 10%) deleterious mutation in *B2M* (p.M1I). This mutation was not found in subsequent biopsy specimens from this patient. After progression on second-line chemotherapy, copy number analysis revealed heterozygous *B2M* loss, and finally homozygous *B2M* loss in the

ICI-resistant specimen. Multiplex quantitative immunofluorescence confirmed reduction in cell surface B2M and HLA Class I in the ICI-resistant sample compared to the pre-immunotherapy tumor sample. A patient derived xenograft (PDX) was additionally established from the ICI resistant tumor specimen. This model demonstrated absence of tumor B2M protein expression by western blot as well as absence of cell surface B2M and HLA Class I by flow cytometry. This persisted after intra-tumoral provocation with interferon-γ (IFN-γ) injection used to exclude IFN-γ signaling defects and show that upregulation could not be induced.

Patient derived xenografts were established from ICI-resistant specimens in 2 other patients from this cohort and analyzed along with PDXs generated from two patients with primary resistance to ICI (5 total). All 5 PDX models had intact IFN- γ signaling (measured by STAT1 phosphorylation), while only 3/5 PDX models had both normal upregulation in B2M and HLA class I antigen in response to IFN-γ. One PDX had evidence of intact IFN-γ signaling but poor upregulation of HLA Class I suggestive of an intervening defect in the antigen presentation pathway between these steps.

This data, and additional QIF analysis demonstrating downregulation of HLA Class 1 or B2M in the 5/8 paired pre-/ post ICI AR, alludes to a mechanism in which cancer cells can acquire resistance to ICIs through modification of antigen presentation machinery. Though this can occur by genomic loss of elements of the antigen presentation pathway, like B2M, other mechanisms that lead to downregulation of MHC I antigen presentation appear to be additionally involved here.

To functionally study the role of antigen presentation defects and acquired resistance, investigators used a murine NSCLC cell line (UNSCC680AJ) previously shown to have sensitivity to anti-PD-1 therapy [109]. Mice were engrafted with tumors with WT (+/+) or KO (−/−) B2M UNSCC680AJ cells. Mice with B2M −/− tumors progressed on anti-PD-1 therapy whereas those with B2M +/+ tumors demonstrated predictable disease control. Moreover, UNSCC680AJ tumor-specific CD8 T-cells were shown to be defective at killing the B2M (−/−) tumor cells even at the highest effector T-cell/target cell ratio of 1:1.

6 Uncovering Mechanisms of IO-Acquired Resistance in Other Tumor Types

6.1 Acquired Defects in Interferon-Gamma (IFN- γ) Signaling and Antigen Presentation

Much can be learned from studies evaluating immunotherapy acquired resistance mechanisms in melanoma and other diseases, as these mechanisms are likely to be shared across tumor types. Using paired specimens from four metastatic melanoma patients with acquired resistance to PD-1 axis inhibitors, Zaretsky and colleagues identified potential genomic defects mediating acquired resistance [110]. Acquired loss-of-function mutations in JAK1/2, genes encoding kinases associated with the

IFN-γ pathway, were seen in the post-progression biopsy specimens from two separate patients. These mutations resulted in loss of heterozygosity and ultimately a lack of response to IFN- γ with abrogation of the antiproliferative effects of IFN-γ on malignant cells. Another patient was found to have two *B2M* truncating mutations resulting in loss of heterozygosity at two unique sites of progression. Functional loss of MHC I expression was confirmed by immunohistochemistry at one site of progression. Aberrations in *B2M* and response to IFN-γ in the microenvironment have also been implicated in other patients with acquired resistance to checkpoint inhibitor treatment. Loss of B2M protein expression was seen in sequential biopsies in 3/5 patients with acquired resistance to checkpoint blockade in one melanoma cohort [111]. This mechanism has additionally been demonstrated in several patients with colorectal cancer and in melanoma patients treated with other forms of immunotherapy [112–114].

In another report, a patient with metastatic colorectal cancer was treated with an expanded population of polyclonal CD8+ HLA-C*08:02–restricted tumor infiltrating lymphocytes (TILs) directed at an epitope specific for the tumor's *KRAS* G12D mutation [115]. The patient had initial response of 7 lung metastases followed by eventual progression at one site. The progressing lesion was resected and whole exome and transcriptome sequencing showed preservation of mutated *KRAS*. However, the resistant site contained several genetic abnormalities distinct from other pre-cell-therapy resected lesions including a copy-neutral loss of heterozygosity at chromosome 6, encoding the HLA-C*08:02 MHC Class I molecule. The genetic loss of the HLA-locus required for recognition by the *KRAS* mutation-reactive T cells was suspected to be the culprit mediator of acquired resistance.

HLA loss was has also been implicated in patients with merkel cell carcinoma (MCC) who developed acquired resistance to immunotherapy [116]. Two patients with MCC treated with autologous Merkel cell polyomavirus-specific CD8+ T cells in combination with immune-checkpoint inhibitors had initial response then developed resistance 22 and 18 months after initiation of therapy. Pretreatment and post-progression biopsies were subjected to whole exome sequencing which did not reveal a genetic event to explain acquired resistance. However, using single cell RNA sequencing, investigators demonstrated apparent transcriptional downregulation of the HLA restricting the targeted tumor-specific epitope. Though this was posited to be a transcription-level change leading to acquired resistance in these patients, it was not determined whether these post-progression findings stemmed from outgrowth of a pre-existing sub clonal cell population or from acquired transcriptional suppression in response to immunotherapy.

Transcriptional downregulation mediating acquired resistance raises the possibility that epigenetic modifications may be an underappreciated source of tumor immune-escape. One protein pertaining to broad epigenetic modification, Ezh2, was shown to be upregulated in melanoma models of acquired resistance to CTLA-4 and IL-2 treatment. Ezh2 upregulation led to dedifferentiation of melanoma cells, loss of dominant tumor antigens, silencing of the antigen-processing and presenting machinery, and ultimate loss of tumor immunogenicity. Ezh2 blockade led to restored presentation of dominant melanoma antigens and downregulation of PD-1 axis signaling therefore restoring anti-tumor immune function [117].

6.2 Immune-Suppressive Changes in the Tumor Microenvironment

MHC-II expression characterizes a subset of tumors exhibiting a T-cell inflamed phenotype, which tend to be particularly responsive to PD-1 axis inhibitors [118, 119]. LAG-3 is an alternative immune checkpoint that competes with CD4 as a ligand for MHC-II, leading to suppression of antigen presentation [120, 121]. Using patient samples from MHC II-expressing tumors, Johnson and colleagues demonstrated TIL upregulation of LAG-3 in acquired resistance samples compared to pretreatment samples [119]. Fc receptor-like 6 (FCRL6) is another ligand of MHC II expressed by cytotoxic NK cells and CD8+ T effector memory cells [122, 123]. In lung and melanoma tumor samples, expression of FCRL6 correlated with LAG-3 expression and was elevated in PD-1 axis inhibitor post-progression samples relative to untreated samples at both the mRNA and protein levels. Upregulation of these alternative checkpoints, LAG-3 and FCRL6, may drive resistance in MHC II-expressing tumors exposed to PD-1 axis inhibitors, and this may have therapeutic implications for combination strategies targeting these proteins. Similarly, another immune checkpoint protein, VISTA, was shown to be upregulated by immunohistochemistry on T-cells from sites of PD-1 inhibitor acquired resistance in unselected melanoma patients [124].

6.3 PTEN Loss

Oncogenic alterations in genes other than *B2M*, *JAK1/2* and *HLA* may mediate resistance in a subset of patients with PD-1 axis inhibitor acquired resistance. One patient with melanoma and acquired resistance to combination checkpoint inhibitor therapy was found to have biallelic loss of *PTEN* [125]. Loss of *PTEN*, a tumor suppressor gene, promotes activation of the PI3K-AKT pathway. Additionally, it has been demonstrated that *PTEN* loss leads to decreased CD8+ t-cell infiltration in tumors and induction of immunosuppressive cytokines including VEGF [126]. By these mechanisms, acquired PTEN loss likely contributes to immunotherapy resistance not only in melanoma, but in other tumor types as well [127].

6.4 Novel Experimental Discoveries

In addition to studies using acquired resistance patient specimens, novel experimental approaches can be used to shed light on potential mechanisms of resistance to immunotherapy. Genetic studies, like CRISPR-Cas9 screens, may allow us to simultaneously look at defects in antigen presentation as well as other genome-level alterations that mediate immunosuppressive changes in the tumor microenvironment. CRISPR technology can be used to perturb genes in tumor cells to mimic loss-of-function mutations, in this case to identify mediators of immunotherapy resistance. In one study, a CRISPR- Cas9 mutagenesis screen in human melanoma cells was used to systematically identify genes essential for T-cell effector function [128]. A "two cell-type" (2CT) CRISPR assay was designed using human T-cells as effectors and melanoma cells as targets. As expected, genes known to be involved in effector T-cell mediated anti-tumor activity such as *HLA-A, B2M, TAP1, TAP2,* and *TAPBP* were among the most highly enriched genes in the CRISPR-Cas9 screen. Additionally, several other genes were found to be capable of modulating melanoma growth when targeted by T-cells, including *SOX10, CD58, MLANA, PSMB5, RPL23 and APLNR.* The protein product of one of these genes, *APLNR,* was shown to modulate IFN-γ responses in tumors through interactions with JAK1. Its functional loss reduced the efficacy of adoptive T-cell transfer and checkpoint inhibition in melanoma mouse models, suggesting that genomic events or other expression-level changes may play a role in acquired resistance to immunotherapy. Another group developed a CRISPR-Cas9 screen to identify genes that increase sensitivity to immunotherapy in a transplantable melanoma model [129]. The screen identified *ADAR1,* which encodes an adenosine deaminase that binds to and limits the sensing of endogenous double-stranded RNA (dsRNA) [130–134]. In the context of tumor immunity, this protein serves as a checkpoint that restrains sensing of IFN-inducible dsRNA ultimately attenuating tumor inflammation. Investigators showed that in *B2M*-deleted IO-resistant tumors, loss of *ADAR1* restored sensitivity to immunotherapy, and was associated with a significant increase in immune cell infiltration. In addition to establishing the role of *ADAR1,* these results also demonstrate that loss of antigen presentation can be overcome if sufficient inflammation can be elicited in an IFN-sensitive tumor.

Identifying specific mechanisms of acquired resistance to immunotherapy may eventually lead to an individualized therapeutic approach to re-engaging anti-tumor immunity. For instance, loss of *ADAR1* restores IO-sensitivity despite persistent defects in antigen presentation, therefore serving as a potential target for *B2M*-deficient tumors. Recently, one group identified IL-18 Binding Protein as a potential target for tumors that develop acquired resistance via similar mechanisms [135]. IL-18 is a member of the IL-1 cytokine family that stimulates lymphocytes, and recombinant IL-18 has been shown to synergize with ICIs in tumor models [136–138]. However, clinical efficacy of rIL-18 has not matched its pre-clinical promise [139]. This is likely related to a "secreted immune checkpoint," IL-18 Binding Protein (IL-18BP), which is a high affinity IL-18 antagonist shown to be induced upon treatment with the recombinant cytokine [140–142]. Investigators engineered a "decoy-resistant" IL-18 (DR-18) which maintained IL-18 signaling but resisted IL-18BP inhibition [135]. The protein was shown to enhance anti-tumor T-cell function, but especially pertinent to acquired resistance models, it was also shown to enhance the activity of NK cells in MHC Class I-deficient tumors. Tumor regression was seen in ICI-resistant models (including a *B2M*-null tumor) and antibody depletion studies indicated that NK cell activity was essential to the anti-tumor activity of DR-18. Augmenting anti-tumor NK cell activity in MHC Class I deficient tumors represents another possible strategy to restore tumor sensitivity to immunotherapy in acquired resistance.

6.5 Conclusions and Future Visions

Despite more durable responses to immunotherapy than chemotherapy, with some indefinite responses, the majority of patients with PD-1 axis inhibitor-responsive advanced NSCLC will develop resistance. Case series have shown that local therapy can be effective for oligoprogressive sites of immune escape, but these local therapy interventions are sometimes not feasible, are often exhausted, and mostly fail to impact systemic progression. When next-line systemic therapy is needed, we typically use traditional cytotoxic chemotherapy or enroll patients in clinical trials investigating empirically applied immunotherapy combinations. Though there are many ongoing clinical trials for patients that progress on PD-1 axis inhibitors, we have yet to identify effective biomarker-driven strategies or a go-to "salvage" immunotherapy combination for unselected patients experiencing acquired resistance.

As more patients with diverse tumor types are treated with and respond to immunotherapy, we will continue to learn about new mechanisms of acquired resistance that develop under pressure from these agents. In NSCLC, human translational studies and experimental mouse models have uncovered specific mechanisms such as tumor-associated neoantigen loss and acquired loss of antigen presentation [107, 108]. In melanoma and other tumor types, other mechanisms have been shown to mediate acquired resistance including genome- and expression-level IFN-γ signaling and antigen presentation changes, upregulation of other suppressive signals in the tumor microenvironment, and acquisition of new oncogenic drivers [110, 124, 125, 143].

Properly elucidating mechanisms of resistance requires rigorous translational methodology. Investigators must acquire and compare pretreatment patient samples to anatomically consistent samples harvested after initial response and subsequent development of acquired resistance to immunotherapy. To achieve this, considerable efforts to attain post-progression samples must be made, which will require additional biopsies or surgical procedures. Though conventional strategies have been employed to detect genome-, transcriptome-, or proteome-level changes that drive resistance, novel approaches such as genome-wide CRISPR/Cas9 assays have more recently been invoked to identify such mechanisms. Parallel studies using modified autologous T-cell assays, patient derived xenografts, and other engineered tumor models continue to be effective strategies to further investigate these mechanisms.

Collaborative efforts would undoubtedly enhance this process. An interinstitutional consortium on acquired resistance to immunotherapy would allow for centralized collection of more paired patient samples across a variety of tumor types, and institutions with specific experimental expertise would have access to these samples. Moreover, these highly sophisticated experimental techniques could be run in parallel, cutting down significantly on cost and time. With more samples for study, mechanistically-grouped patient subsets could be identified that may be treated using biomarker-driven approaches, increasing the likelihood for favorable response in trial populations. Ultimately, further directed investigation will allow for development of personalized therapeutic strategies, which we hope will translate into more durable responses and improved patient outcomes.

References

1. Brahmer J et al (2015) Nivolumab versus docetaxel in advanced squamous-cell non-small-cell lung cancer. N Engl J Med 373(2):123–135
2. Borghaei H et al (2015) Nivolumab versus docetaxel in advanced nonsquamous non-small-cell lung cancer. N Engl J Med 373(17):1627–1639
3. Gettinger SN et al (2015) Overall survival and long-term safety of Nivolumab (anti-programmed death 1 antibody, BMS-936558, ONO-4538) in patients with previously treated advanced non-small-cell lung cancer. J Clin Oncol 33(18):2004–2012
4. Antonia SJ et al (2017) Durvalumab after Chemoradiotherapy in stage III non-small-cell lung cancer. N Engl J Med 377(20):1919–1929
5. Reck M et al (2016) Pembrolizumab versus chemotherapy for PD-L1-positive non-small-cell lung cancer. N Engl J Med 375(19):1823–1833
6. Gandhi L et al (2018) Pembrolizumab plus chemotherapy in metastatic non-small-cell lung cancer. N Engl J Med 378(22):2078–2092
7. Paz-Ares L et al (2018) Pembrolizumab plus chemotherapy for squamous non-small-cell lung cancer. N Engl J Med 379(21):2040–2051
8. Socinski MA et al (2018) Atezolizumab for first-line treatment of metastatic nonsquamous NSCLC. N Engl J Med 378(24):2288–2301
9. Mok TSK et al (2019) Pembrolizumab versus chemotherapy for previously untreated, PD-L1-expressing, locally advanced or metastatic non-small-cell lung cancer (KEYNOTE-042): a randomised, open-label, controlled, phase 3 trial. Lancet 393(10183):1819–1830
10. West H et al (2019) Atezolizumab in combination with carboplatin plus nab-paclitaxel chemotherapy compared with chemotherapy alone as first-line treatment for metastatic non-squamous non-small-cell lung cancer (IMpower130): a multicentre, randomised, open-label, phase 3 trial. Lancet Oncol 20(7):924–937
11. Hellmann MD et al (2019) Nivolumab plus Ipilimumab in advanced non-small-cell lung cancer. N Engl J Med 381(21):2020–2031
12. Reck M et al (2020) Nivolumab (NIVO) + ipilimumab (IPI) + 2 cycles of platinum-doublet chemotherapy (chemo) vs 4 cycles chemo as first-line (1L) treatment (tx) for stage IV/recurrent non-small cell lung cancer (NSCLC): CheckMate 9LA. J Clin Oncol 38(15_suppl):9501–9501
13. Herbst RS et al (2020) Atezolizumab for first-line treatment of PD-L1-selected patients with NSCLC. N Engl J Med 383(14):1328–1339
14. Topalian SL et al (2019) Five-year survival and correlates among patients with advanced melanoma, renal cell carcinoma, or non-small cell lung cancer treated with Nivolumab. JAMA Oncol 5:1411
15. Antonia SJ et al (2019) Four-year survival with nivolumab in patients with previously treated advanced non-small-cell lung cancer: a pooled analysis. Lancet Oncol 20(10):1395–1408

16. Gettinger S et al (2018) Five-year follow-up of Nivolumab in previously treated advanced non-small-cell lung cancer: results from the CA209-003 study. J Clin Oncol 36(17):1675–1684

17. von Pawel J et al (2019) Long-term survival in patients with advanced non-small-cell lung cancer treated with atezolizumab versus docetaxel: results from the randomised phase III OAK study. Eur J Cancer 107:124–132

18. Garon EB et al (2019) Five-year overall survival for patients with advanced nonsmall-cell lung cancer treated with Pembrolizumab: results from the phase I KEYNOTE-001 study. J Clin Oncol 37(28):2518–2527

19. Brahmer JR, R-AD, Robinson AG (2020) KEYNOTE-024 5-year OS update: first-line (1L) pembrolizumab (pembro) vs platinum-based chemotherapy (chemo) in patients (pts) with metastatic NSCLC and PD-L1 tumour proportion score (TPS) ≥50%. Ann Oncol 31:S1142–S1215

20. Herbst RS et al (2018) Long-term survival in patients (pts) with advanced NSCLC in the KEYNOTE-010 study overall and in pts who completed two years of pembrolizumab (pembro). Ann Oncol 29 Suppl 8:viii749

21. Reck M et al (2019) Updated analysis of KEYNOTE-024: Pembrolizumab versus platinum-based chemotherapy for advanced non-small-cell lung Cancer with PD-L1 tumor proportion score of 50% or greater. J Clin Oncol 37(7):537–546

22. Gettinger S et al (2019) OA14.04 five-year outcomes from the randomized, phase 3 trials CheckMate 017/057: Nivolumab vs docetaxel in previously treated NSCLC. J Thorac Oncol 14(10):S244–S245

23. Schoenfeld AJ, Hellmann MD (2020) Acquired resistance to immune checkpoint inhibitors. Cancer Cell 37(4):443–455

24. Kluger HM et al (2020) Defining tumor resistance to PD-1 pathway blockade: recommendations from the first meeting of the SITC immunotherapy resistance taskforce. J Immunother Cancer 8(1):e000398

25. Eisenhauer EA et al (2009) New response evaluation criteria in solid tumours: revised RECIST guideline (version 1.1). Eur J Cancer 45(2):228–247

26. Brahmer JLH, Hossein B, Ramalingam S, Pluzanski A, Burgio MA, Garassino MC, Chow LQM, Gettinger S, Crino L, Planchard D, Butts C, Drilon A, Wojcik-Tomaszewska J, Otterson G, Agrawal S, Li A, Penrod JR, Antonia SJ, Bautista Y (2019) Long-term survival outcomes with Nivolumab (NIVO) in patients with previously treated advanced non-small cell lung Cancer (NSCLC): impact of early disease control and response. J Thorac Oncol 14(11):S1152–S1153

27. Brahmer JR et al (2010) Phase I study of single-agent anti-programmed death-1 (MDX-1106) in refractory solid tumors: safety, clinical activity, pharmacodynamics, and immunologic correlates. J Clin Oncol 28(19):3167–3175

28. Gettinger SN et al (2018) Clinical features and management of acquired resistance to PD-1 Axis inhibitors in 26 patients with advanced non-small cell lung cancer. J Thorac Oncol 13(6):831–839

29. Shah S et al (2018) Clinical and molecular features of innate and acquired resistance to anti-PD-1/PD-L1 therapy in lung cancer. Oncotarget 9(4):4375–4384

30. Weickhardt AJ et al (2012) Local ablative therapy of oligoprogressive disease prolongs disease control by tyrosine kinase inhibitors in oncogene-addicted non-small-cell lung cancer. J Thorac Oncol 7(12):1807–1814

31. Tan DS et al (2016) The International Association for the study of lung cancer consensus statement on optimizing management of EGFR mutation-positive non-small cell lung cancer: status in 2016. J Thorac Oncol 11(7):946–963

32. Mu Y et al (2019) Clinical modality of resistance and subsequent management of patients with advanced non-small cell lung cancer failing treatment with Osimertinib. Target Oncol 14(3):335–342

33. Basler L, Kroeze SG, Guckenberger M (2017) SBRT for oligoprogressive oncogene addicted NSCLC. Lung Cancer 106:50–57

34. Becker K, Xu Y (2014) Management of tyrosine kinase inhibitor resistance in lung cancer with EGFR mutation. World J Clin Oncol 5(4):560–567

35. Suh YG, Cho J (2019) Local ablative radiotherapy for oligometastatic non-small cell lung cancer. Radiat Oncol J 37(3):149–155
36. Ko EC, Raben D, Formenti SC (2018) The integration of radiotherapy with immunotherapy for the treatment of non-small cell lung cancer. Clin Cancer Res 24(23):5792–5806
37. Bergsma DP et al (2017) Radiotherapy for Oligometastatic lung cancer. Front Oncol 7:210
38. Shaverdian N et al (2017) Previous radiotherapy and the clinical activity and toxicity of pembrolizumab in the treatment of non-small-cell lung cancer: a secondary analysis of the KEYNOTE-001 phase 1 trial. Lancet Oncol 18(7):895–903
39. Deng L et al (2014) Irradiation and anti-PD-L1 treatment synergistically promote antitumor immunity in mice. J Clin Invest 124(2):687–695
40. Gong X et al (2017) Combined radiotherapy and anti-PD-L1 antibody synergistically enhances antitumor effect in non-small cell lung cancer. J Thorac Oncol 12(7):1085–1097
41. Kroon P et al (2016) Concomitant targeting of programmed death-1 (PD-1) and CD137 improves the efficacy of radiotherapy in a mouse model of human BRAFV600-mutant melanoma. Cancer Immunol Immunother 65(6):753–763
42. Dovedi SJ et al (2017) Fractionated radiation therapy stimulates antitumor immunity mediated by both resident and infiltrating polyclonal T-cell populations when combined with PD-1 blockade. Clin Cancer Res 23(18):5514–5526
43. Theelen W et al (2019) Effect of Pembrolizumab after stereotactic body radiotherapy vs Pembrolizumab alone on tumor response in patients with advanced non-small cell lung cancer: results of the PEMBRO-RT phase 2 randomized clinical trial. JAMA Oncol 5:1276
44. Bauml JM et al (2019) Pembrolizumab after completion of locally ablative therapy for Oligometastatic non-small cell lung cancer: a phase 2 trial. JAMA Oncol 5:1283
45. Goldberg SB et al (2020) Pembrolizumab for management of patients with NSCLC and brain metastases: long-term results and biomarker analysis from a non-randomised, open-label, phase 2 trial. Lancet Oncol 21(5):655–663
46. Singh C et al (2019) Local tumor response and survival outcomes after combined stereotactic radiosurgery and immunotherapy in non-small cell lung cancer with brain metastases. J Neurosurg 132(2):512–517
47. Shepard MJ et al (2019) Stereotactic radiosurgery with and without checkpoint inhibition for patients with metastatic non-small cell lung cancer to the brain: a matched cohort study. J Neurosurg:1–8
48. Colaco RJ et al (2016) Does immunotherapy increase the rate of radiation necrosis after radiosurgical treatment of brain metastases? J Neurosurg 125(1):17–23
49. Spigel D, FDM, Giaccone G, Reinmuth N, Vergnenegre A, Barrios CH, Morise M, Felip E, Andric ZG, Geater S, Özgüroğlu M, Mocci S, McCleland M, Enquist I, Komatsubara KM, Deng Y, Kuriki H, Wen X, Jassem J, Herbst RS (2019) IMPOWER110: interim overall survival (OS) analysis of a phase III study of Atezolizumab (Atezo) vs. platinum-based chemotherapy (chemo) as first-line (1L) treatment (Tx) in PD-L1-selected NSCLC. In: ESMO 2019 congress, Barcelona, Spain
50. Waterhouse DM et al (2020) Continuous versus 1-year fixed-duration Nivolumab in previously treated advanced non-small-cell lung Cancer: CheckMate 153. J Clin Oncol 38:3863
51. Sheth S et al (2020) Durvalumab activity in previously treated patients who stopped durvalumab without disease progression. J Immunother Cancer 8(2):e000650
52. Reck M et al (2019) OA14.01 KEYNOTE-024 3-year survival update: Pembrolizumab vs platinum-based chemotherapy for advanced non–small-cell lung cancer. J Thorac Oncol 14(10, Supplement):S243
53. Dolladille C et al (2020) Immune checkpoint inhibitor Rechallenge after immune-related adverse events in patients with cancer. JAMA Oncol 6:865
54. Simonaggio A et al (2019) Evaluation of Readministration of immune checkpoint inhibitors after immune-related adverse events in patients with cancer. JAMA Oncol 5:1310

55. Mouri A et al (2019) Clinical difference between discontinuation and retreatment with nivolumab after immune-related adverse events in patients with lung cancer. Cancer Chemother Pharmacol 84(4):873–880
56. Giaj Levra M et al (2020) Immunotherapy rechallenge after nivolumab treatment in advanced non-small cell lung cancer in the real-world setting: a national data base analysis. Lung Cancer 140:99–106
57. Girard N et al (2009) Third-line chemotherapy in advanced non-small cell lung cancer: identifying the candidates for routine practice. J Thorac Oncol 4(12):1544–1549
58. Fujita K et al (2018) Retreatment with pembrolizumab in advanced non-small cell lung cancer patients previously treated with nivolumab: emerging reports of 12 cases. Cancer Chemother Pharmacol 81(6):1105–1109
59. Buchbinder EI, Desai A (2016) CTLA-4 and PD-1 pathways: similarities, differences, and implications of their inhibition. Am J Clin Oncol 39(1):98–106
60. Keir ME et al (2008) PD-1 and its ligands in tolerance and immunity. Annu Rev Immunol 26:677–704
61. Intlekofer AM, Thompson CB (2013) At the bench: preclinical rationale for CTLA-4 and PD-1 blockade as cancer immunotherapy. J Leukoc Biol 94(1):25–39
62. Garon EB, Spira AI, Goldberg SB, Awad MM et al (2018) Safety and activity of durvalumab + tremelimumab in immunotherapy (IMT)-pretreated advanced NSCLC patients. J Clin Oncol 36(No 15_suppl):9041
63. Wrangle JM et al (2018) ALT-803, an IL-15 superagonist, in combination with nivolumab in patients with metastatic non-small cell lung cancer: a non-randomised, open-label, phase 1b trial. Lancet Oncol 19(5):694–704
64. Diab A et al (2018) NKTR-214 (CD122-biased agonist) plus nivolumab in patients with advanced solid tumors: preliminary phase 1/2 results of PIVOT. J Clin Oncol 36(15_suppl):3006–3006
65. Bentebibel SE et al (2019) A first-in-human study and biomarker analysis of NKTR-214, a novel IL2Rbetagamma-biased cytokine, in patients with advanced or metastatic solid tumors. Cancer Discov 9(6):711–721
66. Ordentlich P et al (2019) Abstract CT041: identification of gene signatures associated with response in a phase II trial of entinostat (ENT) plus pembrolizumab (PEMBRO) in non-small cell lung cancer (NSCLC) patients whose disease has progressed on or after anti-PD-(L)1 therapy. Cancer Res 79(13 Supplement):CT041–CT041
67. Hellmann M et al (2018) OA05.01 efficacy/safety of Entinostat (ENT) and Pembrolizumab (PEMBRO) in NSCLC patients previously treated with anti-PD-(L)1 therapy. J Thorac Oncol 13(10):S330
68. Gray JE et al (2019) Phase I/Ib study of Pembrolizumab plus Vorinostat in advanced/metastatic non-small cell lung cancer. Clin Cancer Res 25(22):6623–6632
69. Johnson MEK, Halmos B, Patel M et al (2018) Phase 2 trial of mocetinostat in combination with durvalumab in NSCLC patients with progression on prior checkpoint inhibitor therapy. In: 2018 annual meeting of SITC, Washington, DC
70. Emens L et al (2017) Abstract CT119: CPI-444, an oral adenosine A2a receptor (A2aR) antagonist, demonstrates clinical activity in patients with advanced solid tumors. Cancer Res 77(13 Supplement):CT119–CT119
71. Willingham SB et al (2018) A2AR antagonism with CPI-444 induces antitumor responses and augments efficacy to anti-PD-(L)1 and anti-CTLA-4 in preclinical models. Cancer Immunol Res 6(10):1136–1149
72. Leal TA et al (2017) PS02.08 evidence of clinical activity of Sitravatinib in combination with Nivolumab in NSCLC patients progressing on prior checkpoint inhibitor therapy: topic: medical oncology. J Thorac Oncol 12(11):S1567
73. Davar D, Boasburg PD, LoRusso P et al (2018) A phase 1 study of TSR-022, an anti-TIM-3 monoclonal antibody, in combination with TSR-042, an anti-PD-1 antibody (AMBER). In: 2018 SITC annual meeting, Washington, D.C

74. Shafique MR et al (2020) Interim results from a phase Ib/II study of pepinemab in combination with avelumab in advanced NSCLC patients following progression on prior systemic and/or anti-PDx therapies. J Clin Oncol 38(5_suppl):75
75. Morgensztern D et al (2019) Viagenpumatucel-L (HS-110) plus nivolumab in patients with advanced non-small cell lung cancer (NSCLC) after checkpoint inhibitor treatment failure. J Clin Oncol 37(15_suppl):9109
76. Senko C et al (2019) P2.04-11 overcoming resistance to immunotherapy using CVA21: initial results from a phase II study. J Thorac Oncol 14(10):S711
77. Barlesi FIN, Felip E, Gulley J (2017) O14. Initial results from phase 1 trial of M7824 (MSB0011359C), a bifunctional fusion protein targeting PD-L1 and TGF-β, in patients with NSCLC refractory or resistant to prior anti–PD1/anti–PD-L1 agents. In: 2017 annual meeting of SITC, National Harbor, MD
78. Xu W et al (2013) Efficacy and mechanism-of-action of a novel superagonist interleukin-15: interleukin-15 receptor alphaSu/Fc fusion complex in syngeneic murine models of multiple myeloma. Cancer Res 73(10):3075–3086
79. Rhode PR et al (2016) Comparison of the superagonist complex, ALT-803, to IL15 as cancer immunotherapeutics in animal models. Cancer Immunol Res 4(1):49–60
80. Romee R et al (2018) First-in-human phase 1 clinical study of the IL-15 superagonist complex ALT-803 to treat relapse after transplantation. Blood 131(23):2515–2527
81. Margolin K et al (2018) Phase I trial of ALT-803, a novel recombinant IL15 complex, in patients with advanced solid tumors. Clin Cancer Res 24(22):5552–5561
82. Hurwitz ME et al (2017) Effect of NKTR-214 on the number and activity of CD8+ tumor infiltrating lymphocytes in patients with advanced renal cell carcinoma. J Clin Oncol 35(6_suppl):454
83. Kim K et al (2014) Eradication of metastatic mouse cancers resistant to immune checkpoint blockade by suppression of myeloid-derived cells. Proc Natl Acad Sci U S A 111(32):11774–11779
84. Orillion A et al (2017) Entinostat neutralizes myeloid-derived suppressor cells and enhances the antitumor effect of PD-1 inhibition in murine models of lung and renal cell carcinoma. Clin Cancer Res 23(17):5187–5201
85. Zheng H et al (2016) HDAC inhibitors enhance T-cell chemokine expression and augment response to PD-1 immunotherapy in lung adenocarcinoma. Clin Cancer Res 22(16):4119–4132
86. Beavis PA et al (2015) Adenosine receptor 2A blockade increases the efficacy of anti-PD-1 through enhanced antitumor T-cell responses. Cancer Immunol Res 3(5):506–517
87. Allard B et al (2013) Targeting CD73 enhances the antitumor activity of anti-PD-1 and anti-CTLA-4 mAbs. Clin Cancer Res 19(20):5626–5635
88. Fong L et al (2017) Safety and clinical activity of adenosine A2a receptor (A2aR) antagonist, CPI-444, in anti-PD1/PDL1 treatment-refractory renal cell (RCC) and non-small cell lung cancer (NSCLC) patients. J Clin Oncol 35(15_suppl):3004
89. Willingham S, HA, Hsieh J, Munneke B, Kwei L, Mobasher M, Buggy J, Miller R (2019) Adenosine and AMP gene expression profiles predict response to adenosine pathway therapies and indicate a need for dual blockade of CD73 and A2AR with CD73 inhibitors. In: 2019 Society for Immunotherapy of Cancer (SITC) 34th annual meeting, S.f.I.o.C. (SITC), National Harbor, MD
90. Leal TA et al (2018) Stage 2 enrollment complete: Sitravatinib in combination with nivolumab in NSCLC patients progressing on prior checkpoint inhibitor therapy. Ann Oncol 29:viii400–viii401
91. Du W et al (2018) Sitravatinib potentiates immune checkpoint blockade in refractory cancer models. JCI Insight 3(21):e124184
92. Sakuishi K et al (2010) Targeting Tim-3 and PD-1 pathways to reverse T cell exhaustion and restore anti-tumor immunity. J Exp Med 207(10):2187–2194
93. Hu X et al (2016) Synthetic RORgamma agonists regulate multiple pathways to enhance antitumor immunity. Onco Targets Ther 5(12):e1254854

94. Mahalingam D et al (2019) Phase 1 open-label, multicenter study of first-in-class RORgamma agonist LYC-55716 (Cintirorgon): safety, tolerability, and preliminary evidence of antitumor activity. Clin Cancer Res 25(12):3508–3516

95. Demaria S et al (2005) Immune-mediated inhibition of metastases after treatment with local radiation and CTLA-4 blockade in a mouse model of breast cancer. Clin Cancer Res 11(2 Pt 1):728–734

96. Hirano F et al (2005) Blockade of B7-H1 and PD-1 by monoclonal antibodies potentiates cancer therapeutic immunity. Cancer Res 65(3):1089–1096

97. Camidge DR et al (2018) RORγ agonist LYC-55716 in combination with pembrolizumab to treat metastatic non-small cell lung cancer: an open-label, multicenter phase Ib trial. Ann Oncol 29:viii417

98. Shiono A et al (2019) Improved efficacy of ramucirumab plus docetaxel after nivolumab failure in previously treated non-small cell lung cancer patients. Thorac Cancer 10(4):775–781

99. Schvartsman G et al (2017) Response rates to single-agent chemotherapy after exposure to immune checkpoint inhibitors in advanced non-small cell lung cancer. Lung Cancer 112:90–95

100. Garon EB et al (2014) Ramucirumab plus docetaxel versus placebo plus docetaxel for second-line treatment of stage IV non-small-cell lung cancer after disease progression on platinum-based therapy (REVEL): a multicentre, double-blind, randomised phase 3 trial. Lancet 384(9944):665–673

101. Park SE et al (2018) Increased response rates to salvage chemotherapy administered after PD-1/PD-L1 inhibitors in patients with non-small cell lung cancer. J Thorac Oncol 13(1):106–111

102. Leighl NB (2012) Treatment paradigms for patients with metastatic non-small-cell lung cancer: first-, second-, and third-line. Curr Oncol 19(Suppl 1):S52–S58

103. Shepherd FA et al (2000) Prospective randomized trial of docetaxel versus best supportive care in patients with non-small-cell lung cancer previously treated with platinum-based chemotherapy. J Clin Oncol 18(10):2095–2103

104. Hanna N et al (2004) Randomized phase III trial of pemetrexed versus docetaxel in patients with non-small-cell lung cancer previously treated with chemotherapy. J Clin Oncol 22(9):1589–1597

105. Kim ES et al (2008) Gefitinib versus docetaxel in previously treated non-small-cell lung cancer (INTEREST): a randomised phase III trial. Lancet 372(9652):1809–1818

106. Rizvi NA et al (2015) Cancer immunology. Mutational landscape determines sensitivity to PD-1 blockade in non-small cell lung cancer. Science 348(6230):124–128

107. Anagnostou V et al (2017) Evolution of Neoantigen landscape during immune checkpoint blockade in non-small cell lung cancer. Cancer Discov 7(3):264–276

108. Gettinger S et al (2017) Impaired HLA class I antigen processing and presentation as a mechanism of acquired resistance to immune checkpoint inhibitors in lung cancer. Cancer Discov 7(12):1420–1435

109. Azpilikueta A et al (2016) Successful immunotherapy against a transplantable mouse squamous lung carcinoma with anti-PD-1 and anti-CD137 monoclonal antibodies. J Thorac Oncol 11(4):524–536

110. Zaretsky JM et al (2016) Mutations associated with acquired resistance to PD-1 blockade in melanoma. N Engl J Med 375(9):819–829

111. Sade-Feldman M et al (2017) Resistance to checkpoint blockade therapy through inactivation of antigen presentation. Nat Commun 8(1):1136

112. Restifo NP et al (1996) Loss of functional beta 2-microglobulin in metastatic melanomas from five patients receiving immunotherapy. J Natl Cancer Inst 88(2):100–108

113. Le DT et al (2017) Mismatch repair deficiency predicts response of solid tumors to PD-1 blockade. Science 357(6349):409–413

114. Sucker A et al (2017) Acquired IFNgamma resistance impairs anti-tumor immunity and gives rise to T-cell-resistant melanoma lesions. Nat Commun 8:15440

115. Tran E et al (2016) T-cell transfer therapy targeting mutant KRAS in cancer. N Engl J Med 375(23):2255–2262
116. Paulson KG et al (2018) Acquired cancer resistance to combination immunotherapy from transcriptional loss of class I HLA. Nat Commun 9(1):3868
117. Zingg D et al (2017) The histone methyltransferase Ezh2 controls mechanisms of adaptive resistance to tumor immunotherapy. Cell Rep 20(4):854–867
118. Johnson DB et al (2016) Melanoma-specific MHC-II expression represents a tumour-autonomous phenotype and predicts response to anti-PD-1/PD-L1 therapy. Nat Commun 7:10582
119. Johnson DB et al (2018) Tumor-specific MHC-II expression drives a unique pattern of resistance to immunotherapy via LAG-3/FCRL6 engagement. JCI Insight 3(24):e120360
120. Baixeras E et al (1992) Characterization of the lymphocyte activation gene 3-encoded protein. A new ligand for human leukocyte antigen class II antigens. J Exp Med 176(2):327–337
121. Huard B et al (1994) Lymphocyte-activation gene 3/major histocompatibility complex class II interaction modulates the antigenic response of CD4+ T lymphocytes. Eur J Immunol 24(12):3216–3221
122. Wilson TJ et al (2007) FcRL6, a new ITIM-bearing receptor on cytolytic cells, is broadly expressed by lymphocytes following HIV-1 infection. Blood 109(9):3786–3793
123. Schreeder DM et al (2008) FCRL6 distinguishes mature cytotoxic lymphocytes and is upregulated in patients with B-cell chronic lymphocytic leukemia. Eur J Immunol 38(11):3159–3166
124. Kakavand H et al (2017) Negative immune checkpoint regulation by VISTA: a mechanism of acquired resistance to anti-PD-1 therapy in metastatic melanoma patients. Mod Pathol 30(12):1666–1676
125. Trujillo JA et al (2019) Secondary resistance to immunotherapy associated with beta-catenin pathway activation or PTEN loss in metastatic melanoma. J Immunother Cancer 7(1):295
126. Peng W et al (2016) Loss of PTEN promotes resistance to T cell-mediated immunotherapy. Cancer Discov 6(2):202–216
127. George S et al (2017) Loss of PTEN is associated with resistance to anti-PD-1 checkpoint blockade therapy in metastatic uterine Leiomyosarcoma. Immunity 46(2):197–204
128. Patel SJ et al (2017) Identification of essential genes for cancer immunotherapy. Nature 548(7669):537–542
129. Manguso RT et al (2017) In vivo CRISPR screening identifies Ptpn2 as a cancer immunotherapy target. Nature 547(7664):413–418
130. Mannion NM et al (2014) The RNA-editing enzyme ADAR1 controls innate immune responses to RNA. Cell Rep 9(4):1482–1494
131. Liddicoat BJ, Chalk AM, Walkley CR (2016) ADAR1, inosine and the immune sensing system: distinguishing self from non-self. Wiley Interdiscip Rev RNA 7(2):157–172
132. Ahmad S et al (2018) Breaching self-tolerance to Alu duplex RNA underlies MDA5-mediated inflammation. Cell 172(4):797–810. e13
133. Chung H et al (2018) Human ADAR1 prevents endogenous RNA from triggering translational shutdown. Cell 172(4):811–824. e14
134. Ishizuka JJ et al (2019) Loss of ADAR1 in tumours overcomes resistance to immune checkpoint blockade. Nature 565(7737):43–48
135. Zhou T et al (2020) IL-18BP is a secreted immune checkpoint and barrier to IL-18 immunotherapy. Nature 583:609
136. Mantovani A et al (2019) Interleukin-1 and related cytokines in the regulation of inflammation and immunity. Immunity 50(4):778–795
137. Guo L, Junttila IS, Paul WE (2012) Cytokine-induced cytokine production by conventional and innate lymphoid cells. Trends Immunol 33(12):598–606
138. Ma Z et al (2016) Augmentation of immune checkpoint Cancer immunotherapy with IL18. Clin Cancer Res 22(12):2969–2980
139. Tarhini AA et al (2009) A phase 2, randomized study of SB-485232, rhIL-18, in patients with previously untreated metastatic melanoma. Cancer 115(4):859–868

140. Robertson MJ et al (2006) Clinical and biological effects of recombinant human interleukin-18 administered by intravenous infusion to patients with advanced cancer. Clin Cancer Res 12(14 Pt 1):4265–4273
141. Dinarello CA et al (2013) Interleukin-18 and IL-18 binding protein. Front Immunol 4:289
142. Robertson MJ et al (2008) A dose-escalation study of recombinant human interleukin-18 using two different schedules of administration in patients with cancer. Clin Cancer Res 14(11):3462–3469
143. Chen L et al (2018) CD38-mediated immunosuppression as a mechanism of tumor cell escape from PD-1/PD-L1 blockade. Cancer Discov 8(9):1156–1175

Chapter 6
Management of Brain Metastases

Emily F. Collier, Veronica Chiang, and Sarah B. Goldberg

Abstract Brain metastases account for the majority of malignant brain tumors and as newer cancer treatments improve patient survival, the reported incidence of brain metastases is increasing. Lung cancer is the most frequent origin of metastases to the brain, and this diagnosis is associated with significant morbidity as well as decreased quality of life and a worse prognosis. The treatment for brain metastases in NSCLC has historically been local therapy, either surgery or radiation, as many chemotherapies have limited efficacy in the brain. These strategies are highly effective but can be a source of morbidity themselves. Newer systemic therapies, including targeted small molecule drugs and immunotherapy, have shown promise in treating NSCLC associated CNS disease either alone or in combination with local therapies. Increasing evidence for this strategy is accumulating as more clinical trials allow the inclusion of patients with untreated asymptomatic brain metastases. This chapter summarizes the current use of systemic therapy in the treatment of brain metastases in NSCLC.

Keywords Brain metastases · NSCLC · Systemic therapy · Targeted therapy · Immunotherapy

E. F. Collier
Department of Medicine (Medical Oncology), Yale School of Medicine/Yale Cancer Center, Smilow Cancer Hospital Care Center at Saint Francis,
Hartford, CT, USA

S. B. Goldberg (✉)
Department of Medicine (Medical Oncology), Yale School of Medicine/Yale Cancer Center, New Haven, CT, USA
e-mail: sarah.goldberg@yale.edu

V. Chiang
Department of Neurosurgery, Yale School of Medicine/Yale Cancer Center, New Haven, CT, USA

© Springer Nature Switzerland AG 2021
A. C. Chiang, R. S. Herbst (eds.), *Lung Cancer*, Current Cancer Research,
https://doi.org/10.1007/978-3-030-74028-3_6

1 Introduction

Brain metastases account for about 90% of malignant brain tumors and as newer cancer treatments improve patient survival, the reported incidence of brain metastases is increasing [1]. The presence of metastatic disease in the brain carries a poor prognosis across all cancer types and can be associated with significant morbidity and decreased quality of life [2, 3]. Lung cancer is the most frequent origin of metastases to the brain [4], occurring in 10% of NSCLC patients at diagnosis [5] and developing in up to 20% of patients over the course of their disease [6].

The standard first line approach to the treatment of brain metastases in NSCLC has long been local therapy, either in the form of surgery or radiotherapy. While chemotherapy has been effective in systemic disease, most agents have shown reduced activity in the CNS. Local approaches are effective for palliating symptoms and decreasing death from neurological causes, but they are not without morbidity in and of themselves. Treatments such as whole brain radiation, once standard for a majority of patients with CNS metastases, have been shown to cause long lasting cognitive effects which are increasingly apparent as patients live longer [7]. As the treatment of NSCLC has moved to include small molecule targeted therapies, biologics and immunotherapies, it has been shown that many of these drugs have activity in the central nervous system. This chapter will address the most recent strategies for systemic treatment of brain metastases.

2 Local Treatments for Brain Metastases: The Historical Standard of Care

For many years the main treatment modalities for brain metastases were radiation or surgery. Neurosurgery for brain metastasis has been practiced as far back as the nineteenth century [8]. Case series from the early 1920s demonstrated surgery could significantly palliate symptoms, though it did not improve survival [9]. However, as better imaging was developed and surgical techniques were refined, it became clear that surgery for brain metastases could provide both symptom relief and better outcomes, with improvements in overall survival, quality of life, and preservation of functional independence in patients [10–14]. These benefits are generally greater for patients that are younger, have a good performance status and fewer comorbidities, and whose lesions are large, symptomatic and in non-eloquent regions of the brain [15].

The development of radiation therapy in the 1950s provided a non-surgical option for patients who were poor surgical candidates or who had multiple or unresectable lesions [7, 16]. Prior to that, the mainstay of treatment for patients who could not undergo brain surgery was steroids and best supportive care. In this setting, the median survival after diagnosis of brain metastases was in the range of weeks to a month or two [11]. A landmark study from 1954 showed that whole brain radiation (WBRT) could be used to improve symptom burden in patients with brain metastases, with symptomatic relief achieved in 63% of patients within their cohort

[17]. As WBRT was used more widely through the 1960s and 1970s, a survival benefit was also noted, with improvement in median overall survival (OS) from 1 month up to 6 months [3, 18–20].

Techniques for neurosurgery and radiation have continued to be refined in the years since, leading to improved benefits and decreased toxicity. More targeted radiation techniques such as stereotactic radiosurgery (SRS) in which high doses of ionizing radiation are delivered to defined areas via multiple crossing radiation beams, offer excellent efficacy with less toxicity than WBRT [16]. SRS has also been used as an alternative to surgery in patients who are poor surgical candidates, or whose tumors are in a location that make surgery impractical or impossible [21]. These treatments have continued to be the first-line for most patients presenting with metastatic disease in the brain.

Unfortunately, these treatments are not without drawbacks. While WBRT is both safe and well tolerated in most patients, for some severe fatigue and neurocognitive deficits can develop and persist for weeks and months after the end of treatment [7]. As systemic treatments have improved and patients are living longer, more long term effects of WBRT are being noted, with some patients experiencing neurocognitive decline that is progressive and irreversible [22]. Another downside to WBRT is that it may delay the initiation of systemic therapy, which can be detrimental in rapidly progressing disease. Because it can be arranged and performed quickly, and has fewer neurocognitive toxicities [23], SRS is now chosen as first line treatment over WBRT for most patients with NSCLC. SRS can also lead to toxicity however, most commonly radionecrosis [24, 25]. In small cell lung cancer (SCLC), WBRT continues to play an important role as prophylaxis for limited stage disease (prophylactic cranial irradition, PCI), and the main radiation modality for the majority of patients with multiple or recurrent brain lesions in extensive stage disease [26].

While historically, local therapies have been the mainstay of treatment for brain metastases, there is increasing investigation into the use of systemic therapies alone or in conjunction with local therapies.

3 Challenges in the Use of Systemic Treatment for Brain Metastases

There are multiple theoretical and practical challenges associated with the use of systemic therapies in the treatment of brain metastases. One significant issue is the inability of many drugs to achieve therapeutic levels in the CNS due to the presence of the blood-brain barrier. In order to maintain the complex microenvironment necessary for chemical and electrical signaling in the brain, strict homeostasis in the CNS must be sustained. Multiple historical experiments as early as the 1880s demonstrated that substances such as dyes and drugs could not enter the brain after being injected into the blood stream [27, 28]. This "barrier" was recognized to be at the level of the brain vasculature and was named the blood brain barrier by E. Goldman in 1913 [28]. Today we recognize that the blood-brain barrier (BBB) is made up of the microvascular network of the CNS and its associated structures, which serve to regulate the passage of substances from the blood stream into the brain. The capillaries of the BBB are comprised of specialized endothelial cells which are bound together with tight junctions, lacking the fenestrations seen in peripheral capillaries. These specialized endothelial cells are enmeshed with pericytes (contractile cells that help regulate blood flow), and the foot processes of astrocytes, all embedded together in a basement membrane and forming a semipermeable barrier between the CNS and the rest of the body [29].

While many drugs are being designed specifically with the intention of crossing the BBB, even drugs which could not ordinarily cross may reach therapeutic levels in the CNS under certain circumstances. Permeability of the blood brain barrier can be affected by multiple physiologic and pathologic factors. Disruption of the barrier is seen in inflammatory states such as infection, malignancy or trauma [30]. These disruptions are important in the treatment of brain metastases, as they allow penetration of the CNS by drugs which might otherwise be excluded. Even with this disruption, many drugs do not achieve optimal levels, complicating the selection of treatments for patients with CNS metastatic disease and making in vivo analysis of the drugs in clinical trials essential (Table 6.1).

Another challenging aspect of the brain microenvironment, especially in the age of immunotherapy, is the status of the CNS as an "immune privileged" site. As discussed above, the regulation of material in and out of the CNS is tightly controlled by the blood brain barrier and blood-CSF barrier, and the elements of the immune system are no exception. This means that the central nervous system is fairly isolated from systemic/peripheral immune responses, allowing maintenance of the strict homeostasis that is required for the brain to function. Beyond the strict regulation in the trafficking of antibodies, immune mediators, and immune cells into the CNS, there are other notable differences in the CNS immune response [31]. There are very few antigen presenting cells in the brain parenchyma, as well as low levels of major histocompatibility complex and resident T-cells. In addition, there is no classic lymphoid tissue in the brain, although it is now known that there is a lymphatic system of sorts in the meninges [32] allowing for drainage of CNS antigens into the deep cervical nodes [33, 34]. These unique characteristics of the CNS may contribute to a sluggish immune response and the presence of a relatively immunosuppressive microenvironment [35].

As our understanding of the immune system has grown, a more nuanced model of CNS immunity has arisen, making clear that the previous model of "strict immune privilege" is likely too simple. There is passage of antigens and immune cells from CNS to periphery and vice versa, as well as some form of immune surveillance even under normal physiologic conditions [32]. In addition, there are changes in the trafficking of immune cells caused by different pathologies, including brain metastases. The finding that there are high levels of tumor infiltrating lymphocytes in brain metastases was taken to suggest that the modulation of the immune system via immunotherapy might be possible [36]. Although the mechanisms by which these drugs act on the brain is yet unclear, data from a variety of trials suggests that they do have activity in the CNS [37–39].

Table 6.1 Selected Trials of CNS Outcomes with Systemic Therapy[a]

	Drug	Trial	Outcomes
Targeted Therapy			
EGFR	Osimertinib	**FLAURA (Soria et al. 2018)** Osimertinib versus erlotinib/gefitib 116 patients with CNS disease	iRR: 91% (vs 68%) CNS progression: 6% (vs 15%)
ALK	Alectinib	**ALEX (Peters et al. 2017)** Alectinib versus crizotinib 122 patients with CNS disease (21 measurable)	iRR: 81% (vs 50%) ICDOR response: 17.3 m (vs 5.5 m)
	Brigatinib	**ALTA-1L (Camidge et al. 2018)** Brigatinib versus crizotinib 90 patients with CNS disease (39 measurable)	iRR: 78% (vs 28%) Rate of IC progression: 9% (vs 19%)
	Lorlatinib	**CROWN Interim Analysis (Solomon et al. 2020)** Lorlatinib versus crizotinib 30 patients with CNS disease	iRR: 82% (vs 23%)
ROS-1	Entrectinib	**ALKA-372-001/STARTRK-1/ STARTRK-2 Integrated Analysis (Drilon et al. 2020)** Entrectinib, single arm 20 patients with CNS disease	iRR: 55% ICDOR 12.9 m Median ICPFS 7.7 m
RET	Selpercatinib	**LIBRETTO-001 (Velcheti et al. 2017)** Selpercatinib, single arm 11 patients with measurable CNS disease	iRR: 91% ICDOR: 10.1 m
Immunotherapy			

(continued)

Table 6.1 (continued)

Drug	Trial	Outcomes
Pembrolizumab	**Goldberg et al (Goldberg et al. 2020)** Pembrolizumab, single arm (all with CNS disease) Cohort 1 PD-L1 ≥ 1%: 37 patients evaluated	iRR: 29.7% ICDOR: 5.7 m 2 year OS: 34%
Nivolumab	**Italian Expanded Access Program** Nivolumab, single arm	
	Non-squamous cohort (Crino et al. 2019) 409 patients with CNS disease (29% on low dose steroids, 18% on steroids + XRT)	Subgroup ORR: 17% 1 year subgroup OS: 43% (48% for all patients)
	Squamous cohort (Cortinovis et al. 2019) 37 patients with CNS disease (22% on low dose steroids, 57% prior XRT)	iRR: 19% ICDCR: 49%
Atezolizumab	**OAK Subgroup Analysis (Lukas et al. 2017)** Atezolizumab versus Docetaxol 85 patients with CNS disease	Subgroup OS: 20 m (vs 11.9 m) Time to development of new CNS lesions: Not reached (vs 9.5 m)

Abbreviations: *iRR* intracranial response rate, *ICDOR* intracranial duration of response, *IC* intracranial, *ICPFS* intracranial progression free survival, *ORR* objective response rate, *OS* overall survival, *CNS* central nervous system, *m* months
[a]This table is not comprehensive; it includes representative and/or important trials and results

4 Systemic Therapies for Brain Metastases in NSCLC

4.1 Chemotherapy

In both NSCLC and SCLC there are several traditional chemotherapy agents that have been shown to have activity in the CNS. Prospective trials have evaluated the intracranial response rates with different cytotoxic chemotherapy drugs and regimens in the first line setting, typically in patients with small and asymptomatic brain metastases. Intracranial response rates (iRR) vary widely with different combinations: a 30% iRR has been seen with cisplatin and etoposide [40], 30% with carboplatin/pemetrexed [41], 38% with carboplatin/paclitaxel combined with either gemcitabine or vinorelbine [42], 55% for combination of cisplatin, ifosfamide and irinotecan [43], and 86% with cisplatin/gemcitabine [44]. Efficacy is generally lower with single agents and in pretreated patients, but pemetrexed has shown single agent activity in that setting [45]. Topotecan has excellent CNS penetration and has demonstrated CNS activity in patients with SCLC, with iRR ranging from 33% to as high as 57% [46, 47]. Chemotherapy has also been used in combination with radiotherapy as a sensitizer. Although this strategy resulted in a PFS benefit and increased ORR, there was no difference in survival compared with WBRT alone and an unacceptable increase in toxicity was observed [48].

Traditional chemotherapies have also been combined with anti-angiogenic drugs such as bevacizumab, a strategy which has been previously shown to have benefit for extracranial disease [49]. CNS activity of this regimen was evaluated in a phase II non-randomized study, the BRAIN trial, which examined the use of bevacizumab + carboplatin/paclitaxel as first line treatment in patients with NSCLC and asymptomatic untreated brain metastases [50]. In this trial the objective response rate in intracranial lesions (iORR) was 61%, comparable to the response seen in extracranial sites.

In summary, some cytotoxic chemotherapies do have activity in the CNS, with response rates in the 30–50% range. However, in most cases patients should be treated with local therapy prior to the initiation of systemic therapy.

4.2 Targeted Therapies

Systemic therapy has a very significant role in the treatment of brain metastases for patients with oncogene-addicted NSCLC. Around 30% of patients with adenocarcinoma are found to have a targetable mutation [51]. This number can be even higher in certain populations, including non-smokers and those of Asian descent. There has been an explosion in the number of drugs targeting the most common mutations, including EGFR, ALK, ROS1, MET and others. A number of these drugs have shown penetration into the CNS and efficacy in the treatment of brain metastasis from NSCLC. As such, the strategy for treatment of brain lesions in patients with targetable driver mutations has shifted in recent years to include consideration of first line systemic therapy, rather than local therapy in certain populations; specifically, this approach is useful in patients with small lesions in non-critical locations, without significant mass effect or CNS symptoms, and in those for whom the delay of local therapy would not change local therapy options. Importantly, as patients are living longer, this may have a significant impact on quality of life, avoiding some of the long-term morbidity of local strategies like WBRT.

4.2.1 EGFR Mutations

EGFR (epidermal growth factor receptor) gene mutations are among the most common driver mutations found in NSCLC, occurring at rates as high as 15% of North American/European populations (higher in non-smokers) [52] and up to 60% of Asian populations [53]. These mutations are associated with high rates of de novo brain metastases compared with patients that express wild type EGFR [54, 55], and patients with these mutations also have a higher risk for developing brain metastases over the course of their disease [55]. Some reports place the overall risk of developing brain metastases in the course of disease as high as 60% in patients with *EGFR* mutant lung cancer, compared with 30% in those expressing the wild type gene [56].

CNS penetration and efficacy for the first generation TKIs (tyrosine kinase inhibitors) erlotinib and gefitinib have been looked at both retrospectively and prospectively. Studies of erlotinib demonstrated moderate concentrations of the drug and its active metabolites in the CSF of patients with NSCLC [57, 58]. Multiple studies have demonstrated that erlotinib has efficacy in treating brain metastases. In a 2011 retrospective study including 17 patients with *EGFR* driver mutations, an intracranial response rate (iRR) of 82.4% was observed in patients treated with erlotinib (compared with no responses in the patients with wild type *EGFR*) [59]. A similar iRR was seen in the CTONG-0803 study, a phase II including 48 patients with lung adenocarcinoma treated with erlotinib after progression of brain metastases on chemotherapy [60]. This study demonstrated an intracranial PFS (iPFS) of 10.1 months and a 1-year survival of 73% with erlotinib alone, similar to patients whose brain metastases had been treated with radiation [60]. Another prospective study of 28 patients with brain metastasis from EGFR mutated NSCLC showed an objective response rate (ORR) of 83% and a disease control rate (DCR) of 93% when treated with first generation TKI (either gefitinib or erlotinib) [61]. Interestingly, there was no difference seen between erlotinib and gefitinib in this study, despite evidence showing low CNS penetration for gefitinib [62]. Several additional studies, both prospective and retrospective, have likewise demonstrated that gefitinib has activity in CNS disease despite the drug's poor CNS levels [63–67].

One third of patients develop new brain metastases while on a first generation EGFR TKI. Interestingly these lesions often lack the acquired resistance mutation T790M, which is commonly observed in progressing systemic disease [68]. This suggests that perhaps inadequate drug levels in the brain may be responsible for progression in the CNS rather than development of actual drug resistance. Several strategies have been suggested to improve the levels of these drugs in the CNS with the hope of increasing efficacy in the brain. Multiple small studies have looked at the use of a high dose "pulsatile" erlotinib schedule, giving 1500 mg once weekly or twice per week (as opposed to the standard 150 mg daily) [69, 70]. In a small retrospective study it was demonstrated that 6 of 9 patients with EGFR mutant lung cancer and brain metastases had a partial response when treated with this pulsed dose schedule [69]. A phase I study treated 34 patients (11 with brain metastases) with twice weekly 1200 mg erlotinib and saw one complete and 24 partial responses (iRR not documented) and no patients had CNS progression during the course of the study [70]. In that study, however, several of the patients still needed to undergo treatment for their brain metastases with local therapy. Another Phase I study enrolled 19 patients with EGFR mutated NSCLC and untreated brain metastases, and treated them with the same pulsed dose schedule. They found a 75% iRR with only 16% of patients showing CNS progression, although they did not see an improvement in PFS or a delay in the emergence of resistance mutations [71].

The second generation EGFR TKI afatinib has also been shown to have activity in the CNS. In the LUX-Lung 3 phase III study of frontline afatinib for EGFR mutant NSCLC (versus chemotherapy), there was a predefined subgroup analysis of 42 patients with asymptomatic brain metastases [72]. These patients had an improved PFS compared with chemotherapy (11 months vs 5.3 months), similar to those patients without brain metastases, although these results were not statistically significant. Similar results were seen in LUX-Lung 6, which looked at an unselected Asian population of NSCLC patients, including 49 with brain metastases [73]. Combined analysis of these two trials did yield a statistically significant improvement in PFS for patients with brain metastases, the magnitude of which was similar to that for patients without brain metastases [74]. This benefit however, was significantly greater in patients that had been treated previously with WBRT (13.8 vs 4.7 months HR 0.37). Another study looking at the use of afatinib after progression on chemotherapy and first generation TKI included 100 patients with brain metastases (including leptomeningeal disease). In this study there was a 35% CNS response rate with a 66% disease control rate [75].

Although there is evidence of CNS activity in these first and second generation TKIs, there is data demonstrating that early use of local therapy may still confer survival benefit. One retrospective study looked at *EGFR* mutant lung cancer patients with newly diagnosed brain metastases and compared those getting WBRT or SRS with those treated with erlotinib alone [76]. Overall survival was similar between erlotinib and WBRT group (26 vs 35 months p 0.62), but the group treated with SRS had a significantly longer OS (64 months p 0.006). Additionally, there was a longer time to intracranial progression in the WBRT group compared with the erlotinib group (24 vs 16 months) and the 2-year intracranial PFS (iPFS) was also significantly higher in WBRT (52% versus 26%). A later meta-analysis of 12 observational studies showed improved 4-month intracranial PFS and improved 2-year overall survival in patients that underwent upfront cranial irradiation [77]. The authors acknowledged serious methodologic concerns with the component studies, limiting conclusions from the meta-analysis. However, a later retrospective study looking at patients treated with SRS, WBRT and TKI demonstrated similar results [78]. In that study, median OS was 46, 30 and 25 months for patients treated with initial SRS+TKI, WBRT+TKI and TKI alone respectively. The inferior outcomes in the TKI alone group were seen despite the radiation groups having patients with lower Graded Prognostic Assessment scores, larger and more brain metastases, and more symptomatic lesions. Prospective studies are therefore needed to determine the benefit of upfront radiotherapy in these patients.

The approval of the drug osimertinib, a third generation TKI which targets the resistance mutation T790M, has changed clinical practice with respect to systemic therapy in *EGFR* mutant lung cancer. Results of the FLAURA phase III trial showed significant improvement in PFS (18.9 vs 10.2 months HR 0.46) for patients treated with osimertinib versus first generation TKIs erlotinib or gefitinib [79]. The results of this trial have made osimertinib the preferred frontline choice for treatment of patients with *EGFR* mutated NSCLC [80]. Preclinical data suggested that osimertinib had superior CNS penetration compared with earlier generation EGFR TKIs [81]. Early studies of osimertinib in the second line setting showed efficacy of the drug in the CNS [82], with pooled data from phase I and II studies of 50 patients with asymptomatic brain metastases showing an intracranial ORR of 54% with complete response (CR) in 12% [83]. Further, in a phase I trial including 32 patients with confirmed leptomeningeal disease, a form of CNS disease which is quite difficult to treat, 10 patients had responses and 13 had stable disease [84]. Subset analysis of the patients with CNS disease in the FLAURA trial (21% of 556 patients), showed iORR of 91% in the osimertinib group versus 68% with first generation TKIs [79]. In addition, PFS for patients with brain metastases was longer with osimertinib versus erlotinib or gefitinib (15.2 vs 9.6 months, HR 0.47) and the rate of CNS progression in the overall population was significantly lower with osimertinib (6% versus 15%). The use of osimertinib upfront in treating brain metastases is now standard of care because of its excellent CNS penetration and high RR and PFS.

4.2.2   *ALK* Rearrangements

Anaplastic lymphoma kinase (*ALK*) rearrangements are found in 5% of NSCLC patients [85]. As in patients with *EGFR* driver mutations, *ALK* positive patients have an increased risk of brain metastases compared to patients without driver mutations; around 20% have de novo brain metastasis and up to 58% develop them by 2 years [86]. Initial trials of crizotinib included significant numbers of patients with brain metastases – around 31% in a pooled analysis from the PROFILE 1005 Phase II and PROFILE 1007 Phase III (with 60% having undergone prior radiation therapy) [87]. Treatment with crizotinib was associated with similar rates of intracranial disease control regardless of prior radiation (62% vs 56%), although the ORR was improved if the patient had been previously radiated as was the time to intracranial progression. In the PROFILE 1014 trial, 79 patients with treated brain metastases showed better ORR and PFS with crizotinib versus chemotherapy, with a 12-week intracranial disease control rate of 85% [88]. Ultimately however, over 60% of patients eventually develop brain metastases during the course of their treatment with crizotinib [87], possibly due to poor penetration of the blood brain barrier and insufficient levels of drug in the CNS [89].

Alectinib is another ALK inhibitor which, in addition to showing excellent activity in patients with crizotinib resistance, also showed good CNS penetration in preclinical models [90]. A pooled analysis from two phase II studies of alectinib in pretreated *ALK* positive patients included 136 patients with brain metastases, 50 of whom had measurable disease [91]. For the patients with measurable CNS disease, there was an iORR of 64% (22% CRs), CNS DCR of 90%, and a median duration of response of 10.8 months. For patients with measurable and unmeasurable disease the iORR was 42% with 27% CRs. These numbers were similar between patients who had and had not received prior CNS radiation. The ALUR trial, a phase III study of *ALK* positive patients with crizotinib resistance, showed that alectinib had an iORR of 54% compared with 0% for chemotherapy among the 24 patients with measurable brain disease [92]. The ALEX trial demonstrated the superiority of alectinib to crizotinib in the front-line treatment of ALK positive NSCLC patients [93].

This study cohort included 122 patients with brain metastases, including 21 patients with measurable disease. In subset analysis of these patients there was an iORR 81% with alectinib compared to 50% with crizotinib, and a longer duration of intra-cranial response (17.3 months vs. 5.5 months). All of these studies excluded patients with symptomatic brain metastases, but a retrospective study looking at 19 patients with large or symptomatic brain metastases in *ALK* positive NSCLC patients dem-onstrated some efficacy in that population as well [94]. They found an iORR of 72%, CNS DCR of 100%, and duration of response of 17 months in patients treated with alectanib. Ceritinib, a second generation ALK inhibitor, has also been demon-strated to have CNS activity, though it has not been directly compared to either crizotinib or alectinib. Studies have demonstrated intracranial RR ranging from 35–73% [95–97].

Other agents have also shown promise in the CNS for ALK positive NSCLC patients. Brigatinib was demonstrated to be effective in CNS disease for patients with crizotinib resistant *ALK* positive NSCLC [98]. This study found an iORR of 67% with standard dosing and a median iPFS of greater than 1 year. The ALTA-1L phase III trial demonstrated efficacy of brigatinib over crizotinib in the first line set-ting for *ALK* positive NSCLC [99]. This study included 90 patients with brain metastases at baseline, 39 with measurable disease, and showed an iORR of 78% for brigatinib versus 28% for crizotinib. Brigatinib was also associated with decreased rates of intracranial disease progression: 9% versus 19% with crizotinib. Lorlatinib is a third generation ALK/ROS1 inhibitor which was specifically designed to have CNS penetration. In a Phase I trial of pretreated *ALK* and *ROS1* positive NSCLC patients, lorlatinib demonstrated an intracranial response rate of 46% in the 24 patients with measurable CNS disease (CR in 24%) [100]. In the Phase II of this study, the intracranial response rate for lorlatinib in treatment-naive *ALK* positive patients was 75% and 39% in the most heavily pretreated populations (3 prior TKIs + chemotherapy) [101]. Interim analysis of data from the phase III CROWN trial showed improvement in iRR for patients treated with lorlatinib versus crizotinib in the first line setting (82% versus 23%), although the number of patients with CNS disease was small. This study also showed an improvement in the median time to CNS progression, as well as a trend towards improvement in overall survival for this subset of patients (though OS data not yet mature) [102, 103]. Ensartinib, another novel ALK TKI, has also shown promise in the interim analysis of a Phase III trial of patients treated with ensartinib versus crizotinib in the first line setting [104]. There was an improvement in iRR (54% versus 19%) for patients with measurable CNS disease, and a delayed time to treatment failure in the brain for patients with-out de novo CNS disease (4% versus 24% at 12 months).

In summary, most of the ALK inhibitors have some activity in CNS disease. However, patients on crizotinib frequently progress in the brain and it is therefore not the agent of choice for patients with de novo CNS metastases. Alectinib can be used for frontline treatment of patients with low-risk CNS disease as well as for patients who have had CNS progression on crizotinib. Brigatinib, ceritinib, lorlati-nib and ensartinib also have good CNS activity.

4.2.3   Other Driver Mutations (*ROS1, RET, BRAF, MET, NTRK*)

For the rarer oncogenic driver mutations seen in NSCLC, less is known with regards to the best first-line therapy for both systemic and CNS disease. *ROS-1* alterations have been treated with ceritinib and lorlatinib, with intracranial response rates appearing comparable to those seen in *ALK* positive patients [100, 105, 106]. Entrectinib, a ROS1/TRK inhibitor with good CNS penetration, has been FDA approved for the treatment of NSCLC patients with *ROS-1* alterations. In an inte-grated analysis of three phase 1/2 trials, iRR was 55% among 20 patients with CNS disease [107]. In patients with *RET* fusions, accounting for only 1–2% of unselected NSCLC patients, some intracranial responses were seen with cabozantinib and alec-tinib [108, 109]. Early clinical results/case studies with RET inhibitor LOXO-292 (now selpercatinib) suggested good CNS activity and data from the LIBERETTO-001 study demonstrated an iRR of 91% in pre-treated patients with NSCLC positive for *RET* fusion [110–112]. *BRAF* mutations are uncommon in lung cancer (2–4% of patients), but quite common in melanoma and as such the studies evaluating effi-cacy of BRAF inhibitors in the CNS have mainly been in melanoma patients. In that population both single agent BRAF inhibition with dabrafenib and combined ther-apy with dabrafenib and the MET inhibitor trametinib have demonstrated CNS activity [113, 114]. This combination is effective for the systemic treatment of V600E-*BRAF* mutated NSCLC [115–117], though there is little data beyond case studies on the effectiveness in the CNS in this population [118, 119].

In summary, there is not yet consensus on the best agents for use in patients with the less common driver mutations and CNS metastases.

4.3   Immunotherapy – Checkpoint Inhibitors

With the increasing use of checkpoint inhibitors for the treatment of many cancers, including NSCLC, there has been interest in their efficacy for treating metastatic CNS disease. These drugs work by disrupting so-called immune checkpoint path-ways, the inhibitory signals that normally regulate the body's immune response [120]. These pathways are now known to be important in the process by which cancer cells evade immune surveillance and are able to grow and metastasize. By targeting these pathways, checkpoint inhibitors are thought to lead to activation of T-cell mediated immunity, restoring the ability of T-cells to recognize and destroy tumor cells [120]. The two main targets of current drugs are the programmed cell death protein 1 (PD-1)/programmed cell death protein ligand -1 (PDL-1) axis and cytotoxic T-lymphocyte associated antigen 4 (CTLA-4). Multiple checkpoint inhib-itors are FDA approved for the treatment of NSCLC, including nivolumab and pem-brolizumab (PD-1 inhibitors) and atezolizumab and durvalumab (PD-L1 inhibitors) [121]. All of these drugs have demonstrated benefit in the treatment of NSCLC, and those data will not be addressed in this chapter. In addition, recent trials have dem-onstrated the efficacy of ipilimumab/nivolumab and ipilimumab/nivolumab +

chemotherapy in NSCLC, leading to FDA approvals for these combination regimens [122, 123].

Because of the status of the brain as an "immune-privileged" site, it was initially unclear if these drugs would have any CNS activity, although preclinical data in mouse models of GBM suggested that they did [124]. Multiple conceptual challenges exist regarding the possible efficacy of these drugs in the CNS: the ability of the monoclonal antibodies to cross the blood brain barrier, the low number of T-cells in the normal brain parenchyma, and the widespread use of steroids for treatment of symptomatic brain lesions [125]. Because of these theoretical challenges, many of the initial trials of checkpoint inhibitors in NSCLC and other cancers excluded patients with brain metastases, or required local therapy prior to initiation of systemic therapy, thus limiting interpretation of the intracranial activity of the drugs.

To date, only one prospective study has evaluated the use of immune checkpoint inhibitors as frontline treatment in NSCLC with untreated brain metastases [38, 39]. This phase 2 non-randomized, open label study included patients with melanoma or NSCLC who had asymptomatic brain metastases treated with pembrolizumab. Early analysis showed that of 18 NSCLC patients, 6 (33%) had intracranial responses, with four complete responses and two partial responses. These response rates were similar to those seen in extracranial disease [38]. Final analysis of this trial showed iRR of 29.7% in patients with PD-L1 > 1% and 2 year OS was 34% (versus historical OS in this population of 14.3%) [39]. Of note, this trial allowed only patients with asymptomatic brain metastases which were <20 mm in size, without symptoms or corticosteroid requirement.

Although most other trials of checkpoint inhibitors in lung cancer excluded patients with untreated brain metastases, several of the initial trials evaluating systemic efficacy of nivolumab, pembrolizumab and atezolizumab included analysis of patients with stable locally treated brain metastases. In these studies, they were able to perform subgroup analyses to see if the same PFS and OS benefits were seen in the population with brain metastases. The Checkmate 057 Phase 3 trial of nivolumab versus docetaxel in the second line setting included 68 patients with treated brain metastases out of 582 non-squamous NSCLC patients [126]. In this analysis, intracranial responses were not assessed but there was no OS benefit in this subgroup (HR 1.04). An analysis of pooled data from the phase II and III CheckMate 057, 063 and 017 trials of nivolumab versus docetaxel in previously treated advanced NSCLC, also did not find an OS benefit in the subgroup of patients with brain metastases but did note that at the time of progression, 33% of patients had no evidence of CNS progression [127].

The KEYNOTE 024 Phase 3 study of front line pembrolizumab versus platinum-based chemotherapy in NSCLC (PD-L1 expression >50%) included 128 patients (out of 305) with stable treated brain metastasis and had a planned subgroup analysis [128]. Again, intracranial response was not assessed but the subgroup analysis showed a trend towards PFS benefit with pembrolizumab compared to chemotherapy (HR 0.55 but CI 0.2–1.56). The KEYNOTE 189, a phase 3 trial of pembrolizumab and platinum doublet versus chemotherapy alone for non-squamous NSCLC, included one the largest preplanned subgroups of patients with brain metastases, and was one of the few to allow patients with untreated brain metastases [129]. Of 616 patients enrolled, 109 patients (17%) had brain metastases (treated and untreated). In this subset analysis a significant OS benefit was found in the subgroup with CNS disease, with a hazard ratio of 0.36 for triplet therapy versus chemotherapy alone. A subgroup analysis of patients from KEYNOTE-189 with liver or brain metastases confirmed benefit in those populations, with improved PFS and OS that was similar to the benefit observed in patients without brain metastases [130].

The OAK trial, a phase 3 study of atezolizumab versus docetaxel in pre-treated NSCLC patients also included a pre-planned subgroup analysis of the 123 patients with stable or treated brain metastases [131, 132]. In this study there was a trend towards OS benefit in patients with CNS disease with median OS of 16.0 months in the atezolizumab group versus 11.9 in the docetaxel group (HR 0.75, p = 0.1633) [132]. They also observed a longer median time to development of new CNS lesions in patients with baseline brain metastases (median not reached versus 9.5 months) as well as a higher probability of being free of new brain lesions at 6,12 and 24 months (85% vs 64%, 76% vs 42% and 76% vs 0 respectively). An analysis of pooled data from OAK and 4 other trials also evaluated efficacy and safety in patients with CNS disease treated with atezolizumab [133]. Efficacy analyses in this study were conducted on the 85 patients with CNS disease from the OAK trial, and safety analyses were conducted on 79 patients with CNS disease in the pooled safety cohort . There was an OS benefit for patients treated with atezolizumab (HR 0.54), with a median OS of 20.1 months versus 11.9 months with docetaxel. The risk of developing new lesions was lower in the atezolizumab group (HR 0.42) with time to develop new lesions not reached versus 9.5 months for docetaxel. Safety assessments did show a slight increase in the number of neurologic adverse effects in patients with brain metastases, but no grade 3–5 neurologic toxicities were observed [133].

Some of the largest study cohorts for checkpoint inhibitors that included patients with brain metastases were the Italian and French expanded access programs for nivolumab treatment of non-squamous NSCLC patients. In the Italian expanded access program 409 out of 1588 patients with pre-treated non-squamous NSCLC had asymptomatic brain metastases [134]. Of note, in that group 117 patients (29%) were being treated with low dose steroids (<10 mg/day prednisone) and 74 (18%) were getting low dose steroids and radiotherapy. The ORR was 17% in CNS metastasis patients, which was similar to that seen in the general population (CR in 4 patients and PR in 64 patients). One-year OS was 43% in patients with brain metastases compared with 48% for all patients in the cohort. In this group, nivolumab toxicity was similar in the groups with and without CNS disease. There was also a squamous NSCLC cohort as part of the Italian expanded access program, and separate analysis was done looking at patients with CNS metastases in this group as well [135]. In this cohort a subgroup of 37 out of 371 patients had brain metastases, of which 22% were on low dose steroids and 57% had received prior radiotherapy. Similar to the non-squamous group, OS and PFS benefits were similar between patients with and without brain metastases. Intracranial ORR was 19% and intracranial DCR 49%. Safety was found to be comparable between groups, with no grade

3–5 CNS toxicities. The French expanded access program for Nivolumab included 130 patients with brain metastases out of 600 patients with pre-treated advanced NSCLC. In this cohort partial response rate was 16%, with stable disease in 33%, which was comparable to the overall population of patients [136]. Overall survival in patients with brain metastases was 6.6 months compared with 9.9 months in patients without CNS disease.

Results from a large observational study looking at a cohort of 1025 patients with NSCLC treated with immune checkpoint inhibitors in 5 European centers, included 255 patients with brain metastases at the start of treatment [137]. In this study ORR was similar between those with and without brain metastases – 20% versus 22%. Intracranial ORR was 27%, with intracranial DCR of 60%. This was also one of the few studies to look at the impact of PD-L1 status, showing that in the 14 patients where this information was available, patients with PD-L1 expression 1% or higher had improved intracranial response (35%) compared with PD-L1 negative patients (11%). Median PFS was similar at 1.7 months for those with brain metastases and 2.1 months for those without. Median OS was worse in patients with CNS disease at 8.6 months versus 11.4 months for those without (p 0.035).

Another line of inquiry which has been explored is the combination of immuno-therapy and radiotherapy. There has been speculation about a possible additive effect, as radiation itself produces an immune response and has been postulated to potentially unmask neoantigens [138] and lead to improved tumor specific T-cell responses [139–141]. Preclinical studies have suggested that this may lead to a synergistic effect of treatment with both radiation and immunotherapy in lung cancer [142]. Secondary analysis of data from the KEYNOTE 001 trial showed that patients who had previously received radiation (intra- or extra-thoracic) had significantly longer PFS and OS on pembrolizumab compared with those who had not been radiated [143]. Several retrospective studies, case series, and one prospective study evaluated this approach in patients with melanoma and brain metastases and showed that the combination of immune checkpoint inhibitors with CNS radiation appeared safe and potentially beneficial [144–149]. Two additional retrospective studies evaluating this combination included patients with lung cancer, and again appeared to show that this approach was safe and potentially beneficial [144, 150]. Only one retrospective study looking at 180 patients who underwent GKRS for brain metastasis, including 71 lung cancer patients, showed that patients treated with immunotherapy had a higher rate of radiation necrosis compared with those that received cytotoxic chemotherapy or targeted therapy [151]. In this study, 39 out of 180 patients developed radiation necrosis or "treatment related imaging changes" (the imaging equivalent of radiation necrosis): 37% (12/32) on immunotherapy alone, 25% (5/20) in patients treated with targeted therapy only and 16.9% (14/83) treated with cytotoxic chemotherapy alone. Interestingly, receiving any chemotherapy in the course of treatment (including patients also treated with immunotherapy or targeted therapy) was associated with a decreased risk of developing radiation necrosis.

Increasing evidence suggests the safety and efficacy of checkpoint inhibitors in NSCLC patients with brain metastases. In selected cases, patients may be able to forgo local treatment for small and asymptomatic CNS lesions in non-critically located parts of the brain, especially in those who have a higher likelihood of benefit from immunotherapy (i.e. those with high PD-L1 expression). For patients with large or symptomatic brain metastases, particularly those requiring high doses of steroids, upfront local therapy remains the recommended first-line treatment. The use of radiation and immunotherapy either concurrently or sequentially may increase responses in the CNS, but may also increase the risk of radiation necrosis. The optimal approach has yet to be determined and additional studies are underway.

5 Conclusions

CNS disease is an important cause of morbidity and mortality in patients with NSCLC. While local therapy remains the treatment of choice for most patients, there is increasing evidence that some patients can be treated with systemic therapy upfront along with close surveillance of the brain. Checkpoint inhibitors and many targeted therapies for NSCLC have demonstrated efficacy and safety in the CNS. For some, this may provide effective disease control without the toxicities that can occur with local therapies such as radiation and surgery.

References

1. Svokos KA, Salhia B, Toms SA (2014) Molecular biology of brain metastasis. Int J Mol Sci 15(6):9519–9530
2. Peters S et al (2016) The impact of brain metastasis on quality of life, resource utilization and survival in patients with non-small-cell lung cancer. Cancer Treat Rev 45:139–162
3. Laurie Gaspar, C.S.M, Rotman M, Asbell S, Phillips T, Wasserman T, McKenna WG, Byhardt R (1997) Recursive Partition Analysis (RPA) of prognostic factors in three Radiation Therapy Oncology Group (RTOG) brain metastases trials. Int J Radiat Oncol Biol Phys 37:745–751
4. Cagney DN et al (2017) Incidence and prognosis of patients with brain metastases at diagnosis of systemic malignancy: a population-based study. Neuro-Oncology 19(11):1511–1521
5. Kromer C et al (2017) Estimating the annual frequency of synchronous brain metastasis in the United States 2010-2013: a population-based study. J Neuro-Oncol 134(1):55–64
6. Barnholtz-Sloan JS et al (2004) Incidence proportions of brain metastases in patients diagnosed (1973 to 2001) in the Metropolitan Detroit Cancer Surveillance System. J Clin Oncol 22(14):2865–2872
7. Brown PD, MSA, Kahn OH, Asher AL, Wefel JS, Gondi V (2018) Whole brain radiotherapy for brain metastases: evolution or revolution. J Clin Oncol 36:483
8. <Weinberg2001_Article_SurgicalManagementOfBrainMetas.pdf>
9. Grant FC (1926) Concerning Intrcranial malignant metastases: their frequency and the value of surgery in their treatment. Ann Surg 84:635–646
10. Narayan Sundaresan JHG (1985) Surgical treatment of brain metastases. Cancer 55:1382–1388
11. Markesbery WR, Brooks WH, Gupta GD, Young AB (1978) Treatment for patients with cerebral metastases. JAMA Neurol 35:754–756
12. Mandell L et al (1986) The treatment of single brain metastasis from non-oat cell lung carcinoma. Surgery and radiation versus radiation therapy alone. Cancer 58(3):641–649

13. White KT, Fleming TR, Laws ER Jr (1981) Single metastasis to the brain. Surgical treatment in 122 consecutive patients. Mayo Clin Proc 56(7):424–428
14. Bindal RK et al (1993) Surgical treatment of multiple brain metastases. J Neurosurg 79(2):210–216
15. Mintz AH et al (1996) A randomized trial to assess the efficacy of surgery in addition to radiotherapy in patients with a single cerebral metastasis. Cancer 78(7):1470–1476
16. Brown PD et al (2016) Effect of radiosurgery alone vs radiosurgery with whole brain radiation therapy on cognitive function in patients with 1 to 3 brain metastases: a randomized clinical trial. JAMA 316(4):401–409
17. Jen-Hung Chao, RP, Nickson JJ (1954) Roentgen-ray therapy of cerebral metastases. Cancer 7:682–689
18. Borgelt BGR, Kramer S, Brady LW, Chang CH, Davis LW, Perez CA, Hendrickson FR (1980) The palliation of brain metastases: final results of the first two studies by the Radiation Therapy Oncology Group. Int J Radiat Oncol Biol Phys 6:1
19. Sneed PK, Larson DA, Wara WM (1996) Radiotherapy for cerebral metastases. Neurosurg Clin N Am 7(3):505–516
20. Katz HR (1981) The relative effectiveness of radiation therapy, corticosteroids, and surgery in the management of melanoma metastatic to the central nervous system. Int J Radiat Oncol Biol Phys 7(7):897–906
21. Hussain A et al (2007) Stereotactic radiosurgery for brainstem metastases: survival, tumor control, and patient outcomes. Int J Radiat Oncol Biol Phys 67(2):521–524
22. Tallet AV et al (2012) Neurocognitive function impairment after whole brain radiotherapy for brain metastases: actual assessment. Radiat Oncol 7:77
23. Schimmel WCM et al (2018) Cognitive effects of stereotactic radiosurgery in adult patients with brain metastases: a systematic review. Adv Radiat Oncol 3(4):568–581
24. Minniti G et al (2011) Stereotactic radiosurgery for brain metastases: analysis of outcome and risk of brain radionecrosis. Radiat Oncol 6:48
25. Chin LS, Ma L, DiBiase S (2001) Radiation necrosis following gamma knife surgery: a case-controlled comparison of treatment parameters and long-term clinical follow up. J Neurosurg 94(6):899–904
26. Network, N.C.C. Small cell lung cancer (version 1.2021. 2020 November 15, 2020]; Available from: https://www.nccn.org/professionals/physician_gls/pdf/sclc_blocks.pdf
27. Ribatti D et al (2006) Development of the blood-brain barrier: a historical point of view. Anat Rec B New Anat 289(1):3–8
28. Saunders NR et al (2014) The rights and wrongs of blood-brain barrier permeability studies: a walk through 100 years of history. Front Neurosci 8:404
29. Fricker G et al (2014) The Blood Brain Barrier (BBB). Springer, Berlin, Heidelberg
30. Stamatovic SM, Keep RF, Andjelkovic AV (2008) Brain endothelial cell-cell junctions: how to "open" the blood brain barrier. Curr Neuropharmacol 6(3):179–192
31. Galea I, Bechmann I, Perry VH (2007) What is immune privilege (not)? Trends Immunol 28(1):12–18
32. Louveau A et al (2015) Structural and functional features of central nervous system lymphatic vessels. Nature 523(7560):337–341
33. Cserr HF, Harling-Berg CJ, Knopf PM (1992) Drainage of brain extracellular fluid into blood and deep cervical lymph and its immunological significance. Brain Pathol 2(4):269–276
34. Kida S, Pantazis A, Weller RO (1993) CSF drains directly from the subarachnoid space into nasal lymphatics in the rat. Anatomy, histology and immunological significance. Neuropathol Appl Neurobiol 19(6):480–488
35. Wekerle H, Sun DM (2010) Fragile privileges: autoimmunity in brain and eye. Acta Pharmacol Sin 31(9):1141–1148
36. Berghoff AS et al (2016) Tumor infiltrating lymphocytes and PD-L1 expression in brain metastases of small cell lung cancer (SCLC). J Neuro-Oncol 130(1):19–29

37. Kamath SD, Kumthekar PU (2018) Immune checkpoint inhibitors for the treatment of Central Nervous System (CNS) metastatic disease. Front Oncol 8:414
38. Goldberg SB et al (2016) Pembrolizumab for patients with melanoma or non-small-cell lung cancer and untreated brain metastases: early analysis of a non-randomised, open-label, phase 2 trial. Lancet Oncol 17(7):976–983
39. Goldberg SB et al (2020) Pembrolizumab for management of patients with NSCLC and brain metastases: long-term results and biomarker analysis from a non-randomised, open-label, phase 2 trial. Lancet Oncol 21(5):655–663
40. Vittorio Franciosi GCM, Michiara M, Di Constanzo F, Fosser V, Tonato M, Carlini P, Boni C, Di Sarra S (1999) Front-line chemotheraphy with Cisplatin and Etoposide for patients with brain metastases from breast carcinoma, nonsmall cell lung carcinoma, or malignant melanoma. Cancer 85:1599–1605
41. Bailon O et al (2012) Upfront association of carboplatin plus pemetrexed in patients with brain metastases of lung adenocarcinoma. Neuro-Oncology 14(4):491–495
42. Cortes J et al (2003) Front-line paclitaxel/cisplatin-based chemotherapy in brain metastases from non-small-cell lung cancer. Oncology 64(1):28–35
43. Fujita A et al (2000) Combination chemotherapy of cisplatin, ifosfamide, and irinotecan with rhG-CSF support in patients with brain metastases from non-small cell lung cancer. Oncology 59(4):291–295
44. Quadvlieg V et al (2004) Frontline gemcitabine and cisplatin based chemotherapy in patients with NSCLC inoperable brain metastases. J Clin Oncol 22(14_suppl):7117
45. Bearz A et al (2010) Activity of Pemetrexed on brain metastasis from non-small cell lung cancer. Lung Cancer 68(2):264–268
46. Ardizzoni A et al (1997) Topotecan, a new active drug in the second-line treatment of small-cell lung cancer: a phase II study in patients with refractory and sensitive disease. The European Organization for research and treatment of cancer early clinical studies group and new drug development office, and the lung cancer cooperative group. J Clin Oncol 15(5):2090–2096
47. Korfel A, O.C, von Pawel J, Keppler U, Deppermann M, Kaubitsch S, Thiel E (2002) Response to topotecan of symptomatic brain metastases of small-cell lung cancer also after whole-brain irradiation. A multicentre phase II study. Eur J Cancer 38:1724–1729
48. Qin H et al (2014) Whole brain radiotherapy plus concurrent chemotherapy in non-small cell lung cancer patients with brain metastases: a meta-analysis. PLoS One 9(10):e111475
49. Sandler A et al (2006) Paclitaxel-carboplatin alone or with bevacizumab for non-small-cell lung cancer. N Engl J Med 355(24):2542–2550
50. Besse B et al (2015) Bevacizumab in patients with nonsquamous non-small cell lung cancer and asymptomatic, untreated Brain metastases (BRAIN): a nonrandomized, phase II study. Clin Cancer Res 21(8):1896–1903
51. Barlesi F et al (2016) Routine molecular profiling of patients with advanced non-small-cell lung cancer: results of a 1-year nationwide programme of the French Cooperative Thoracic Intergroup (IFCT). Lancet 387(10026):1415–1426
52. Kris MG et al (2014) Using multiplexed assays of oncogenic drivers in lung cancers to select targeted drugs. JAMA 311(19):1998–2006
53. Shi Y et al (2014) A prospective, molecular epidemiology study of EGFR mutations in Asian patients with advanced non-small-cell lung cancer of adenocarcinoma histology (PIONEER). J Thorac Oncol 9(2):154–162
54. Iuchi T et al (2015) Frequency of brain metastases in non-small-cell lung cancer, and their association with epidermal growth factor receptor mutations. Int J Clin Oncol 20(4):674–679
55. Shin DY et al (2014) EGFR mutation and brain metastasis in pulmonary adenocarcinomas. J Thorac Oncol 9(2):195–199
56. Omuro AM et al (2005) High incidence of disease recurrence in the brain and leptomeninges in patients with nonsmall cell lung carcinoma after response to gefitinib. Cancer 103(11):2344–2348

57. Deng Y et al (2014) The concentration of erlotinib in the cerebrospinal fluid of patients with brain metastasis from non-small-cell lung cancer. Mol Clin Oncol 2(1):116–120
58. Masuda T et al (2011) Erlotinib efficacy and cerebrospinal fluid concentration in patients with lung adenocarcinoma developing leptomeningeal metastases during gefitinib therapy. Cancer Chemother Pharmacol 67(6):1465–1469
59. Porta R et al (2011) Brain metastases from lung cancer responding to erlotinib: the importance of EGFR mutation. Eur Respir J 37(3):624–631
60. Wu YL et al (2013) Erlotinib as second-line treatment in patients with advanced non-small-cell lung cancer and asymptomatic brain metastases: a phase II study (CTONG-0803). Ann Oncol 24(4):993–999
61. Park SJ et al (2012) Efficacy of epidermal growth factor receptor tyrosine kinase inhibitors for brain metastasis in non-small cell lung cancer patients harboring either exon 19 or 21 mutation. Lung Cancer 77(3):556–560
62. Zhao J et al (2013) Cerebrospinal fluid concentrations of gefitinib in patients with lung adenocarcinoma. Clin Lung Cancer 14(2):188–193
63. Zhang Q et al (2016) Effects of epidermal growth factor receptor-tyrosine kinase inhibitors alone on EGFR-mutant non-small cell lung cancer with brain metastasis. Thorac Cancer 7(6):648–654
64. Ma S et al (2009) Treatment of brain metastasis from non-small cell lung cancer with whole brain radiotherapy and Gefitinib in a Chinese population. Lung Cancer 65(2):198–203
65. Iuchi T et al (2013) Phase II trial of gefitinib alone without radiation therapy for Japanese patients with brain metastases from EGFR-mutant lung adenocarcinoma. Lung Cancer 82(2):282–287
66. Ceresoli GL et al (2004) Gefitinib in patients with brain metastases from non-small-cell lung cancer: a prospective trial. Ann Oncol 15(7):1042–1047
67. Wu C et al (2007) Gefitinib in the treatment of advanced non-small cell lung cancer with brain metastasis. Zhonghua Zhong Liu Za Zhi 29(12):943–945
68. Hata A et al (2015) Spatiotemporal T790M heterogeneity in individual patients with EGFR-mutant non-small-cell lung cancer after acquired resistance to EGFR-TKI. J Thorac Oncol 10(11):1553–1559
69. Grommes C et al (2011) "Pulsatile" high-dose weekly erlotinib for CNS metastases from EGFR mutant non-small cell lung cancer. Neuro-Oncology 13(12):1364–1369
70. Yu HA et al (2017) Phase 1 study of twice weekly pulse dose and daily low-dose erlotinib as initial treatment for patients with EGFR-mutant lung cancers. Ann Oncol 28(2):278–284
71. Arbour KC et al (2018) Twice weekly pulse and daily continuous-dose erlotinib as initial treatment for patients with epidermal growth factor receptor-mutant lung cancers and brain metastases. Cancer 124(1):105–109
72. Sequist LV et al (2013) Phase III study of afatinib or cisplatin plus pemetrexed in patients with metastatic lung adenocarcinoma with EGFR mutations. J Clin Oncol 31(27):3327–3334
73. Wu Y-L et al (2014) Afatinib versus cisplatin plus gemcitabine for first-line treatment of Asian patients with advanced non-small-cell lung cancer harbouring EGFR mutations (LUX-Lung 6): an open-label, randomised phase 3 trial. Lancet Oncol 15(2):213–222
74. Schuler M et al (2016) First-line Afatinib versus chemotherapy in patients with non-small cell lung cancer and common epidermal growth factor receptor gene mutations and brain metastases. J Thorac Oncol 11(3):380–390
75. Hoffknecht P et al (2015) Efficacy of the irreversible ErbB family blocker afatinib in epidermal growth factor receptor (EGFR) tyrosine kinase inhibitor (TKI)-pretreated non-small-cell lung cancer patients with brain metastases or leptomeningeal disease. J Thorac Oncol 10(1):156–163
76. Gerber NK et al (2014) Erlotinib versus radiation therapy for brain metastases in patients with EGFR-mutant lung adenocarcinoma. Int J Radiat Oncol Biol Phys 89(2):322–329

77. Soon YY et al (2015) EGFR tyrosine kinase inhibitors versus cranial radiation therapy for EGFR mutant non-small cell lung cancer with brain metastases: a systematic review and meta-analysis. Radiother Oncol 114(2):167–172
78. Magnuson WJ et al (2017) Management of brain metastases in tyrosine kinase inhibitor-naive epidermal growth factor receptor-mutant non-small-cell lung cancer: a retrospective multi-institutional analysis. J Clin Oncol 35(10):1070–1077
79. Soria JC et al (2018) Osimertinib in untreated EGFR-mutated advanced non-small-cell lung cancer. N Engl J Med 378(2):113–125
80. Network, N.C.C. Lung cancer (Version 7.2019). August 15., 2019]; Available from: https://www.nccn.org/professionals/physician_gls/pdf/nscl_blocks.pdf
81. Ballard P et al (2016) Preclinical comparison of Osimertinib with other EGFR-TKIs in EGFR-mutant NSCLC brain metastases models, and early evidence of clinical brain metastases activity. Clin Cancer Res 22(20):5130–5140
82. Mok TS et al (2017) Osimertinib or platinum-Pemetrexed in EGFR T790M-positive lung cancer. N Engl J Med 376(7):629–640
83. Goss G et al (2018) CNS response to osimertinib in patients with T790M-positive advanced NSCLC: pooled data from two phase II trials. Ann Oncol 29(3):687–693
84. Yang JC-H et al (2017) Osimertinib for patients (pts) with leptomeningeal metastases (LM) from EGFR-mutant non-small cell lung cancer (NSCLC): updated results from the BLOOM study. J Clin Oncol 35(15_suppl):2020
85. Rodig SJ et al (2009) Unique clinicopathologic features characterize ALK-rearranged lung adenocarcinoma in the western population. Clin Cancer Res 15(16):5216–5223
86. Rangachari D et al (2015) Brain metastases in patients with EGFR-mutated or ALK-rearranged non-small-cell lung cancers. Lung Cancer 88(1):108–111
87. Costa DB et al (2015) Clinical experience with Crizotinib in patients with advanced ALK-rearranged non-small-cell lung cancer and brain metastases. J Clin Oncol 33(17):1881–1888
88. Solomon BJ et al (2016) Intracranial efficacy of Crizotinib versus chemotherapy in patients with advanced ALK-positive non-small-cell lung cancer: results from PROFILE 1014. J Clin Oncol 34(24):2858–2865
89. Costa DB et al (2011) CSF concentration of the anaplastic lymphoma kinase inhibitor crizotinib. J Clin Oncol 29(15):e443–e445
90. Kodama T et al (2014) Antitumor activity of the selective ALK inhibitor alectinib in models of intracranial metastases. Cancer Chemother Pharmacol 74(5):1023–1028
91. Gadgeel SM et al (2016) Pooled analysis of CNS response to Alectinib in two studies of pre-treated patients with ALK-positive non-small-cell lung cancer. J Clin Oncol 34(34):4079–4085
92. Novello S et al (2018) Alectinib versus chemotherapy in crizotinib-pretreated anaplastic lymphoma kinase (ALK)-positive non-small-cell lung cancer: results from the phase III ALUR study. Ann Oncol 29(6):1409–1416
93. Peters S et al (2017) Alectinib versus Crizotinib in untreated ALK-positive non-small-cell lung cancer. N Engl J Med 377(9):829–838
94. Lin JJ et al (2019) Efficacy of Alectinib in patients with ALK-positive NSCLC and symptomatic or large CNS metastases. J Thorac Oncol 14(4):683–690
95. Kim D-W et al (2016) Activity and safety of ceritinib in patients with ALK-rearranged non-small-cell lung cancer (ASCEND-1): updated results from the multicentre, open-label, phase 1 trial. Lancet Oncol 17(4):452–463
96. Shaw AT et al (2017) Ceritinib versus chemotherapy in patients with ALK-rearranged non-small-cell lung cancer previously given chemotherapy and crizotinib (ASCEND-5): a randomised, controlled, open-label, phase 3 trial. Lancet Oncol 18(7):874–886
97. Soria J-C et al (2017) First-line ceritinib versus platinum-based chemotherapy in advanced ALK-rearranged non-small-cell lung cancer (ASCEND-4): a randomised, open-label, phase 3 study. Lancet 389(10072):917–929

98. Kim DW et al (2017) Brigatinib in patients with Crizotinib-refractory anaplastic lymphoma kinase-positive non-small-cell lung cancer: a randomized, multicenter phase II trial. J Clin Oncol 35(22):2490–2498

99. Camidge DR et al (2018) Brigatinib versus Crizotinib in ALK-positive non-small-cell lung cancer. N Engl J Med 379(21):2027–2039

100. Shaw AT et al (2017) Lorlatinib in non-small-cell lung cancer with ALK or ROS1 rearrangement: an international, multicentre, open-label, single-arm first-in-man phase 1 trial. Lancet Oncol 18(12):1590–1599

101. Solomon BJ et al (2018) Lorlatinib in patients with ALK-positive non-small-cell lung cancer: results from a global phase 2 study. Lancet Oncol 19(12):1654–1667

102. Solomon B et al (2020) LBA2 Lorlatinib vs crizotinib in the first-line treatment of patients (pts) with advanced ALK-positive non-small cell lung cancer (NSCLC): results of the phase III CROWN study. Ann Oncol 31:S1180–S1181

103. Goodman A Lorlatinib improves outcomes over Crizotinib in first-line setting of ALK-positive NSCLC: CROWN trial. In: The ASCO post 2020. HSP News Service, L.L.C

104. Selvaggi G et al (2020) ID:1882 phase III randomized study of Ensartinib vs Crizotinib in anaplastic lymphoma kinase (ALK) POSITIVE NSCLC patients: eXalt3. J Thorac Oncol 15(10):e41–e42

105. Solomon B et al (2017) OA 05.06 phase 2 study of Lorlatinib in patients with advanced ALK+/ROS1+ non-small-cell lung cancer. J Thorac Oncol 12(11):S1756

106. Lim SM et al (2017) Open-label, multicenter, phase II study of Ceritinib in patients with non-small-cell lung cancer harboring ROS1 rearrangement. J Clin Oncol 35(23):2613–2618

107. Drilon A et al (2020) Entrectinib in ROS1 fusion-positive non-small-cell lung cancer: integrated analysis of three phase 1–2 trials. Lancet Oncol 21(2):261–270

108. Drilon A et al (2018) Frequency of brain metastases and multikinase inhibitor outcomes in patients with RET-rearranged lung cancers. J Thorac Oncol 13(10):1595–1601

109. Lin JJ et al (2016) Clinical activity of Alectinib in advanced RET-rearranged non-small cell lung Cancer. J Thorac Oncol 11(11):2027–2032

110. Velcheti V et al (2017) OA 12.07 LOXO-292, a potent, highly selective RET inhibitor, in MKI-resistant RET fusion-positive lung cancer patients with and without brain metastases. J Thorac Oncol 12(11):S1778

111. Guo R et al (2019) Response to selective RET inhibition with LOXO-292 in a patient with RET fusion-positive lung cancer with leptomeningeal metastases. JCO Precis Oncol 3:1

112. Drilon A et al (2020) Efficacy of Selpercatinib in RET fusion-positive non-small-cell lung cancer. N Engl J Med 383(9):813–824

113. Falchook GS et al (2012) Dabrafenib in patients with melanoma, untreated brain metastases, and other solid tumours: a phase 1 dose-escalation trial. Lancet 379(9829):1893–1901

114. Davies MA et al (2017) Dabrafenib plus trametinib in patients with BRAFV600-mutant melanoma brain metastases (COMBI-MB): a multicentre, multicohort, open-label, phase 2 trial. Lancet Oncol 18(7):863–873

115. Planchard D et al (2016) Dabrafenib in patients with BRAFV600E-positive advanced non-small-cell lung cancer: a single-arm, multicentre, open-label, phase 2 trial. Lancet Oncol 17(5):642–650

116. Planchard D et al (2016) Dabrafenib plus trametinib in patients with previously treated BRAFV600E-mutant metastatic non-small cell lung cancer: an open-label, multicentre phase 2 trial. Lancet Oncol 17(7):984–993

117. Planchard D et al (2017) Dabrafenib plus trametinib in patients with previously untreated BRAFV600E-mutant metastatic non-small-cell lung cancer: an open-label, phase 2 trial. Lancet Oncol 18(10):1307–1316

118. Robinson SD et al (2014) BRAF V600E-mutated lung adenocarcinoma with metastases to the brain responding to treatment with vemurafenib. Lung Cancer 85(2):326–330

119. Yamamoto G et al (2019) Response of BRAF(V600E)-mutant lung adenocarcinoma with brain metastasis and leptomeningeal dissemination to Dabrafenib plus Trametinib treatment. J Thorac Oncol 14(5):e97–e99

120. Pardoll DM (2012) The blockade of immune checkpoints in cancer immunotherapy. Nat Rev Cancer 12(4):252–264

121. Drugs FDA approved for lung cancer (2019, Sept 18) [cited 2019 October 10, 2019]; Available from: https://www.cancer.gov/about-cancer/treatment/drugs/lung#1

122. Hellmann MD et al (2019) Nivolumab plus Ipilimumab in advanced non-small-cell lung Cancer. N Engl J Med 381(21):2020–2031

123. Reck M et al (2020) Nivolumab (NIVO) + ipilimumab (IPI) + 2 cycles of platinum-doublet chemotherapy (chemo) vs 4 cycles chemo as first-line (1L) treatment (tx) for stage IV/recurrent non-small cell lung cancer (NSCLC): CheckMate 9LA. J Clin Oncol 38(15_suppl):9501

124. Reardon DA et al (2016) Glioblastoma eradication following immune checkpoint blockade in an orthotopic, immunocompetent model. Cancer Immunol Res 4(2):124–135

125. Berghoff AS, Preusser M (2018) New developments in brain metastases. Ther Adv Neurol Disord 11:1756286418785502

126. Borghaei H et al (2015) Nivolumab versus docetaxel in advanced nonsquamous non–small-cell lung cancer. N Engl J Med 373(17):1627–1639

127. Goldman JW et al (2016) Nivolumab (nivo) in patients (pts) with advanced (adv) NSCLC and central nervous system (CNS) metastases (mets). J Clin Oncol 34(15_suppl):9038

128. Reck M et al (2016) Pembrolizumab versus chemotherapy for PD-L1–positive non–small-cell. Lung Cancer 375(19):1823–1833

129. Gandhi L et al (2018) Pembrolizumab plus chemotherapy in metastatic non-small-cell lung cancer. N Engl J Med 378(22):2078–2092

130. Garassino MC et al (2019) Abstract CT043: outcomes among patients (pts) with metastatic nonsquamous NSCLC with liver metastases or brain metastases treated with pembrolizumab (pembro) plus pemetrexed-platinum: results from the KEYNOTE-189 study. 79(13 Supplement):CT043

131. Rittmeyer A et al (2017) Atezolizumab versus docetaxel in patients with previously treated non-small-cell lung cancer (OAK): a phase 3, open-label, multicentre randomised controlled trial. Lancet 389(10066):255–265

132. Gadgeel SM et al (2019) Atezolizumab in patients with advanced non-small cell lung cancer and history of asymptomatic, treated brain metastases: exploratory analyses of the phase III OAK study. Lung Cancer 128:105–112

133. Lukas RV et al (2017) Safety and efficacy analyses of atezolizumab in advanced non-small cell lung cancer (NSCLC) patients with or without baseline brain metastases. Ann Oncol 28:1128

134. Crino L et al (2019) Nivolumab and brain metastases in patients with advanced non-squamous non-small cell lung cancer. Lung Cancer 129:35–40

135. Cortinovis D et al (2019) Italian cohort of the Nivolumab EAP in squamous NSCLC: efficacy and safety in patients with CNS metastases. Anticancer Res 39(8):4265–4271

136. Molinier O et al (2017) OA 17.05 IFCT-1502 CLINIVO: real-life experience with Nivolumab in 600 patients (pts) with advanced Non-Small Cell Lung Cancer (NSCLC). J Thorac Oncol 12(11):S1793

137. Hendriks LEL et al (2019) Outcome of patients with non-small cell lung Cancer and brain metastases treated with checkpoint inhibitors. J Thorac Oncol 14:1244

138. Demaria S, Formenti SC (2012) Role of T lymphocytes in tumor response to radiotherapy. Front Oncol 2:95

139. Sharabi AB et al (2015) Radiation and checkpoint blockade immunotherapy: radiosensitisation and potential mechanisms of synergy. Lancet Oncol 16(13):e498–e509

140. Demaria S, Golden EB, Formenti SC (2015) Role of local radiation therapy in cancer immunotherapy. JAMA Oncol 1(9):1325

141. Gupta A et al (2012) Radiotherapy promotes tumor-specific effector CD8+ T cells via dendritic cell activation. J Immunol 189(2):558–566
142. Herter-Sprie GS et al (2016) Synergy of radiotherapy and PD-1 blockade in Kras-mutant lung cancer. JCI Insight 1(9):e87415
143. Shaverdian N et al (2017) Previous radiotherapy and the clinical activity and toxicity of pembrolizumab in the treatment of non-small-cell lung cancer: a secondary analysis of the KEYNOTE-001 phase 1 trial. Lancet Oncol 18(7):895–903
144. Ahmed KA et al (2017) Outcomes targeting the PD-1/PD-L1 axis in conjunction with stereotactic radiation for patients with non-small cell lung cancer brain metastases. J Neuro-Oncol 133(2):331–338
145. Williams NL et al (2017) Phase 1 study of Ipilimumab combined with whole brain radiation therapy or radiosurgery for melanoma patients with brain metastases. Int J Radiat Oncol Biol Phys 99(1):22–30
146. Anderson ES et al (2017) Melanoma brain metastases treated with stereotactic radiosurgery and concurrent pembrolizumab display marked regression; efficacy and safety of combined treatment. J Immunother Cancer 5(1):76
147. Lehrer EJ et al (2018) Stereotactic radiosurgery and immune checkpoint inhibitors in the management of brain metastases. Int J Mol Sci 19(10):3054
148. Lehrer EJ et al (2019) Treatment of brain metastases with stereotactic radiosurgery and immune checkpoint inhibitors: an international meta-analysis of individual patient data. Radiother Oncol 130:104–112
149. Schoenfeld JD et al (2015) Ipilmumab and cranial radiation in metastatic melanoma patients: a case series and review. J Immunother Cancer 3:50
150. Chen L et al (2018) Concurrent immune checkpoint inhibitors and stereotactic radiosurgery for brain metastases in non-small cell lung cancer, melanoma, and renal cell carcinoma. Int J Radiat Oncol Biol Phys 100(4):916–925
151. Colaco RJ et al (2016) Does immunotherapy increase the rate of radiation necrosis after radiosurgical treatment of brain metastases? J Neurosurg 125(1):17–23

Chapter 7
Spectrum and Management of Immune Related Adverse Events Due to Immune Checkpoint Inhibitors

Marianne Davies and Armand Russo

Abstract The use of immune checkpoint inhibitors (ICPIs) is expanding rapidly to many cancer subtypes. Clinical practice is dominated by the use of these agents. The spectrum of immune-related adverse events (irAEs) due to ICPIs during cancer treatment is vast. Both anti-PD-1/PD-L1 and anti-CTLA-4 checkpoint inhibitors can have off target effects leading to immune system to attack any organ system. The timing of the toxicity is difficult to predict. The degree of severity is variable but can be fatal. Toxicity therefore needs to be evaluated for early and often during the course of treatment and managed at the earliest present signs to avoid life-threatening organ failure. It is vitally important that practitioners of modern oncology know the underlying basis of toxicity, how to identify and grade severity, and manage organ pathophysiology. In this chapter, a review of the incidence, mechanisms of immune related adverse events, and risk factors will be explored. The focus will be the in-depth review of features and management of toxicity by organ system.

Keywords Immunotherapy related toxicities (IRAES) · Immunosuppression · Corticosteroids · Autoimmune disease · Pneumonitis · Colitis · Endocrinopathy · Myocarditis · Dermatitis · Nephritis · Hepatitis · Hypothyroidism · Toxicity · Inflammation · Neuropathy

1 Introduction

FDA approvals for immune checkpoint inhibitors have increased rapidly in the first decade of the twentieth century. There are nine disease areas with more than one FDA approved indication in the first line of therapy and beyond [142]. By therapy, for instance, the anti-PD1 agent pembrolizumab has 20 approvals for diseases as

M. Davies (✉) · A. Russo
Department of Medicine (Medical Oncology), Yale School of Medicine/Yale Cancer Center,
New Haven, CT, USA
e-mail: marianne.davies@yale.edu

© Springer Nature Switzerland AG 2021
A. C. Chiang, R. S. Herbst (eds.), *Lung Cancer*, Current Cancer Research,
https://doi.org/10.1007/978-3-030-74028-3_7

heterogeneous as squamous head and neck cancer, melanoma, relapsed/refractory Hodgkin's lymphoma, primary mediastinal B cell lymphoma, and non-small cell lung cancer. In addition, ICPI approval for mismatch repair deficiency/microsatellite instability high (MMRd/MSI-H) tumors is agnostic to disease and has been used in recent years in colon cancer and ovarian cancer that harbor acquired or hereditary loss of mismatch repair proteins and microsatellite stability. It is clear that ICPIs have tied together disparate diseases by exploiting a common mechanism for treatment. Due to the ubiquitous use of ICPIs in modern cancer therapy, the need for education and appropriate management of toxicities is paramount.

1.1   Clinical Scenario

A 61-year old man with 50-pack-year smoking history presented to clinic with a right-upper lobe lesion measuring 2.5 cm, with 2 cm enlargement of several ipsilateral paratracheal lymph nodes as well as left axillary lymph nodes, and a destructive C4 vertebral lesion requiring surgical stabilization. These lesions were avid on PET/CT imaging. The surgical specimen from the cervical spine fixation showed adenocarcinoma, consistent with lung primary. PDL1 was 90% in tumor cells from the vertebral surgical biopsy. The patient enrolled on clinical trial and as part of his trial therapy, he received pembrolizumab with flat dosing of 200 mg every 3 weeks. Unfortunately, after the third dose, 9 weeks from beginning therapy, the patient experienced nausea, vomiting, severe fatigue, abdominal discomfort, and diarrhea (four liquid stools per day). The ALT and AST had increased to 4-times the upper limit of normal, with concomitant 4-fold increase in alkaline phosphatase. The patient had to discontinue trial therapy due to his toxicities.

International oncology organizations such as the NCCN, ASCO, SITC, and ESMO each have contributed to expert guidance on the management of ICPI toxicity. The Journal of the NCCN [140], Journal of Clinical Oncology [21], Journal of Immunology of Cancer [111] and Annals of Clinical Oncology [53] contain expert written guidance for practitioners. These will be reviewed throughout this chapter.

In what follows, we will review the diagnosis, grading and management of organ-specific toxicities from ICPIs. The goal of this review is to provide a universal resource for identifying and managing potentially life-threatening toxicities in all clinical settings. The case above will be discussed in the conclusion.

1.2 Mechanism of Immune Related Adverse Events Due to Immune Checkpoint Inhibitors

Tumorigenesis is a multiphase process that unleashes cellular growth and metastasis. One process that supports tumorigenesis is the tumor's ability to evade surveillance of the body's immune system by exploiting checkpoint pathways. Immune checkpoints *in vivo* prevent T-cell activation, proliferation and mediated inflammation. Tumors can exploit these natural checkpoints, preventing recognition by and promoting exhaustion of T-cells. Immune checkpoint inhibitors (ICPI), such as anti-CTLA-4 and anti-PD-1/L1 inhibitors, block these exhaustion pathways, allowing for anti-tumor immune response [58]. In the process, collateral uncontrolled inflammation of any body tissue and development of adverse events can occur. In other words, the activation of the immune system for anti-tumor response is not only confined to the tumor. ICPIs can lead to off-target tissue damage. These result in irAEs due to unwanted strength and breadth of T cell activation. Many studies have noted clinically meaningful anti-tumor targeting and concurrent burden of irAEs [11].

The pathophysiology of off-target immune effects of ICPIs is not fully elucidated but requires multistep processes linking the reversal of immune cell exhaustion and activation to normal body tissues. Several concepts help guide thinking about immune activation and toxicity. Amplification of the T cell response; increase in pre-existing auto-antibodies; production of new auto-antibodies; enhanced complement mediated activation with inhibition of CTLA-4; epitope spreading whereby primed T cells begin to recognize a wider swath of antigens from the initial T cell response; and dysbiosis with exposure of microbiome antigens that spur self-directed immunity are examples of these guiding concepts [89, 109, 128, 133]. Underlying HLA polymorphisms are also thought to contribute to pathophysiology [71, 72]. Anti-CTLA4 expression in the hypothalamus serves as a target for antibody, cell-mediated cytotoxicity with use of ipilimumab [64]. Vitiligo occurs in melanoma patients being treated with ICPIs as an example of T-cell cross-reactivity of malignant antigens with normal melanocytic antigens [106, 155]. The gut microbiome, particularly with *Bacteroides* genus in anti-CTLA-4 blockade and *Bifidobacterium* in anti-PD-L1 blockade, enhances tumor killing [127, 144]. Antibiotic exposure prior to and during ICPI therapy attenuates the normal gut microbiome, impacting negatively on progression free survival, overall survival and reduced response rates in patients with NSCLC compared to patients not receiving antibiotics [49, 108, 116].

1.3   Incidence of IRAEs by Agent and in Combination

Immune-related adverse events (irAEs) occur in up to 90% of patients treated with ICPI, with more severe toxicities occurring in up to 13% [77]. IrAEs occur more frequently and with greater severity with anti-CTLA-4 inhibitors that act in the primary lymphatic tissue, compared with anti-PD1/L-1 inhibitors that are active in the peripheral tissue and tumor microenvironment, with the highest irAE with combination blockade [10, 20, 39, 46, 55, 109].

The incidence of all grade irAEs reported is 60–90% for anti-CTLA-4 inhibitors versus 39–70% with anti-PD-1/L-1 [20, 28]. The rate of grade ≥3 reported is 14% with anti-PD-1/L1 inhibitors, 34% with anti-CTLA-4 inhibitors, 55% with combination ICPI and 46% with combination ICPI and chemotherapy [10, 50]. Higher grade irAEs can lead to severe morbidity and fatality [69, 89]. GI toxicity described as diarrhea, for instance, is higher with anti-CTLA-4 inhibitors than for anti-PD-1 (35% vs 13%) [128]. The leading causes of fatality are gastrointestinal, pulmonary, cardiac and hepatic toxicity, with higher fatal toxicity associated with the anti-CTLA-4 inhibitor ipilimumab versus anti-PD-1 inhibitors [66, 149]. Fatality rates with anti-PD-1, anti-CTLA-4 and anti-PD-1+CTLA-4 are from 0.25% to 1% for each [99]. IrAEs usually present within weeks to months after initiation of treatment, however, some can develop even after cessation of therapy [39, 68, 109].

Resumption of ICPI after toxicity requires clinical judgment. IrAEs are expected in about 28% of patients being re-challenged [45]. The risk appears higher for resumption after hepatitis (OR 3.38; CI, 1.31–8.74; $P = .01$), colitis (OR 1.77; CI, 1.14–2.75; $P = .01$) and pneumonitis (OR 2.26; CI, 1.18–4.32; $P = .01$). Time to re-appearance of the toxicity was similar to the time to initial appearance. Re-challenge was much more frequent after endocrine toxicities than other toxicities such as pneumonitis or colitis, given the higher risk of fatal outcomes of these toxicities when they do recur.

1.4   Biomarkers to Identify Patients at Risk for Developing IRAEs

Currently no predictive markers are used routinely to anticipate irAEs [61]. Age is not a predictive factor for toxicity as demonstrated in a study of 254 patients with metastatic melanoma treated with anti-PD-1 therapy [18]. In a study of 184 non-small cell lung cancer patients, the occurrence of any irAE was associated with low baseline blood neutrophil-lymphocyte ratio (L-NLR) and platelet-to-lymphocyte ratio (L-PLR) [105]. Among patients with L-PLR, the percentage that developed irAE was 42.9% versus 21.3% among patients with high-PLR. L-PLR was also associated with improved PFS.

2 Management of Immune-Related Adverse Events Due to Immune Checkpoint Inhibitors (ICPIs)

Effective management of irAEs depends on early recognition and intervention. Expert consensus clinical practice guidelines (CPGs), extrapolated from treatment of autoimmune diseases, clinical trials and case reports, have been developed by professional organizations as recommendations for the management of irAEs [1, 21, 53, 54, 109, 111, 140]. The Common Terminology Criteria for Adverse Events (CTCAE) tool is used as a reference to describe and grade the severity of each irAE [141]. Guideline interventions are based on the severity or grade of irAE. The goal of the intervention is to resolve the irAE without negating the therapeutic benefit of the ICPI therapy. Mild (grade 1) irAEs can be managed with supportive and symptomatic measures, close monitoring and in most cases, continuation of ICPI therapy. ICPI therapy is held for moderate (grade 2) irAEs and permanently discontinued for severe (grade 3–4) irAEs.

Corticosteroid immunosuppressant therapy with methylprednisolone (0.5–2.0 mg/kg/day) is the foundation of treatment of grade 2 and higher irAEs because of the rapid onset and anti-inflammatory effects [39, 86, 114]. Dosing continues until the irAE is improved to grade 1. Corticosteroids are then tapered down slowly over a minimum of 4 weeks to prevent relapse of the irAE. In some cases, the taper may take weeks to months [126, 140]. Patients will require ongoing assessment of potential side-effects from the corticosteroids such as weight gain, hyperglycemia, hypertension, gastritis, opportunistic infections, muscle atrophy and skin fragility and mood disturbances.

Gastritis and indigestion can be reduced by taking the steroid with food and with a H2 blocker. Anti-microbial prophylaxis with trimethoprim/sulfamethoxazole DS TIW can reduce the risk of opportunistic infections such as pneumocystis jiroveci prophylaxis (PJP) [13]. If patients have a sulfa allergy, atovaquone may be prescribed. The use of PPIs and trimethoprim/sulfamethoxazole carry a risk for acute interstitial nephritis, so kidney function must be monitored closely [126]. Proton pump inhibitors should be avoided, as some studies suggest that use of PPIs may negatively impact overall survival of patients with NSCLC treated with ICPI therapy [27]. Antiviral and antifungal coverage may be recommended in patients requiring long term steroid therapy. Calcium and vitamin D are recommended to reduce the risk of osteoporosis.

Re-initiation of ICPI therapy can be considered cautiously for grade 2 irAEs, as there is a risk for recurrence of the irAE upon rechallenge [121, 125]. If an irAE is refractory to corticosteroid therapy, additional or alternative immunosuppressant therapy may be required. Hyperactivated regulatory T cells may release additional cytokines, such as tumor necrosis factor-alpha (TNF-α), which induce additional proflammatory cytokines that contribute to the inflammatory response in tissues and organs [104]. TNF-α has been found in high concentrations in patients that have developed refractory CTLA-4 induced colitis [30]. Infliximab, an TNF-α inhibitor, is generally the recommended treatment, with the exception of certain contraindications including hepatitis, active tuberculosis infection, gastrointestinal perforation, and congestive heart failure [21, 39, 53, 54, 109, 111, 114, 124, 140]. Infliximab is dosed at 5 mg/kg/IV and may be repeated in 2 weeks if symptoms persist. Corticosteroid administration continues until the irAE is grade 1 or less. If time allows, testing for TB, HIV, hepatitis A & B is recommended in patients at high risk for those infections. Additional immunomodulating agents include mycophenolate mofetil (MMF), IVIG, cyclophosphamide, methotrexate, antithymocyte globulin (ATG), tocilizumab, rituximab and others [21, 86, 140, 147].

Corticosteroid use after the onset of irAEs does not interfere with response rates or overall survival [62, 80, 122]. Nor does the use of additional immunosuppressive agents for steroid refractory irAEs negatively impact survival benefit [23, 62, 147]. However, baseline use of steroids > prednisone 10 mg/day or the use of steroids for cancer-related symptoms is associated with decreased ORR, PFS and overall survival in patients with NSCLC [9, 43]. Specific management algorithms for each organ specific irAE, will be outlined in more detail below.

3 Organ Specific Immune-Related Adverse Events

3.1 Dermatologic

Dermatologic symptoms are the most common irAE reported, occurring in 8–21% receiving ipilimumab, 18% PD-1/PD-L1 inhibitors and 40% combination [79, 114], with median onset of 4–8 weeks [39, 153]. Dermatologic irAEs can include maculopapular rash, pruritis, erythema, mucositis, vitiligo and lichenoid eruptions [34]. Pruritis typically precedes rash or it may present alone. Other causes of dermatologic toxicities should be evaluated. These include: contact dermatitis, flare of eczema/psoriasis, viral illness, infection and other drug toxicity (ie, due to combination chemotherapy, targeted therapies, antibiotics). A complete skin exam should be performed including mucosal areas to define the body surface area (BSA) affected. Grade 1 rash is described as <10% of BSA distribution and can be treated with mild to moderate strength topical steroids. Grade 2 rash covers 10–30% BSA, should be treated with moderate strength topical steroids, with consideration of systemic oral steroids. ICPI therapy can be continued for low grade dermatologic toxicities. However, ICPI therapy should be held for grade 3–4, with initiation of systemic intravenous steroids and referral to dermatologist. Antihistamines, GABA agonists, NK-1 receptor inhibitors, antidepressants or omalizumab may be used for severe pruritis [139]. Severe and potentially life-threatening dermatologic reactions, though rare, require permanent discontinuation of ICPI and aggressive medical intervention. These include Steven-Johnson syndrome, toxic epidermal necrolysis (TEN), drug induced rash with eosinophilia and systemic symptoms (DRESS) and acute febrile neutrophilic dermatosis (Sweet syndrome) [15, 111].

Grade based recommendation for rash and pruritis management are outlined in Table 7.1.

3.2 Gastrointestinal

Gastrointestinal irAEs include diarrhea, colitis, anorexia, nausea, mucositis, esophagitis, gastritis and pancreatic dysfunction. Diarrhea and/or colitis are the second most commonly reported irAEs, with median time to onset at 6–8 weeks of treatment [39, 153]. Colitis may develop or recur even after the discontinuation of ICPI therapy [31]. Diarrhea occurs in 20–32% of NSCLC patients receiving ICPI [8, 56, 78]. Diarrhea/colitis occur more frequently with anti-CTLA-4 monotherapy (54%) than with PD-1/PD-L1 inhibitors (11–19%), with highest incidence in patients treated with combination anti-CTLA-4 and PD-1/PD-L1 inhibitors [2, 52]. The incidence of colitis, characterized by abdominal pain or endoscopic evidence of colon inflammation, 1–1.9% with anti-PD-1/PD-L1 agents [57, 112], with increase to 3–12% with combination anti-PD-1 and anti-CTLA-4 therapy [8, 56, 78]. The incidence of all grade colitis in patients with non-small cell lung cancer (1.52%) is increased when receiving anti-PD-1/PD-L1 therapy in the first line versus second line setting (1.88% vs 0.78%) [81].

Patients may present with watery stools, abdominal cramping, urgency, abdominal pain, blood and mucous in the stool, increased bloating, abdominal distension, fever. It is important to assess for baseline bowel pattern prior to the start of therapy, as patients with chronic or opioid induced constipation, may present with differing patterns of irAEs. Clinicians should calculate the frequency and volume of stools in 24 hours, including ostomy output and incontinence.

Practitioners should assess for other possible causes of diarrhea including dietary intake, infectious etiology, other inflammatory etiology, medication side-effects (ie, antibiotics, stool softeners and laxatives). The chronic use of non-steroidal anti-inflammatory drugs (NSAIDS), proton pump inhibitors (PPI) and selective serotonin reuptake inhibitors (SSRI) leads to increased risk of microscopic colitis [22, 145]. Laboratory tests of complete blood count, complete metabolic panel, erythrocyte sedimentation rate (ESR), C-reactive protein (CRP). Bacterial and viral stool cultures leucocytes, ova/parasites, viral PCR, Clostridium difficile toxin, CMV and cryptosporidia) should be obtained to rule out infectious causes. Abdominal/pelvic CT scan is useful to evaluate for colonic wall thickening with immune related colitis. Colonoscopy and/or endoscopy are recommended to evaluate the extent and severity of colitis [60, 148]. Fecal lactoferrin and calprotectin, stool inflammatory biomarkers, help to differentiate functional versus inflammatory diarrhea and may help identify patients likely to have mucosal ulceration on endoscopy and predict poor responsiveness to corticosteroid therapy [148].

Mild grade 1 diarrhea/colitis can be treated with antidiarrheal agents such as loperamide and diphenoxylate atropine sulfate. Corticosteroids are recommended for grade 2 or higher diarrhea, with taper over 4–6 weeks after resolution to grade 1.

Table 7.1 Dermatologic toxicity: rash & pruritis

Assessment	Assess for history of prior dermatologic conditions (i.e. eczema, psoriasis) Comprehensive skin exam including mucosa prior to therapy and with each treatment Assess for blistering and lymphedema Documentation of rash with photos Rule out other causes: viral illness, infection, other drug rash, contact dermatitis; flare of eczema, psoriasis Laboratory: CBC, CMP, LFTs, Serologic testing for autoimmune skin disorders If autoimmune disorder suspected, obtain antinuclear antibody test			
Grade	1	2	3	4
	Macules/ papules covering <10% of BSA with or without symptoms (e.g. pruritus, burning, tightness) No impact on quality of life	Macules/papules covering 10–30% of BSA with or without symptoms (e.g. pruritis, burning, tightness) Limiting instrumental activities of daily living (IADLs)	Macules/papules covering >30% BSA with or without symptoms Limiting selfcare ADL	Papulopustular rash associated with life-threatening superinfection Stevens-Johnson syndrome, TEN and bullous dermatitis covering >30% of BSA requiring ICU admission
Medical management	Continue ICPI Topical steroids (mild to moderate strength) cream ± oral or topical antihistamines for pruritis	Consider holding ICPI Topical steroids (moderate strength) ± oral or topical antihistamines for pruritis Consider initiation of prednisone (or equivalent) 0.5–1.0 mg/kg/ day Consider dermatology consult Monitor weekly. If unresponsive, treat as G3	HOLD ICPI Topical high potency steroid cream Initiate IV methylprednisolone 0.5–1.0 mg/kg Consult with dermatology Consider skin biopsy Resume when grade 1	HOLD ICPI Initiate IV methylprednisolone 1.0–2.0 mg/kg Urgent dermatology consultation Consider inpatient admission Consider resuming ICPI when grade 1 and steroids have been reduced to prednisone equivalent ≤10 mg/day
Supportive interventions	Avoid skin irritants Avoid sun exposure Topical emollients GABA agonists, aprepitant or omalizumab for pruritis Oral/IV antibiotics for superinfection			

Data from: AIMwithImmunotherapy Essentials [1], Brahmer [21], Haanen [53, 54], Thompson [139, 140], and US Dept. HHS [141]
Abbreviations: *BSA* Body Surface Area, *TEN* Toxic Epidermal Necrolysis, *CBC* Complete Blood Count, *CMP* Complete Metabolic Panel, *LFTs* Liver Function Tests

If diarrhea is refractory to corticosteroid therapy, additional immunosuppressant therapy with infliximab is recommended with repeat dosing 2 weeks following the first if needed [21, 139]. Initiation of infliximab within 10 days of colitis may shorten the duration of symptoms, reduce hospitalizations and steroid taper failure [4]. Vedolizumab, a monoclonal antibody immunosuppressant that targets the gastrointestinal tract is recommended for patients' refractory to infliximab [16]. Emerging data suggests earlier initiation ($\leq$10 days) of alternative immunosuppressant agents (e.g. infliximab, vedolizumab), without waiting for failure of steroid therapy, leads to more favorable outcomes including shorter duration of symptoms, hospitalization stay and steroid use, as well as reduced rate of steroid failure [4, 70].

Reported rates of pancreatic dysfunction with > grade 3 serum lipase and/or amylase elevations are 0.9–3% with anti-CTLA-4 agent and 0.5–4% with anti-PD-L/L-1 and 1.2–8% with combination [5, 56, 57, 78, 112, 130]. The median time to observation of laboratory abnormalities is 46 days for anti-PD-L/L-1 and 69 days for anti-CTLA-4 monotherapy. Clinically, patients are typically asymptomatic with normal pancreatic imaging and incidental laboratory abnormalities. Patients with prior history of pancreatitis, type II diabetes and excessive alcohol use may be at higher risk [5]. Lipase levels typically improve to baseline with temporary hold of ICPI therapy [60]. If the toxicity progresses to acute pancreatitis, immunosuppressant therapy is indicated.

Grade based recommendations for diarrhea/colitis management are outlined in Table 7.2.

3.3 Pulmonary

The rates of reported pneumonitis ranges from 5% to 19%, with 1–2% with grade 3 and 4 pneumonitis [48, 57, 96]. The incidence is higher in anti-PD-L1 monotherapy over anti-PD-1 and anti-CTLA-4 monotherapies, and combination anti-PD-1/PD-L1 with anti-CTLA-4 [96–98, 100, 107, 154]. Though relatively rare, pneumonitis is one of the most common causes of irAE related fatalities. Higher rates of pneumonitis occur in patients with history of smoking, pre-existing lung disease, NSCLC and the elderly [74, 93, 98]. Treatment naïve patients develop pneumonitis at higher rates compared with those previously treated (4.3% vs 2.8%) [74]. Patients with NSCLC are at increased risk of high-grade pneumonitis, death from pneumonitis [100] and poorer overall survival [32, 48, 131, 132]. Low serum albumin was shown to be a predictor of pneumonitis in NSCLC in one study [48]. The median time to onset is 2–24 months [97, 100]. Presenting symptoms may be subtle, including new and worsening cough, dyspnea, fever, chest pain, wheezing, worsening hypoxia (oxygen saturation <90% on room air) and increasing supplemental oxygen requirements. In some cases, pneumonitis may appear on CT scan prior to the onset of noticeable symptoms. Symptoms may mimic other pulmonary conditions such as pulmonary metastasis, lymphangitic disease progression, infection, pulmonary embolism and pleural effusion.

Table 7.2 Gastrointestinal-diarrhea ± colitis

Assessment	Calculate frequency and volume of stools in 24 hours, including ostomy output and incontinence. Medication reconciliation to rule out other contributors to diarrhea/colitis: antibiotics, stool softeners, laxatives, NSAIDS, PPI, SSRI Obtain blood (CBC, CMP, LFTs, CRP, TSH) to rule out infection and electrolyte imbalances. Stool lactoferrin and Calprotectin biomarkers Stool cultures to rule out other causes (leucocytes, ova & parasites, viral PCR, *Clostridium Difficile* toxin, CMV and cryptosporidium) Consider abdominal/pelvic CT scan Consider colonoscopy and or endoscopy			
Grade	1	2	3	4
	<4 stools/day or increase in ostomy output over baseline Asymptomatic	4–6 liquid/soft stools/day or moderate increase in ostomy output over baseline Abdominal pain, blood or mucous in stool	≥7 stools/day; In continence; Significant increase in ostomy output over baseline. Interference with ADLs	Peritoneal signs; Life-threatening
Medical management	Observation; Anti-motility agents (loperamide or oral diphenoxylate atropine sulfate) once infection is ruled out Budesonide Anti-spasmodic	HOLD ICPI; Prednisone 1 mg/kg/day; If no response in 2–3 days, increased dose of steroid and consider infliximab Consider gastroenterology consult	Discontinue anti-CTLA-4; PD1/PD-L1 may be resumed after recovery to G1	Permanently discontinue ICPI
			Gastroenterology consult. Consider inpatient care; Intravenous methylprednisolone 1–2 mg/kg/day; If no response in 2–3 days, continue steroids and consider adding infliximab; If refractory, or infliximab is contraindicated, consider vedolizumab	
Supportive interventions	Discontinue stool softeners and laxatives Dietary modifications: bland diet, avoid high fiber/lactose, fats, alcohol, caffeine. NPO if grade 4 Hydration			

Data from: AIMwithImmunotherapy Essentials [1], Brahmer [21], Haanen [53, 54], Thompson [139, 140], and US Dept. HHS [141]

Abbreviations: *CBC* Complete Blood Count, *CMP* Complete Metabolic Panel, *LFTs* Liver Function Tests, *CRP* C-reactive Protein, *ESR* Erythrocyte Sedimentation Rate, *TSH* Thyroid Stimulating Hormone, *CMV* Cytomegalovirus

Pneumonitis can progress rapidly to respiratory failure and death, therefore ICPI should be held for any signs or evidence of pneumonitis, while complete evaluation is undertaken. High-resolution CT scan of chest is recommended when pneumonitis is suspected. The CT scan patterns vary. Diffuse cryptogenic organizing pneumonia pattern is the most common in NSCLC, with reports of unilateral infiltrates, non-specific interstitial pneumonia (NSIP) and hypersensitivity pneumonia (HP) [48,

100]. NSCLC patients with cryptogenic organizing pneumonia pattern have increased likelihood of requiring immunosuppressant therapy [96]. Chronic pneumonitis is described as pneumonitis that persists at end of recommended steroid tapering guidelines, worsens during taper necessitating increased steroid dosing and/or additional immunosuppression and/or necessitates a total duration of immunosuppression of >12 weeks [21, 97, 111, 139, 140] has been reported despite discontinuation of ICPI with down titration of steroids, necessitating a protracted course of immunosuppression. The incidence of chronic pneumonitis in NSCLC is 2% with monotherapy, increased in combination checkpoint therapy, with median duration of steroid taper of 37 weeks [97].

Corticosteroid immunosuppression with methylprednisolone/prednisone 1–2 mg/kg/day should be initiated for grade 2 pneumonitis. Corticosteroid taper can begin when pneumonitis improved to <grade 1. If there is no improvement in 48 hours, increased steroid or additional immunosuppressant therapy with infliximab, mycophenolate mofetil, IVIG or cyclophosphamide should be initiated [21, 97, 111, 139, 140]. Close monitoring of oxygen saturation and CT scan is essential. Pulmonology consult should be initiated when pneumonitis is suspected. An infectious disease consult is warranted if fever, productive cough and suspicion of infection. A bronchoalveolar lavage may be helpful in differentiating irAE pneumonitis from infection or progression of disease [97].

Grade based recommendations for pneumonitis management is outlined in Table 7.3.

3.4 Endocrine

Endocrine irAEs are a unique class toxicity of ICPI therapy affecting thyroid, pituitary and adrenal gland. Thyroid dysfunction occurs more frequently with anti-PD-1/L-1 inhibitors than with anti-CTLA-4 agents (2–10% vs 1.5–6%) and increased in combination therapy (11–23%) in patients with NSCLC [14, 24, 33, 115]. It often begins with thyrotoxicosis (decreased TSH, elevated FT4) and progresses to hypothyroidism within a few weeks, with hypothyroidism the most common endocrine toxicity in patients with NSCLC [42, 57, 112, 115]. Presenting symptoms of thyrotoxicosis/thyroiditis include weight loss, palpitations, heat intolerance, anxiety, diarrhea and other indicators of hypermetabolic activity. Unexplained fatigue, weight gain, cold intolerance, hair loss and depression are noted with hypothyroidism. In patients with NSCLC, treated with pembrolizumab, the median overall survival was significantly longer in patients who developed thyroid dysfunction than those that did not (40 vs 14 months) [103]. The incidence of hypophysitis (inflammation of the pituitary gland) is more prevalent with ipilimumab (1–17%) and combination checkpoint therapy (4–12.8%) over single agent anti-PD-1/L-1 agents (0.2–1.5%) [20, 24, 33, 42]. Hypophysitis may lead to secondary hypothyroidism, secondary adrenal insufficiency and hypogonadism. Primary adrenal insufficiency occurs in <1% with single agent ICPI and 4–8% with combination [33, 57]. Type I

Table 7.3 Pulmonary: pneumonitis

Assessment	Assess for risk factors: prior pulmonary conditions (asthma, COPD, pulmonary hypertension), prior chest radiation, smoking history Monitor pulse oximetry at rest and with ambulation prior to treatment initiation and with each dose of ICPI Rule out other causes: infection, disease progression, lymphangitic spread, pulmonary embolism, pleural effusion, radiation recall, sarcoidosis Laboratory: CBC, sputum culture, screening for viral, bacterial or opportunistic infections Diagnostic Imaging: CXR, CT scan with and without contrast for full differential			
Grade	1	2	3	4
	Radiographic changes only confined to one lobe of lung or <25% of parenchyma; Ground glass opacities, non-specific pneumonia Asymptomatic	Mild/moderate symptoms: dyspnea, chest pain. Involves 25–50% of lung parenchyma Limiting instrumental ADLs Medical intervention indicated	Severe symptoms; New or worsening hypoxia; Involves all lung lobes or >50% of lung parenchyma Limiting self-care ADLs	Life threatening; ARDS Urgent intervention indicated
Medical management	HOLD ICPI Reassess in 1–2 weeks Consider repeat CT in 3–4 weeks; Resume ICPI with radiographic evidence of improvement Monitor pulse oximetry	HOLD ICPI Prednisone 1–2 mg/kg/day and taper by 5–10 mg/week over 4–6 weeks. Pulmonary consult Consider bronchoscopy with bronchoalveolar lavage Consider empiric antibiotics Monitor every 3 days; If no improvement, after 48 hours of prednisone, treat as grade 3	Permanently discontinue ICPI Inpatient admission Methylprednisolone 1–2 mg/kg/day; If no improvement in 48 hours, add infliximab 5 mg/kg or mycophenolate mofetil 1 GM IV BID Pulmonary and infectious disease consult	
Supportive interventions	Provide oxygen support Reduce respiratory irritants Provide smoking cessation support Assure adequate hydration			

Data from: AIMwithImmunotherapy Essentials [1], Brahmer [21], Haanen [53, 54], Thompson [139, 140], and US Dept. HHS [141]

Abbreviations: *COPD* Chronic Obstructive Pulmonary Disease, *ARDS* Acute Respiratory Distress Syndrome, *CBC* Complete Blood Count, *CXR* Chest x-ray diabetes mellitus is a rare irAE, that can present with life-threatening diabetic keto-acidosis [24]. It has been reported in 1.4% of patients treated with ipilimumab, 0.2–0.9% with anti PD-1/L-1 and 5.2–7.6% with combination blockade [33, 42, 90].

The median time to onset of endocrine irAEs is 8–12 weeks. Symptoms may reflect organ specific hormone deficiencies. However, patient may present with vague symptoms of fatigue, weakness, muscle aches, arthralgias, headache, vision changes, heart rate changes, increased sweating, weight gain or loss, increased feelings of hunger or thirst, hair loss, cold or heat intolerance, constipation, diarrhea, nausea, emesis, abdominal discomfort, loss of libido, dizziness, and fainting.

Baseline serum electrolytes, thyroid function tests (TSH, FT4) should be obtained prior to the start of ICPI therapy. Thyroid function tests should then be obtained before each infusion for the first 3 months and then monthly following [21, 53, 139]. If there is suspicion of adrenal or pituitary irAE, additional hormone levels should be obtained (i.e. ACTH, cortisol, FSH, LH, GH, prolactin, estrogen and testosterone). An MRI of the brain with pituitary/sellar cuts is used to diagnose hypophysitis. However, pituitary enlargement is usually seen in the acute phase, but then decreases as loss of function occurs [24, 42].

Endocrine irAEs, especially hypothyroidism and adrenal insufficiency, are chronic, requiring life-time hormone replacement [135]. As these irAEs are usually well controlled with hormone replacement, patients may continue ICPI therapy if deriving clinical benefit and do not require systemic steroids. Patients with diabetes will require insulin support and should be counseled in dietary and life-style modifications. Those with adrenal insufficiency may require mineralocorticoid (fludrocortisone) in addition to glucocorticoid replacement. In the case of adrenal insufficiency and other endocrine IRAEs, steroids must be replaced prior to other hormonal replacement to avoid adrenal crisis [24, 76, 139, 140].

Grade based recommendations for endocrine IRAE management is outlined in Table 7.4.

3.5 Hepatic

The incidence of hepatitis in patients with NSCLC is approximately 2–13% with anti-PD-1/PD-L1 and up to 30% with combination anti-PD-1 plus anti-CTLA-4 [8, 56, 57, 60, 78, 134, 150]. The rate of toxicity may be higher when anti-PD-1/PD-L1 is given in combination with chemotherapy. The range of grade ≥3 is 2–6%. The onset of immune related hepatic dysfunction ranges from 6 to 14 weeks [39, 152].

Immune related hepatic dysfunction is usually detected incidentally on liver function tests with elevation of alanine aminotransferase (ALT) or aspartate aminotransferase (AST) with or without elevation of bilirubin. In the rare severe cases, symptoms may include nausea, emesis, right upper quadrant abdominal pain, drowsiness, jaundice of skin and eyes, dark color urine.

Liver function tests, including ALT, AST, bilirubin and alkaline phosphatase, should be evaluated prior to the start of ICPI therapy and prior to each dose. ICPI

Table 7.4 Endocrine: Thyroid, Pituitary and Adrenal IREA

Hypothyroidism				
Assessment	Laboratory: Obtain baseline thyroid function tests (thyroid stimulating hormone, free T4, free T3) and every 4–6 weeks while on therapy; Once stable, every 6 months Thyroid antibodies Diagnosis: High TSH, normal to low free T4: Primary hypothyroidism Low TSH, low free T4: Secondary to hypophysitis Thyroid antibodies: Thyroid peroxidase (TPO)			
Grade	1	2	3	4
	TSH <10 mIU/L and FT4 normal Asymptomatic	TSH persistent >10 mIU/L Moderate symptoms, able to perform ADLs	Medically significant or life-threatening Severe symptoms Unable to perform ADLs	
Medical management	Observation Continue ICPI Close monitoring of TSH and T4	May hold ICPI until symptoms resolve t baseline Thyroid hormone replacement[a] Consider endocrine consultation	HOLD ICPI until symptoms resolve to baseline with hormone repletion Endocrine consultation May admit for medical management if signs of myxedema (changes in behavior, extreme fatigue, shortness of breath, swelling of hands or feet	
Supportive interventions	[a]For patients with no risk factors, full replacement can be estimate with ideal body weight dosing of 1.6 mcg/kg/day; for elderly or frail with multiple medical comorbidities, titrate dosing starting at 25–50 mcg/day In case of adrenal insufficiency and hypothyroidism, steroids must be given prior to thyroid replacement to prevent adrenal crisis			
Thyrotoxicosis-hyperthyroidism				
Assessment	Laboratory: Baseline thyroid function tests (thyroid stimulating hormone, free T4, free T3) Monitor TSH and FT4 every 4–6 weeks Thyroid antibodies, thyroid stimulating immunoglobulin (TSI), thyroid peroxidase (TPO) antibody Monitor ECG Consider thyroid scan Diagnosis: Low to normal TSH, elevated T4 & T3			
Grade	1	2	3	4
	Asymptomatic or mild symptoms	Moderate symptoms Able to perform ADLs	Severe symptoms Medically significant or life-threatening Unable to perform ADLs	

(continued)

Table 7.4 (continued)

Medical management	Continue ICPI	Consider holding ICPI until symptoms resolve to baseline Consider endocrinology consult	HOLD ICPI until symptoms resolve to baseline with appropriate therapy Endocrinology consult For severe symptoms or concerns for thyroid storm, hospitalize patient and initiate prednisone 1–2 mg/kg/day or equivalent
Supportive interventions	Beta-blockers for symptomatic relief Monitor symptoms closely as thyrotoxicosis usually transitions to hypothyroidism		

Hypophysitis	
Assessment	Evaluate for electrolyte imbalances, specifically hyponatremia; Evaluate for secondary adrenal insufficiency and central hypothyroidism, monitor ACTH, cortisol, TSH, FT4 (low or normal TSH and low free T4; early-morning low ACTH, low cortisol); Evaluate for secondary hypogonadism LH, FSH, prolactin, estradiol in females and testosterone in males. aFull laboratory confirmation cannot be done with morning cortisol if patient is on corticosteroids MRI of brain with pituitary/ sellar cuts

Grade	1	2	3	4
	Asymptomatic or mild symptoms	Moderate symptoms; able to perform ADL	Severe symptoms; medically significant or life-threatening consequences; unable to perform ADL	
Medical management	Consider holding ICPI until patient stabilized on replacement hormone Hormonal supplementation as needed Endocrine consult		HOLD ICPI until patient is stabilized on hormone replacement therapy Hormonal supplementation as needed Endocrine consult Consider initial pulse dose therapy with prednisone 1–2 mg/kg tapered over 2 weeks.	
Supportive interventions	Glucocorticoid and thyroid hormone replacement. Testosterone and estradiol replacement considered In the case of adrenal insufficiency and hypothyroidism, steroids must be given for several days prior to thyroid replacement to avoid adrenal crisis. Instruct patient on stress dosing of steroids for illness; Medical alert bracelet to be worn			

Adrenal insufficiency	

(continued)

Table 7.4 (continued)

Assessment	Assess ACTH and cortisol (low or suppressed morning serum cortisol, high ACTH) monitor for electrolyte disturbances; nausea, vomiting, fatigue, lethargy, confusion or coma. Monitor for adrenal crisis: hypovolemic shock. Consider CT to rule out adrenal metastasis			
Grade	1	2	3	4
	Asymptomatic or mild symptoms	Moderate symptoms Able to perform ADL	Severe symptoms; Medically significant or life-threatening consequences; Unable to perform ALDs	
Medical management	Consider holding ICPI [a]Replacement therapy with prednisone 7.5–10 mg daily (taper to 5 mg daily as able) or hydrocortisone (10–20 mg po every morning, 5–10 mg early afternoon May require fludrocortisone (0.1 mg/d) for mineralocorticoid replacement in primary adrenal insufficiency. Titrate up or down based on blood pressure and symptoms. Endocrine consultation	Consider holding ICPI until patient is stable on replacement hormone Endocrine consult [a]Initiate treatment at 2–3 times maintenance dosing to manage acute symptoms. Taper stress-dosing down over 5–10 days. Maintain maintenance	HOLD ICPI until patient is stabilized on replacement hormone Endocrine consult IV hydration with normal saline and IV stress dose corticosteroids (hydrocortisone 100 mg or dexamethasone 4 mg) Taper stress-dose corticosteroids over 7–10 days. Maintenance therapy as in grade	
Supportive interventions	[a]If symptomatic, and/or low cortisol, high ACTH, administer cortisol replacement If diagnosis already made, stress dosing of corticosteroids can be with hydrocortisone. However, if diagnosis is not yet made, treat with Decadron, as stimulation test can still be done In the case of adrenal insufficiency and hypothyroidism, steroids must be given prior to thyroid replacement to avoid adrenal crisis. Educate patients about stress-dose steroids prior to procedures or in case of infection All patients should wear a medical alert bracelet			

Data from: AIMwithImmunotherapy Essentials [1], Brahmer [21], Haanen [53, 54], Thompson [139, 140], and US Dept. HHS [141]

Abbreviations: *T3* triiodothyroinine, *T4* thyroxine, *ACTH* adrenocorticotropic hormone, *LH* Luteinizing Hormone, *FSH* follicle-stimulating hormone

therapy should be held with elevations of AST or ALT >3× upper limit of normal. Other causes of hepatic dysfunction should be ruled out, including progression of liver metastases, hepatotoxic medications (e.g chemotherapy, acetaminophen, statins, over-the counter medications, herbal supplements), contrast dye, alcohol, thromboembolic events, viral infection (cytomegalovirus, hepatitis A, B, C), cholangitis and portal hypertension. An abdominal ultrasound, CT scan or MRI may assist in evaluating for noninflammatory causes. The timing of onset within the first weeks of combination chemotherapy and ICPI treatment, with recovery of levels to baseline between cycles, is likely due to chemotherapy [117]. Chemotherapy should be held until transaminase levels improve to grade 1, with consideration for dose reduction or permanent discontinuation of the chemotherapy [59]. If no other cause is identified, hepatic irAEs are treated with steroid immunosuppression, methyl-prednisolone/prednisone 1 mg/kg/day. In more severe cases or if refractory, hepatology referral is warranted. If refractory to initial immunosuppressant or recurrence of toxicity, addition of mycophenolate mofetil is the recommended additional immunosuppressant. Infliximab is contradictory as it may induce autoimmune hepatitis and life-threatening acute liver failure [21, 54, 138].

Table 7.5 Hepatic: transaminitis, hepatitis

Assessment	Screen for concomitant hepatotoxic drugs Assess for symptoms: pruritis, change in color of urine or stool, abdominal pain, bruising or bleeding, ascites, change in mental status Laboratory: LFTs (Alk Phos, AST, ALT, Total bilirubin) prior to each infusion; Albumin, INR; If suspected autoimmune hepatitis: CK, GGT, ANA Rule out other causes: viral hepatitis, CMV reactivation, thromboembolic event, liver metastases Consider liver ultrasound or CT of abdomen			
Grade	1	2	3	4
	AST or ALT > ULN to 3 × ULN or total bilirubin > ULN to 1.5 × ULN Asymptomatic	AST or ALT >3 × ULN but ≤5 × ULN or total bilirubin >1.5 × ULN but ≤3 × ULN Asymptomatic	AST or ALT 5–20 × ULN, or total bilirubin 3–10 × ULN Symptomatic	AST or ALT >20 × ULN and/or total bilirubin >10 × ULN Symptomatic
Medical management	Continue ICPI Monitor labs one to two times weekly	HOLD ICPI and resume if decreased to grade 1 or less on prednisone ≤ mg/day Increase frequency of labs (every 3–5 days) Administer corticosteroids 0.5 mg to 1.0 mg/kg/day	Permanent discontinue ICPI Administer corticosteroids 1.0–2.0 mg/kg/day If refractory after 3 days, consider mycophenolate mofetil Monitor LFTs every 1–2 days Referral to hepatologist or gastroenterologist	Permanently discontinue ICPI Administer corticosteroids 2.0 mg/kg/day If refractory after 3 days, consider mycophenolate mofetil Monitor LFTs daily Urgent referral to hepatologist or gastroenterologist May require liver biopsy
Supportive interventions	Discontinue or limit hepatotoxic drugs including over the counter medications, herbal supplements			

Data from: AIMwithImmunotherapy Essentials [1], Brahmer [21], Haanen [53, 54], Thompson [139, 140], and US Dept. HHS [141]
Abbreviations: *LFTS* Liver Function Tests, *AST* Aspartate Aminotransferase, *ALT* Alanine Aminotransferase, *ULN* Upper Limit of Normal, *CMV* Cytomegalovirus, *CK* Creatine Kinase, *ANA* Antinuclear Antibody, *GGT* Gamma-Glutamyl Transferase

Grade based recommendations for hepatic irAE management is outlined in Table 7.5.

3.6 Renal

The most common kidney injury reported is acute interstitial nephritis (AIN). Glomerulonephritis, thrombotic microangiopathy and minimal change disease have also been reported [65, 94]. In a meta-analysis of 48 clinical trials with 11,482 patients, the incidence of acute renal injury ranged from 2% to 4% with anti PD-1/PD-L1, 4.9% anti- CTLA-4, 2.2% combination [85]. Although some institutional studies have reported rates of acute kidney injury as high as 29% [29, 88, 120, 146]. There is an increased risk with concomitant use of NSAIDS and proton-pump-inhibitors [123]. Acute renal injury may not be appreciated if changes in creatinine are subtle and baseline creatinine is low (0.4–0.6 mg/dL) and/or low muscle mass, as a rise in creatinine may still be within institutional normal limits [126, 146]. The median onset is 3–6 months with anti-PD-1/PD-L1 therapy [29, 102]. However, there have been case reports after one dose [123]. Renal toxicity occurs as early as 6–12 weeks with anti-CTLA-4 [102].

Renal toxicities typically present asymptomatically with elevated serum creatine level. In more severe cases patients may experience fatigue, nausea, weakness, hematuria, edema and decreased urine output [29, 60]. Acute kidney injury (AKI) may be identified with routine serum creatinine or BUN, which should be obtained prior to every ICPI therapy. Alterations in serum electrolytes (hypokalemia, hyponatremia) may be seen. Urine tests may reveal sub-nephrotic proteinuria elevated protein: creatinine ratio and eosinophiluria [102]. ICPI therapy should be held for grade ≥2 nephrotoxicity [21, 139]. Other causes of acute renal injury should be excluded. These include dehydration, infection, sepsis, nephrotoxic contrast dye exposure and concomitant drugs (i.e. antibiotics, NSAIDS, ACE inhibitors, diuretics, proton pump inhibitors and chemotherapy) [94, 123]. Platinum-doublet therapy is the mainstay of combination chemotherapy and ICPI therapy in lung cancer, with known risk of renal toxicity. The potential contribution of chemotherapy agents to renal toxicity for patients must be evaluated. The timing of onset within the first weeks of combination treatment, with recovery of levels to baseline between cycles, is likely due to chemotherapy [59]. Chemotherapy should be held until serum creatinine to grade 1, with consideration for dose reduction or permanent discontinuation of the chemotherapy [59]. Mild/ low grade acute renal injury may improve with proper hydration [53]. If no other cause is identified, renal irAEs are treated with steroid immunosuppression, methylprednisolone/prednisone 1 mg/kg/day. If immune related kidney injury is suspected a nephrology consult should be obtained and consideration for renal biopsy. Mycophenolate mofetil, cyclosporin or infliximab can be utilized in steroid refractory cases [84].

Grade based recommendations for renal irAE management is outlined in Table 7.6.

Table 7.6 Renal: Acute kidney injury/nephritis

Assessment	Screen for potential nephrotoxic agents Monitor serum creatinine and BUN prior to start of therapy and prior to each dose Rule out other causes: concomitant chemotherapy, urinary tract infection, urinary obstruction, dehydration			
Grade	1	2	3	4
Serum Cr	>ULN-1.5 × ULN	>1.5–3.0 × baseline >1.5–3.0 × ULN	>3.0 × baseline >3.0–6.0 × ULN	>6.0 × ULN
Proteinuria	Proteinuria 1+, urine protein <1.0 g/24 hours	Proteinuria 2+ and 3+, 1.0–3.5 g/24 ours	Proteinuria 4+, > 3.5 g/24 hours	Life-threatening consequences, dialysis indicated
Medical management	Consider holding ICPI, pending evaluation of other causes Hydration Discontinue nephrotoxic drugs	HOLD ICPI IV hydration Consider inpatient admission Consult nephrology Corticosteroids 0.5–1.0 mg/kd/d; If worsening or no improvement in XX days, 1.0–2.0 mg/kg/day and permanently discontinue ICPI; if improvement, taper over 4–6 weeks. If no recurrence, consider restart of ICPI	Permanently discontinue ICPI Inpatient admission Corticosteroids 1–2 mg/kg/day If improved to grade 1, taper steroids over at least 4 weeks. Grade 3: If elevation persists >3–5 days, add additional immunosuppressant Grade 4: If elevation persists >2–3 days or worsens, additional immunosuppressant Consult nephrology Consider biopsy	
Supportive interventions	Assure adequate hydration Renal dietary restrictions Limit all nephrotoxic agents			

Data from: AIMwithImmunotherapy Essentials [1], Brahmer [21], Haanen [53, 54], Thompson [139, 140], and US Dept. HHS [141]

Abbreviations: *BUN* Blood urea Nitrogen, *ULN* Upper Limit of Normal

3.7 Cardiac

Cardiac IRAEs are extremely rare, with a reported incidence of 1.14% in monotherapy [83]. The incidence is increased in combination anti-PD-1/CTLA-4 therapy [156]. Though the overall incidence may be underestimated as biomarkers of cardiac dysfunction are not routinely monitored on all patients receiving ICPI therapy [143]. Cardiotoxic irAEs includes myocarditis, pericarditis, cardiomyopathy, heart failure, pericardial effusion and arrhythmias [143]. The onset is as early as days after ICPI initiation, with a median onset of 34 days, however, can present after a year of therapy and pose a significant risk for life-threatening consequences [83, 87]. Myocarditis is often associated with concurrent myositis and can be fatal in up to half of patients [67, 92, 119]. Symptoms may be subtle initially with fatigue, weakness and dyspnea and progress to chest pain, palpitations, syncope, lightheadedness, and/or peripheral edema.

An electrocardiogram should be obtained prior to the start of ICPI therapy and if cardiotoxicity is suspected [21, 111, 138]. Diagnostic evaluation with an echocardiogram and/or cardiac MRI, laboratory studies of serum creatinine kinase, serum creatinine kinase myocardial band (CKMB), troponin T. C-reactive protein (elevation) and brain natriuretic peptide (BNP) should be obtained in all patients with suspected cardiotoxicity [21, 54, 111, 138]. Myocardial biopsy may reveal fibrosis, inflammatory cell infiltration and T-cell lymphocytic infiltration [67, 87].

ICPI therapy should be permanently discontinued for grade 2–4 cardiac dysfunction. A multidisciplinary team with referral to cardio-oncology specialist is essential given the risk of rapid progression and potential for fatal outcomes. Corticosteroids should be promptly initiated at a dose of 1 mg/kg/day. In patients that do not respond to corticosteroids within 2 days, additional immunosuppression with infliximab, mycophenolate mofetil, intravenous immunoglobulin or Rituxan should be initiated promptly [21, 138]. Abatacept (a cytotoxic T-lymphocyte-associated antigen 4 {CTLA-4} agonist) has recently demonstrated effect in pre-clinical trials for refractory myocarditis [118].

Grade based recommendations for cardiac irAE management is outlined in Table 7.7.

3.8 Neurologic

Neurologic IRAEs and paraneoplastic neurologic syndromes (PNS), may be peripheral and/or central, including: polyneuropathy, facial nerve palsy, Guillain-Barre syndrome, myasthenia gravis, posterior reversible leukoencephalopathy, encephalitis, aseptic meningitis, neuropathy, and cerebellar ataxia [12, 47, 51, 75]. Neuropathies are the most common irAE, which can be motor or sensory, symmetric or asymmetric, painful or painless. Most neurologic irAEs are mild with an overall incidence is 3.8% with anti-CTLA-4 inhibitors, 6.1% with PD-1 inhibitors and 12% in combination therapy, with rare (<1%) grade 3 or higher [35, 37]. The time to onset is 6–12 weeks, however there have been cases of delayed onset as late as 76 weeks [36]. There are some reports to suggest that patients who experienced neurotoxicity, experienced durable responses to ICPI therapy [129, 156].

Patients should be screened for pre-existing neurologic dysfunction prior to the start of ICPI therapy. Differential evaluation for contribution of concurrent or previous chemotherapy induced peripheral neuropathy should be considered. Neurology consult is recommended for all grade ≥2 neurologic irAE. A full neurologic evaluation is warranted that may include electromyography (EMG), MRI of brain/spine, lumbar puncture, EEG and serum paraneoplastic panel. Corticosteroid immunosuppression should be initiated swiftlyfor any grade 2 or higher IRAE to minimize risk of irreversible neurologic deficits [91]. If there is no improvement in 2–3 days, additional immunosuppressant therapy is warranted. IVIG has been used to help

Table 7.7 Cardiac: pericarditis, myocarditis, cardiomyopathy, ischemia, arrhythmias

Assessment	Assess for preexisting cardiovascular diagnosis and risk factors (hypertension, hyperlipidemia) Assess baseline ECG Assess for signs of heart failure (peripheral edema, dyspnea, effusions) Echocardiogram Laboratory: troponin, BNP, CK, CKMB Rule out myocardial infarction, arrhythmias Consider Cardiac MRI			
Grade	1	2	3	4
	Abnormal cardiac biomarker testing, including abnormal ECG	Abnormal screening tests; Mild symptoms	Moderately abnormal testing or symptoms with mild activity	Moderate to severe decompensation IV medication or intervention required; Life threatening consequences
Medical management	HOLD ICPI	Permanently discontinue ICPI Inpatient admission Cardiology consult High dose methylprednisolone 1.2 mg/kg/day initiated rapidly. If no response in 1–2 days, additional immunosuppressant therapy with infliximab or anti-thymocyte globulin (ATG) Management of cardiac symptoms per ACC/AHA			
Supportive interventions	Encourage smoking cessation Monitor ECG			

Data from: AIMwithImmunotherapy Essentials [1], Brahmer [21], Haanen [53, 54], Thompson [139, 140], and US Dept. HHS [141]

Abbreviations: *ECG* Electrocardiogram, *BNP* Brain Natriuretic Peptide, *ACC/AHA* American College of Cardiology/American Heart Association

mitigate the progress of severe PNS [17, 21]. In most cases, ICPI therapy is permanently discontinued.

Grade based recommendations for peripheral neuropathy irAE management is outlined in Table 7.8.

3.9   Musculoskeletal-Rheumatologic

Musculoskeletal and rheumatologic irAES include arthralgias, myalgias, myositis, sicca syndrome, polymyalgia rheumatica, Sjögren's syndrome and vasculitis [26]. Arthralgias are the most common reported in up to 43% of patients. Myalgias reported less frequently in up to 20% of patients [25, 26, 95]. Arthralgias and myalgias occur more frequently with anti-PD-1/PD-L1 agents than anti CTLA-4 therapy, and higher in combination regimens. The severity of is typically mild, with only 1–7% experiencing more severe symptoms [26]. The onset ranges from one to 24 months from start of therapy [26, 110].

Table 7.8 Neurologic: neuropathy

Assessment	Screen for pre-existing autoimmune neurologic conditions Screen for pre-existing peripheral neuropathy in high risk patients (e.g diabetes, pervious chemotherapy, other medications) Rule out CNS metastasis or progression, CVA, seizure, infection, metabolic abnormalities, diabetes, medications Laboratory assessment: serum glucose, B12/folate, TSH, ALT, CK, CKMB, paraneoplastic panel, CRP, ESR. Consider need for MRI/MRA of brain and spine Consider need for EMG and/or EEG Lumbar puncture for CSF evaluation			
Grade	1	2	3	4
	Mild; no interference with function; Symptoms not concerning to patient	Moderate Interference with ADLs Symptoms concerning t patient	Severe; limiting self-care and aides warranted; weakness limiting walking or respiratory problems (leg weakness, foot drop, rapidly progressing sensory changes); severe may be Gullain-Barre syndrome	
Medical management	Close observation Low threshold to hold ICPI and monitor symptoms for a week. If to continue ICPI, close observation	HOLD ICPI and resume once G1; Initiate prednisone 0.5–1.0 mg/kg Neurology consult Neurontin, pregabalin or duloxetine for pain	Permanent discontinuation of ICPI Admit patient to hospital Neurology consult Initiate methylprednisolone 2–4 mg/kg Severe or refractory: IVIG	
Supportive interventions	Safety initiatives Multidisciplinary care: Physical therapy, occupational and speech therapy			

Data from: AIMwithImmunotherapy Essentials [1], Brahmer [21], Haanen [53, 54], Thompson [139, 140], and US Dept. HHS [141]

Abbreviations: *CNS* Central Nervous System, *CVA* Cardiovascular Accident, *TSH* Thyroid Stimulating Hormone, *ALT* aminotransaminase, *CK* Creatine Kinase, *CKMB* Creatine Kinase muscle/brain, *CRP* C-reactive Protein, *ESR* Erythrocyte Sedimentation Rate, *CSF* Cerebral Spinal Fluid, *EMG* Electromyography, *EEG* Electroencephalogram, *IVIG* Intravenous Immune Globulin

Arthralgias (inflammation of joints) may affect one joint or many, with mild discomfort to disabling limitations on activities of daily living (ADLS) and independent activities of daily living (IADLs) [6, 26]. Patients with underlying autoimmune rheumatic disease may be at risk for flare of their disease and symptoms when treated with ICPI therapy [7, 137]. Clinical workup of arthralgias includes a full rheumatologic examination. Laboratory tests included inflammatory [ie erythrocyte sedimentation rate (ESR), C-reactive protein (CRP), creatinine kinase (CK)] and autoimmune markers [ie rheumatoid factor (RF), anti-nuclear antibody (ANA) and cyclic citullinated peptide antibody (anti-CCP)] [21, 138]. Imaging with plain x-rays should be obtained to assess the degree of joint inflammation.

Myalgias present with general muscle soreness. This may progress to myositis with progressive proximal muscle weakness and inflammation. The diagnosis is based on physical examination, and elevated muscle enzyme levels (CK).

Electromyography (EMG) and muscle magnetic resonance imaging (MRI) may support the diagnosis.

Mild symptoms can be managed with oral non-steroidal anti-inflammatory drugs (NSAIDS). Patients with very mild symptoms may benefit from topical NSAIDS. If arthritic symptoms persist, or in those in whom NSAIDS are contraindicated, low dose corticosteroids (prednisone 10 mg) may be initiated. For grade ≥ 2, corticosteroids are recommended. For more severe cases, Rheumatology consult should be obtained. If symptoms are refractory to corticosteroids, disease modifying antirheumatic drugs (DMARDs), such as hydroxychloroquine or methotrexate, have been used successfully to provide opportunity to taper steroids [7, 73, 113]. Tocilizumab, an IL-6 receptor antibody, has been used in patients in whom TNF inhibitors are contraindicated [73]. Myositis requires more aggressive management, as cardiac myositis can develop and be life-threatening [21, 138].

Grade based recommendations for arthralgia irAE management is outlined in Table 7.9.

3.10   Ocular

Ocular irAEs may affect the entire ocular region, including the conjunctiva, cornea, uvea, retina, optic nerve and eyelids [82]. Toxicities include dry eyes, conjunctivitis, blepharitis, keratitis, retinitis, iritis, uveitis, scleritis and optic neuritis [82]. Dry eyes syndrome is the most common ocular toxicity, occurring in up to 24% of patients in clinical trials [3, 38]. The incidence of more severe inflammation is approximately 1% of patients with more frequency noted with anti-CTLA-4 containing regimens [3, 19]. Anterior uveitis is the most common inflammation reported, but it can progress to posterior or pan-uveitis [63]. Case reports of Vogt-Koyanagi-Harada (VKH) like syndrome, a rare multisystem autoimmune condition targeting melanocytes, that involves bilateral pan-uveitis uveitis, has been reported in NSCLC [136]. Case reports of keratoconjunctivitis sicca resembling Sjögren's syndrome have also been reported [151]. Ocular symptoms include blurred vision, photophobia, tenderness, eye pain, and swelling [82]. The median onset of ophthalmologic toxicities is 2 months [19]. Most ocular IRAEs can be managed with topical or periorbital steroids, with more severe cases requiring systemic steroids [40, 82]. Artificial tears and topical cyclosporin has been used for dry eyes [101]. Ophthalmologist should be consulted immediately for higher grade ocular inflammation, as there is a risk for corneal perforation and permanent vision loss [101].

Grade based recommendations for uveitis irAE management is outlined in Table 7.10.

Table 7.9 Musculoskeletal: arthralgias & myalgias

Assessment	Screen for risk factors: rheumatology history (osteoarthritic, psoriatic arthritis, rheumatoid arthritis, degenerative joint disease) Assess baseline musculoskeletal system for strength and function Consider plain x-rays, ultrasound or MRI to exclude metastases and myositis Laboratory: autoimmune assessment (ANA, rheumatoid factor, anti-CCP), inflammatory markers (CRP, ESR, CK); paraneoplastic autoantibody testing EMG			
Grade	1	2	3	4
	Mild pain with inflammation, erythema or joint swelling Mild weakness, with or without pain	Moderate pain associated with inflammation, erythema or joint swelling Moderate muscle weakness with or without pain Limitation of age appropriate instrumental ADLs	Severe pain; irreversible joint damage Disabling Limits self-care ADLs Severe muscle weakness with or without pain	
Medical management	Continue ICPI Symptom management with acetaminophen and/or NSAIDS (topical and/or oral); If ineffective, may consider low dose prednisone 10 mg/day. If no improvement in 4 weeks, treat as moderate	Consider holding ICPI Prednisone 10–20 mg/day if no improvement If CK elevated >3 × ULN, consider prednisone 0.5–1.0 mg/kg/day Consider rheumatology consult Consider neurology consult	HOLD ICPI Initiate methylprednisolone or prednisone equivalent 0.5–1.0 mg/kg/day Rheumatology consult If no improvement, may consider: Arthritis: biologic DMARD (disease modifying anti-rheumatoid) such as IL-6 receptor inhibitor or TNF-a or synthetic DMARD (methotrexate, hydroxychloroquine) Myositis: plasmapheresis or IVIG, mycophenolate mofetil.	
Supportive interventions	If oligoarthritis, may treat with intra-articular corticosteroids Physical and occupational therapy			

Data from: AIMwithImmunotherapy Essentials [1], Brahmer [21], Haanen [53, 54], Thompson [139, 140], and US Dept. HHS [141]

Abbreviations: *ANA* Antinuclear Antibody, *anti-CCP* anti-cyclic citrullinated peptide, *CRP* C-Reactive Protein, *ESR* Erythrocyte Sedimentation Rate, *CK* Creatine Kinase, *EMG* Electromyography

3.11 Hematologic

Hematologic irAEs are rare, with rate of approximately 0.5% [44]. Hemolytic anemia is the most commonly reported hematologic toxicity, followed by idiopathic

Table 7.10 Ophthalmic toxicity: uveitis, scleritis, iritis, conjunctivitis, episcleritis

Assessment	Assess for at risk patients: history of active uveitis, those with recurrent uveitis requiring systemic immunosuppressant Assess for ocular symptoms Assess for other eye irritants Bilateral visual exam with ophthalmology including fundoscopic evaluation			
Grade	1	2	3	4
	Asymptomatic	Medical intervention; Anterior uveitis	Posterior or pan uveitis	Vision 20/200 or worse
Medical management	Continue ICPI Refer to ophthalmology Artificial tears	HOLD ICPI Urgent ophthalmology consultation Topical corticosteroids, systemic corticosteroids May resume once off systemic corticosteroids or if IRAE improved when dosing is <10 mg/day Retreat after reduced to G1	Permanently discontinue ICPI Urgent ophthalmology evaluation Systemic corticosteroid Consider periocular corticosteroids	Permanently discontinue ICPI Emergent ophthalmology consult Systemic corticosteroids (1–2 mg/kg)
Supportive interventions	Avoid eye irritants: make-up, contact lenses Encourage use of sunglasses, nighttime eye protection to decrease risk of inadvertent eye contact			

Data from: AIMwithImmunotherapy Essentials [1], Brahmer [21], Haanen [53, 54], Thompson [139, 140], and US Dept. HHS [141]
Abbreviations: N/A

thrombocytopenic purpura (ITP) with a fatality rates of 15% and 11% respectively [41]. The onset is usually 1–2 months (40 days) after start of therapy. Toxicities occur earlier with anti-CTLA-4 (monotherapy or combination) versus those associated with anti-PD-1/L-1, though higher rates are reported with anti-PD-1/L1. Additional rare hematologic IRAEs reported include hemophagocytic lymphohistiocytosis, acquired thrombotic thrombocytopenic purpura (TTP), hemolytic uremic syndrome, aplastic anemia, red cell aplasia, neutropenia, immune thrombocytopenia myelodysplasia and hemophilia [41]. It may be challenging to HCPs to attribute cause of the anemia in patients receiving combination chemotherapy and ICPI therapy. Anemia and thrombocytopenia that occurs within 1–2 weeks of combination cytotoxic therapy, is likely attributable to cytotoxic myelosuppression. Immune-mediated hemolytic irAEs should be considered after ruling out other potential causes including bone marrow disease involvement, gastrointestinal bleed, and cytotoxic cytopenia's. Evaluation includes a review of prior history of auto-immune hematologic disease, nutritional evaluation to rule out vitamin deficiency, complete blood count, peripheral blood smear, reticulocyte count, direct antiglobulin test, indirect bilirubin, haptoglobin, lactate dehydrogenase, C-reactive protein, erythrocyte sedimentation rate, immunoglobulin G and immunoglobulin M antibodies, vitamin B12, iron studies and infection panel. A bone marrow examination may be indicated to rule out bone marrow infiltration.

ICPI therapy should be held with grade ≥2 hematologic toxicity until a full differential is considered. If toxicity is attributed to cytotoxic therapy, the management may include dose reduction or discontinuation of the cytotoxic agent. If toxicity is associated with ICPI, therapy should be held until grade ≤1. Corticosteroids should be initiated for grade >2 or higher, with permanent discontinuation of ICPI therapy for grade >3 and 4.

Grade based recommendations for hemolytic anemia irAE management is outlined in Table 7.11.

Table 7.11 Hematologic: hemolytic anemia

Assessment	Baseline CBC prior to initiation of treatment and prior to each dose Screen for other causes of hemolytic anemia: other drugs, insect bites, viral or bacterial infections Laboratory: CBC with peripheral smear, reticulocyte count, free Hgb, haptoglobin, DIC panel; Paroxysmal nocturnal hemoglobinuria screening; Direct and indirect bilirubin, LDH, direct agglutinin; protein electrophoresis, cryoglobulin analysis Rule out bone marrow failure syndrome: B12, folate, copper, Bone marrow biopsy and aspirate may be indicated			
Grade	1	2	3	4
	Hgl <LLN to 10.0 g/dL	Hgb >8.0 to <10.0	Hgl <8.0; transfusion indicated	Life threatening consequences; urgent intervention indicated
Medical management	Continue ICPI Close follow up of labs	HOLD ICPI Consider permanent discontinuation Administer prednisone equivalent 0.5–1.0 mg/kg	Permanently discontinue ICPI Hematology consult Prednisone 1.0–2.0 mg/kg	Permanently discontinue ICPI Inpatient admission Hematology consult
Supportive interventions	RBC transfusion support per institutional guidelines Encourage rest and energy sparing activities			

Data from: AIMwithImmunotherapy Essentials [1], Brahmer [21], Haanen [53, 54], Thompson [139, 140], and US Dept. HHS [141]

Abbreviations: *CBC* complete Blood Count, *Hgl* Hemoglobin, *LLN* Lower Limit of Normal, *DIC* Disseminated intravascular coagulation, *FE* ferritin/ iron, *RBC* Red Blood Cell

4 Summary

The safe and effective use of ICPIs in routine clinical practice requires the use of steroids and other immunosuppressant agents in the outpatient and inpatient settings to counteract the powerful immune-activating effects of ICPIs. As we have seen, ICPIs can activate the immune system against any organ system. Patients will often experience minor off-target immune activation requiring symptomatic management and holding therapy. Many patients will require holding therapy and high dose steroids for management of immune toxicity. A small minority of patients will require hospitalization and advanced medical care in conjunction with the medical oncologist to manage life-threatening side-effects. Unfortunately, some patients will succumb to toxicity. Early and swift management is paramount to limit toxicity and maintain adequate cancer-directed therapy.

For the patient case in the introduction, the trial therapy was discontinued due to grade 4 hepatitis and grade 2 colitis. He started prednisone 1 mg/kg for both indications. The patient completed a prolonged taper of prednisone over 2 months. The symptoms of colitis and fatigue resolved. The lung cancer remains controlled in follow-up without therapy for over 6 months.

References

1. AIMwithImmunotherapy Immuno-Oncology Essentials (IO Essentials). Retrieved from: https://aimwithimmunotherapy.org/. Approved November 2018. Accessed 5 Jun 2020
2. Abdel-Rahman O, El Halawani H, Fouad M (2015) Risk of gastrointestinal complications in cancer patients treated with immune checkpoint inhibitors: a meta-analysis. Immunotherapy 7(11):1213–1227
3. Abdel-Rahman O, Oweira H, Petrausch U et al (2017) Immune-related ocular toxicities in solid tumor patients treated with immune checkpoint inhibitors: a systematic review. Expert Rev Anticancer Ther 17(4):387–394
4. Abu-Sbeih H, Ali FS, Wang X et al (2019) Early introduction of selective immunosuppressive therapy associated with favorable clinical outcomes in patients with immune checkpoint inhibitor-induced colitis. J Immunother Cancer 7:93
5. Abu-Sbeih H, Tang T, Lu Y et al (2019) Clinical characteristics and outcomes of immune checkpoint inhibitor-induced pancreatic injury. J Immunother Cancer 7(1):31
6. Abdul-Wahab N, Tayar JH, Diab A, Sang TK, Lu H, Suarez-Almazor ME (2017) Inflammatory arthritis induced by the use of checkpoint inhibitors for immunotherapy of cancer. J Immunother Cancer 5(Suppl 2):P444. (page 215)
7. Abdul-Wahab N, Shah M, Lopez-Olivo MA, Suarez-Almazor ME (2018) Use of immune checkpoint inhibitors in the treatment of patients with cancer and preexisting autoimmune disease: a systemic review. Ann Intern Med 168(2):121–130
8. Antonia S, Goldberg SB, Balmanoukian A et al (2016) Safety and antitumor activity of durvalumab plus tremelimumab in non-small cell lung cancer : a multicentre, phase 1b study. Lancet Oncol 17:299–308
9. Arbour KC, Mezquita L, Long N et al (2018) Impact of baseline steroids on efficacy of programmed cell death-1 ligand 1 blockade on patients with non-small cell lung cancer. J Clin Oncol 36(28):2872–2878

10. Arnaud-Coffin P, Maillet D, Gan HK et al (2019) A systematic review of adverse events in randomized trials assessing immune checkpoint inhibitors. In J Cancer 145(3):639–648. https://doi.org/10.1002/ijc.32132

11. Aso M, Toi Y, Sugisaka J, Aiba T, Kawana S, Saito R, Ogasawara T, Tsurumi K, Ono K, Shimizu H, Domeki Y, Terayama K, Kawashima Y, Nakamura A, Yamanda S, Kimura Y, Honda Y, Sugawara S (2020) Association between skin reaction and clinical benefit in patients treated with anti-programmed cell death 1 monotherapy for advanced non-small cell lung cancer. Oncologist 25(3):e536–e544. https://doi.org/10.1634/theoncologist.2019-0550. Epub 2019 Nov 7. PMID: 32162801; PMCID: PMC7066688

12. Astaras C, de Micheli R, Moura B, Hundsberger T, Hottinger AF (2018) Neurologic adverse events associated with immune checkpoint inhibitors: diagnosis and management. Curr Neurol Neurosci Rep 18(1):3

13. Baden LR, Bensinger W, Angarone M et al (2012) Prevention and treatment of cancer-related infections. J Natl Compr Cancer Netw 10:1412–1445

14. Barroso-Sousa R, Barry WT, Garido-Castro AC et al (2018) Incidence of endocrine dysfunction following use of different immune checkpoint inhibitor regimens: a systematic review and meta-analysis. JAMA Oncol 4:173–182

15. Belum VR, Benhuri B, Postow M et al (2016) Characterisation and management of dermatologic adverse events to agents targeting the PD-1 receptor. Eur J Cancer 60:12–25

16. Bergqvist V, Hertervig E, Gedeon P et al (2017) Vedolizumab treatment for immune checkpoint inhibitor-induced enterocolitis. Cancer Immunol Immunother 66(5):581–592

17. Berzero G, Karantoni E, Dehais C et al (2018) Early intravenous immunoglobulin treatment in paraneoplastic neurological syndromes with onconeural antibodies. J Neurol Neurosurg Psychiatry 89(7):798–792

18. Betof AS, Nipp RD, Giobbie-Harder A, Johnpulle RAN, Rubin K, Rubinstein SM, Flaherty KT, Lawrence DP, Johnson DB, Sullivan RJ (2017) Impact of age on outcomes with immunotherapy for patients with melanoma. Oncologist 22(8):963–971. https://doi.org/10.1634/theoncologist.2016-0450. Epub 2017 May 5. PMID: 28476944; PMCID: PMC5553960

19. Bitton K, Michot JM, Barreau E et al (2019) Prevalence and clinical pattersn of ocular complications associated with anti-PD-1/PD-L1 anticancer immunotherapy. Am J Ophthalmol 202:109–117

20. Boutros C, Tarhini A, Routier E et al (2016) Safety profiles of anti-CTLA-4 and anti-PD-1 antibodies alone and in combination. Nat Rev Clin Oncol 13(8):473–486

21. Brahmer JR, Lacchetti C, Schneider BJ, et al, in collaboration with the National Comprehensive Cancer Network (2018) Management of immune-related adverse events in patients treated with immune checkpoint inhibitor therapy: American Society of Clinical Oncology clinical practice guidelines. J Clin Oncol 36(17):1714–1768. https://doi.org/10.1200/JCO.2017.77.6385. Epub 2018 Feb 14. PMID: 29442540; PMCID: PMC6481621

22. Brechmann T, Günther K, Neid M, Schmiegel W, Tannapfel A (2019) Triggers of histologically suspected drug induced colitis. World J Gastroenterol 25(8):967–979

23. Burdett N, Hsu K, Xiong L, Tapia-Rico G, Beckmann K, Karapetis C, Brown MP (2020) Cancer outcomes in patients requiring immunosuppression in addition to corticosteroids for immune-related adverse events after immune checkpoint inhibitor therapy. Asia Pac J Clin Oncol 16:e139–e145

24. Byun DJ, Wolchok JD, Rosenberg LM, Girotra M (2017) Cancer immunotherapy-immune checkpoint blockade and associated endocrinopathies. Nat Rev Endocrinol 13:195–207

25. Cappelli LC, Gutierrez AK, Faer AN et al (2016) Inflammatory arthritis and sicca syndrome induced by nivolumab and ipilimumab. Ann Rheum Dis 76(1):43–50

26. Cappelli LC, Gutierrez AK, Bingham CO, Shah AA (2017) Rheumatic and musculoskeletal immune-related adverse events due to immune checkpoint inhibitors: a systemic review of the literature. Arthritis Care Res 69(11):1751–1763

27. Chalabi M, Cardona A, Nagarkar D et al (2020) Efficacy of chemotherapy and atezolizumab patients with non-small-cell lung cancer receiving antibiotics and proton pump inhibitors: pooled post hoc analyses of the OAK and POPLAR trials. Ann Oncol 31(4):525–531
28. Champiat S, Lambotte O, Barreau E et al (2016) Management of immune checkpoint blockade dysimmune toxicities: a collaborative position paper. Ann Oncol 27:559–574
29. Cortazar FB, Marrone KA, Troxell ML et al (2016) Clinical pathological features of acute kidney injury associated with immune checkpoint inhibitors. Kidney Int 90(3):638–647
30. Coutzac C, Adam J, Soularue E et al (2017) Colon immune-related adverse events: anti-CTLA-4 and anti-PD-1 blockade induce distinct immunopathologic entities. J Crohns Colitis 11(10):1238–1246. 20922033
31. Cramer P, Bresalier RS (2017) Gastrointestinal and hepatic complications of immune checkpoint inhibitors. Curr Gastroenterol Rep 19:3
32. Cui P, Huang D, Wu Z et al (2020) Association of immune-related pneumonitis with efficacy of PD-1/PD-L1 inhibitors in non-small cell lung cancer. Ther Adv Med Oncol 12:1–10. https://doi.org/10.1177/17588359
33. Cukier P, Santini FC, Scaranti M, Hoff AO (2017) Endocrine side effects of cancer immunotherapy. Endocr Relat Cancer 24(12):T331–T347
34. Curry JL, Tetzlaff MT, Nagarajan P et al (2017) Diverse types of dermatologic toxicities from immune checkpoint blockade therapy. J Cutan Pathol 44:158–176
35. Cuzzubbo S, Javeri F, Tissier M et al (2017) Neurologic adverse events associated with immune checkpoint inhibitors: review of the literature. Eur J Cancer 73:1–8
36. Daher A, Tummala S (2017) The spectrum of neurological adverse events from immune checkpoint blockade: a comprehensive review of the literature. Neurology 88:174
37. Dalakas MC (2018) Neurologic complications of immune checkpoint inhibitors: what happens when you 'take the breaks off' the immune system. Ther Adv Neurol Disord 11. Published online 2018 Sep 14. https://doi.org/10.1177/175628641879986
38. Dalvin LA, Shields CL, Orloff M, Sato T, Shields JA (2018) Checkpoint inhibitor immune therapy: systemic indications and ophthalmic side effects. Retina 38(6):1063–1078
39. Davies M, Duffield EA (2017) Safety of checkpoint inhibitors for cancer treatments: strategies for patient monitoring and management of immune-mediated adverse events. Immunotargets Ther 6:51–71
40. Davis ME, Francis JH (2017) Cancer therapy with checkpoint inhibitors: establishing a role for ophthalmology. Semin Oncol Nurs 33:415–424
41. Davis EJ, Salem JE, Young A et al (2019) Hematologic complications of immune checkpoint inhibitors. Oncologist 24:584–588. https://doi.org/10.1634/theoncologist.2018-0574
42. De Filette J, Andreescu CE, Cools F, Bravenboer B, Velkeniers B (2019) A systematic review and meta-analysis of endocrine-related adverse events associated with immune checkpoint inhibitors. Horm Metab Res 51:145–156
43. De Giglio A, Mezquita L, Auclin E et al (2020) Impact of intercurrent introduction of steroids on clinical outcomes in advanced non-small-cell lung cancer (NSCLC) patients under immune-checkpoint inhibitors (ICI). Cancers (Basel) 12(10):2827
44. Delanoy N, Michot JM, Comont T et al (2019) Haematological immune-related adverse events induced by anti-PD-1 or anti-PD-L1 immunotherapy: a descriptive observational study. Lancet Haematol 6(1):e48–e57
45. Dolladille C, Ederhy S, Sassier M, Cautela J, Thuny F, Cohen AA, Fedrizzi S, Chrétien B, Da-Silva A, Plane AF, Legallois D, Milliez PU, Lelong-Boulouard V, Alexandre J (2020) Immune checkpoint inhibitor rechallenge after immune-related adverse events in patients with cancer. JAMA Oncol 6(6):865–871. https://doi.org/10.1001/jamaoncol.2020.0726. PMID: 32297899; PMCID: PMC7163782
46. El Osta B, Hu F, Sadek R, Chintalapally R, Tang SC (2017) Not all immune-checkpoint inhibitors are created equal: meta-analysis and systematic review of immune -related adverse events in cancer trials. Crit Rev Oncol Hematol 119:1–12

47. Fellner A, Makranz C, Lotem M et al (2018) Neurologic complications of immune check-point inhibitors. J Neuro-Oncol 137(3):601–609
48. Fukihara J, Sakamoto K, Koyama J et al (2019) Prognostic impact and risk factors of immune-related pneumonitis in patients with non-small cell lung cancer who received programmed death 1 inhibitors. Clin Lung Cancer 20(6):442–450
49. Galli G, Triulzi T, Proto C, Signorelli D, Imbimbo M, Poggi M et al (2019) Association between antibiotic-immunotherapy exposure ratio and outcome in metastatic non-small cell lung cancer. Lung Cancer 132:72–78
50. Gandhi L, Rodriguez-Abreu D, Gadgeel S, et al, KEYNOTE-189 Investigators (2018) Pembrolizumab plus chemotherapy in metastatic non-small cell lung cancer. N Engl J Med 378(22):2078–2092
51. Graus F, Dalmau J (2019) Paraneoplastic neurological syndromes in the era of immune-checkpoint inhibitors. Nat Rev Clin Oncol 16(9):535–548. https://doi.org/10.1038/s41571-019-0194-4
52. Gupta A, De Felice KM, Loftus EV, Khanna S (2015) Systematic review: colitis associated with anti-CTLA-4 therapy. Aliment Pharmacol Ther 42:406–417
53. Haanen JBAG, Carbonnel F, Robert C et al (2017) ESMO Guidelines Committee Management of Toxicities from Immunotherapy: ESMO clinical practice guidelines for diagnosis, treatment and follow-up: corrigendum. Ann Oncol 28(suppl 4):119–142
54. Haanen JBAG, Carbonnel F, Robert C, et al, ESMO Guidelines Committee (2018) Management of toxicities from immunotherapy: ESMO clinical practice guidelines for diagnosis, treatment and follow-up. Ann Oncol 29(suppl 4):264–266
55. Hassel JC, Heinzerling L, Aberle J et al (2017) Combined immune checkpoint blockade (anti-PD-1/anti-CTLA-4): evaluation and management of adverse drug reactions. Cancer Treat Rev 57:36–49
56. Hellman MD, Rizvi NA, Goldman JW et al (2017) Nivolumab plus ipilimumab as first line treatment for advanced non-small cell lung cancer (CheckMate 012): results of an open-label, phase 1, multicohort study. Lancet Oncol 18:31–41
57. Herbst RS, Bass P, Kim DW et al (2016) Pembrolizumab versus docetaxel for previously treated, PD-L1-positive, advanced non-small-cell lung cancer (KEYNOTE-010): a randomized controlled trial. Lancet 387:1540–1550
58. Herbst RS, Morgensztern D, Boshoff C (2018) The biology and management of non-small cell lung cancer. Nature 553:446–454
59. Hoffer B, Leighl NB, Davies M (2020) Toxicity management with combination chemotherapy and programmed death 1/programmed death ligand 1 inhibitor therapy in advanced lung cancer. Cancer Treat Rev 85:101979
60. Hofman L, Forschner A, Loquai C et al (2016) Cutaneous, gastrointestinal, hepatic, endocrine and renal side effects of anti-PD-1 therapy. Eur J Cancer 60:190–209
61. Hopkins AM, Rowland A, Kichenadasse G et al (2017) Predicting response and toxicity to immune checkpoint inhibitors using routinely available blood and clinical markers. Br J Cancer 117:913–920
62. Horvat TZ, Adel NG, Dang TO et al (2015) Immune-related adverse events need for systemic immunosuppression, and effects on survival and time to treatment failure in patients with melanoma treated with ipilimumab at Memorial Sloan Kettering Cancer Center. J Clin Oncol 33(28):3193–3198
63. Huillard O, Bakalian S, Levy C et al (2014) Ocular adverse events of molecularly targeted agents approved in solid tumours: a systematic review. Eur J Cancer 50(3):638–648
64. Iwama S, De Remigis A, Callahan MK, Slovin SF, Wolchok JD, Caturegli P (2014) Pituitary expression of CTLA-4 mediates hypophysitis secondary to administration of CTLA-4 blocking antibody. Sci Transl Med 6(230):230ra45. https://doi.org/10.1126/scitranslmed.3008002
65. Izzedine H, Mathian A, Champiat S et al (2019) Renal toxicities associated with pembrolizumab. Clin Kidney J 12(1):81–88

66. Jiang Y, Zhang N, Pang H, Gao X, Zhang H (2019) Risk and incidence of fatal adverse events associated with immune checkpoint inhibitors: a systematic review and meta-analysis. Ther Clin Risk Manag 15:293–302
67. Johnson DB, Balko JM, Compton ML et al (2016) Fulminant myocarditis with combination checkpoint blockade. N Engl J Med 375(18):1749–1755
68. Johnson DB, Friedman DL, Berry E et al (2015) Survivorship in immune therapy: assessing chronic immune toxicities, health outcomes and functional status among long-term ipilimumab survivors at a single referral center. Cancer Immunol Res 3(5):464–469
69. Johnson DB, Sullivan RJ, Menzies AM (2017) Immune checkpoint inhibitors in challenging populations. Cancer 123(11):1904–1911
70. Johnson DB, Zobniw CM, Trinh VA et al (2018) Infliximab associated with faster symptom resolution compared with corticosteroids alone for the management of immune-related enterocolitis. J Immunother Cancer 6:103
71. Khan Z, Hammer C, Guardino E et al (2019) Mechanisms of immune-related adverse events associated with immune checkpoint blockade: using germline genetics to develop a personalized approach. Genome Med 11:39. https://doi.org/10.1186/s13073-019-0652-8
72. Khan S, Gerber DE (2020) Autoimmunity, checkpoint inhibitor therapy and immune-related adverse events: a review. Semin Cancer Biol 64:93–101. https://doi.org/10.1016/j.semcancer.2019.06.012. Epub 2019 Jul 19. PMID: 31330185; PMCID: PMC6980444
73. Kim ST, Tayar J, Trinh VA et al (2017) Successful treatment of arthritis induced by checkpoint inhibitors with tocilizumab: a case series. Ann Rheum Dis 76:2061
74. Khunger M, Rakshit S, Pasupuleti V et al (2017) Incidence of pneumonitis with use of programmed death 1 and programmed death-ligand 1 inhibitors in non-small cell lung cancer: a systematic review and meta-analysis of trials. Chest 152(2):271–281
75. Kolb NA, Trevino CR, Waheed W et al (2018) Neuromuscular complications of immune checkpoint inhibitor therapy. Muscle Nerve. https://doi.org/10.1002/mus.26070. ePublished online 2018 Jan 17. Accessed 20 May 2020
76. Konda B, Nabhan F, Shah MH (2017) Endocrine dysfunction following immune checkpoint inhibitor therapy. Curr Opin Endocrinol Diabetes Obes 24(5):337–347
77. Kumar V, Chaudhary N, Garg M, Floudas CS, Soni P, Chandra AB (2017) Current diagnosis and management of immune related adverse events (irAEs) induced by immune checkpoint inhibitor therapy. Front Pharmacol 8:49–62
78. Langer CJ, Gadgeel SM, Borghaei H et al (2016) Carboplatin and pemetrexed with or without pembrolizumab for advanced, non-squamous non-small cell lung cancer: a randomized, phase 2 cohort of the open-label KEYNOTE-021 study. Lancet Oncol 17:1497–1508
79. Larkin J, Chiarion-Sileni V, Gonzalez R et al (2015) Combined nivolumab and ipilimumab or monotherapy in untreated melanoma. N Engl J Med 373(1):23–34
80. Leighl N, Gandhi L, Hellman M et al (2015) Pembrolizumab for NSCLC: immune-mediated adverse events and corticosteroid use. J Thorac Oncol 10:S233
81. Lin LL, Lin GF, Luo Q, Chen XQ (2019) The incidence and relative risk of PD-1/PD-L1 inhibitors-related colitis in non-small cell lung cancer: a meta-analysis of randomized controlled trials. Int Immunopharmacol 77:105975. https://doi.org/10.1016/j.intimp.2019.105975
82. Liu X, Wang Z, Zhao C et al (2020) Clinical diagnosis and treatment recommendations for ocular toxicities of targeted therapy and immune checkpoint inhibitor therapy. Thorac Cancer 11(3):810–818
83. Mahmood SS, Fradley MG, Cohen JV et al (2018) Myocarditis in patients treated with immune checkpoint inhibitors. J Am Coll Cardiol 71:1755–1764
84. Mamlouk O, Selamet U, Machado S et al (2019) Nephrotoxicity of immune checkpoint inhibitors beyond tubulointerstitial nephritis: single center experience. J Immunother Cancer 6:7
85. Manhor S, Kompotiatis P, Thongprayoon C et al (2019) Programmed cell death protein inhibition is associated with acute kidney injury and hypocalcemia: a meta-analysis. Nephrol Dial Transplant 34:108–168

86. Martins F, Sofiya L, Sykiotis GP et al (2019) Adverse effects of immune-checkpoint inhibitors: epidemiology, management and surveillance. Nat Rev Clin Oncol 16(9):563–580

87. Matsuo K, Ishiguro T, Najama T et al (2019) Nivolumab induced myocarditis successfully treated with corticosteroid therapy: a case report and review of the literature. Intern Med 58(16):2367–2372

88. Meraz-Muñoz A, Amir E, Ng P et al (2020) Acute kidney injury associated with immune checkpoint inhibitor therapy: incidence, risk factors and outcomes. J Immunother Cancer 8(1):e000467

89. Michot JM, Bigenwald C, Champiat S et al (2016) Immune-related adverse events with immune checkpoint blockade: a comprehensive review. Eur J Cancer 54:139–148. https://doi.org/10.1016/j.ejca.2015.11.016. Epub 2016 Jan 5. PMID: 26765102

90. Mellati M, Eaton KD, Brooks-Worrell BM et al (2015) Anti-PD-1 and anti-PDL-1 monoclonal antibodies causing type 1 diabetes. Diabetes Care 38(9):e137–e138

91. Möhn N, Sühs KW, Gingele S et al (2019) Acute progressive neuropathy-myositis-myasthenia-like syndrome associated with immune checkpoint inhibitor therapy in patients with metastatic melanoma. Melanoma Res 29(4):435–440

92. Moslehi JJ, Salem JE, Sosman JA et al (2018) Increased reporting of fatal immune checkpoint inhibitor associated myocarditis. Lancet 391:933

93. Muchnik E, Loh KP, Strawderman M et al (2019) Immune checkpoint inhibitors in real-world treatment of older adults with non-small cell lung cancer. J Am Geriatr Soc 67:905–912

94. Murakami N, Motwani S, Riella LV (2017) Renal complications of immune checkpoint blockade. Curr Probl Cancer 41(2):100–110

95. Naidoo J, Cappelli LC, Forde PM et al (2017) Inflammatory arthritis: a newly recognized adverse event of immune checkpoint blockade. Oncologist 22(6):627–630

96. Naidoo J, Wang X, Woo KM et al (2017) Pneumonitis in patients treated with anti-programmed death-1/programmed death ligand 1 therapy. J Clin Oncol 35(7):709–717

97. Naidoo J, Cottrell TR, Lipson EJ, Forde PM et al (2020) Chronic immune checkpoint inhibitor pneumonitis. J Immunother Cancer 8:e000840. https://doi.org/10.1136/jitc-2020-000840

98. Naidoo J, Page DB, Li BT et al (2015) Toxicities of the anti-PD-1 and anti-PD-L1 immune checkpoint antibodies. Ann Oncol 26(12):2375–2391

99. Nishijima TF, Shachar SS, Nyrop KA, Muss HB (2017) Safety and tolerability of PD-1/PD-L1 inhibitors compared with chemotherapy in patients with advanced cancer: a meta-analysis. Oncologist 22(4):470–479. https://doi.org/10.1634/theoncologist.2016-0419. Epub 2017 Mar 8. PMID: 28275115; PMCID: PMC5388381

100. Nishino M, Giobbie-Hurder A, Hatabu H, Ramaiya NH, Hodi FS (2016) Incidence of programmed cell death 1 inhibitor-related pneumonitis in patients with advanced cancer: a systematic review and meta-analysis. JAMA Oncol 2(12):1607–1616

101. Nguyen AT, Elia M, Materin MA, Sznol M, Chow J (2016) Cyclosporine for dry eye associated with nivolumab: a case progressing to corneal perforation. Cornea 35(3):399–401

102. Oleas D, Bolufer M, Agraz I et al (2021) Acute interstitial nephritis associated with immune checkpoint inhibitors: a single-centre experience. Clin Kidney J 14(5):1364–1370. https://doi.org/10.1093/ckj/sfaa008

103. Osorio JC, Ni A, Chaft JE et al (2017) Antibody-mediated thyroid dysfunction during T-cell checkpoint blockade in patients with non-small cell lung cancer. Ann Oncol 28:583–589

104. Palladino MA, Gahjat FR, Theodorakis EA, Moldawer LL (2003) Anti-TNF-alpha therapies: the next generation. Nat Rev Drug Discov 2(9):736–746

105. Pavan A, Calvetti L, Dal Maso A, Attili I et al (2019) Peripheral blood markers identify risk of immune-related toxicity in advanced non-small cell lung cancer treated with immune-checkpoint inhibitors. Oncologist 24:1128–1136

106. Phan GQ, Yang JC, Sherry RM, Hwu P, Topalian SL, Schwartzentruber DJ, Restifo NP, Haworth LR, Seipp CA, Freezer LJ, Morton KE, Mavroukakis SA, Duray PH, Steinberg SM, Allison JP, Davis TA, Rosenberg SA (2003) Cancer regression and autoimmunity induced by cytotoxic T lymphocyte-associated antigen 4 blockade in patients with metastatic melanoma.

Proc Natl Acad Sci U S A 100(14):8372–8377. https://doi.org/10.1073/pnas.1533209100. Epub 2003 Jun 25. PMID: 12826605; PMCID: PMC166236

107. Pillai R, Behera M, Owonikoko T et al (2017) Evaluation of toxicity profile of PD-1 versus PD-L1 inhibitors in non-small cell Lung cancer (NSCLC). J Thorac Oncol 12:S253–S254

108. Pinato DJ, Howlett S, Ottaviani D, Urus H, Patel A, Mineo T et al (2019) Association of prior antibiotic treatment with survival and response to immune checkpoint inhibitor therapy in patients with cancer. JAMA Oncol 5(12):1774–1778

109. Postow MA, Sidlow R, Hellman MD (2018) Immune-related adverse events associated with immune checkpoint blockade. N Engl J Med 378(2):158–168

110. Pundole X, Abdel-Wahab N, Suarez-Almazor ME (2019) Arthritis risk with immune checkpoint inhibitor therapy for cancer. Curr Opin Rheumatol 31(3):293–299

111. Puzanov I, Diab A, Abdallah K, et al, Society for Immunotherapy of Cancer Toxicity Management Working Group (2017) Managing toxicities associated with immune checkpoint inhibitors: consensus recommendations from the Society for Immunotherapy of Cancer (SITC) Toxicity Management Working Group. J Immunother Cancer 5(1):1–28

112. Reck M, Rodriguez-Abreu D, Robinson AG et al (2016) Pembrolizumab versus chemotherapy for PD-L1-positive non-small-cell lung cancer. N Engl J Med 375:1823–1833

113. Roberts J, Smylie M, Walker J et al (2019) Hydroxychloroquine is a safe and effective steroid-sparing agent for immune checkpoint inhibitor-induced inflammatory arthritis. Clin Rheumatol 38(5):1513–1519. https://doi.org/10.1007/s10067-019-04451-2

114. Roberts K, Culleton V, Lwin Z, O'Byrne K, Hughes BGM (2017) Immune checkpoint inhibitors: navigating a new paradigm of treatment toxicities. Asia Pac J Clin Oncol 13(4):277–288

115. Rossi E, Sgambato A, DeChiara G et al (2016) Endocrinopathies induced by immune checkpoint inhibitors in advanced non-small cell lung cancer. Expert Rev Clin Pharmacol 9:419–428

116. Routy B, Le Chatelier E, Derosa L, Duong CPM, Alou MT, Daillère R, Fluckiger A, Messaoudene M, Rauber C, Roberti MP, Fidelle M, Flament C, Poirier-Colame V, Opolon P, Klein C, Iribarren K, Mondragón L, Jacquelot N, Qu B, Ferrere G, Clémenson C, Mezquita L, Masip JR, Naltet C, Brosseau S, Kaderbhai C, Richard C, Rizvi H, Levenez F, Galleron N, Quinquis B, Pons N, Ryffel B, Minard-Colin V, Gonin P, Soria JC, Deutsch E, Loriot Y, Ghiringhelli F, Zalcman G, Goldwasser F, Escudier B, Hellmann MD, Eggermont A, Raoult D, Albiges L, Kroemer G, Zitvogel L (2018) Gut microbiome influences efficacy of PD-1-based immunotherapy against epithelial tumors. Science 359(6371):91–97. https://doi.org/10.1126/science.aan3706. Epub 2017 Nov 2 PMID: 29097494.

117. Sakamori Y, Kim YH, Yoshida H et al (2015) Effect of liver toxicity on clinical outcome of patients with non-small cell lung cancer treated with pemetrexed. Mol Clin Oncol 3(2):334–340

118. Salem JE, Allenbach Y, Kerneis M et al (2019) Abatacept for severe immune checkpoint inhibitor-associated myocarditis. N Engl J Med 380(24):2377–2379

119. Salem JE, Manouchhri A, Moey M et al (2018) Cardiovascular toxicities associated with immune checkpoint inhibitors :an observational, restrospective, pharmacovigilance study. Lancet Oncol 19:1579–1589

120. Seethapathy H, Chute D, Oppong Y et al (2018) Acute kidney injury is common in patients receiving checkpoint inhibitors [abstract]. J Am Soc Nephrol 29:124

121. Santini FC, Rivzi H, Wilkins O et al (2017) Safety of retreatment with immunotherapy after immune-related toxicity in patients with lung cancer treated with anti-PD(L)-1 therapy. J Clin Oncol 35(15 suppl):abstract 9012

122. Shafqat H, Gourdin T, Sion A (2018) Immune-related adverse events are linked with improved progression free survival in patients receiving anti-PD-1/PD-L1 therapy. Semin Oncol 45(3):156–163

123. Shirali AC, Perazella MA, Gettinger S (2016) Association of acute interstitial nephritis with programmed cell death 1 inhibitor therapy in lung cancer patients. Am J Kidney Dis 68:287–291

124. Shivaji UN, Jeffery L, Gui X et al (2019) Immune checkpoint inhibitor-associated gastrointestinal and hepatic adverse events and their management. Ther Adv Gastroenterol 12:1756284819884196

125. Simonaggio A, Michot JM, Voisin AL et al (2019) Evaluation of readministration of immune checkpoint inhibitors after immune-related adverse events in patients with cancer. JAMA Oncol 5(9):1310–1317

126. Sise ME, Seethapathy H, Reynolds K (2019) Diagnosis and management of immune checkpoint inhibitor-associated renal toxicity: illustrative case and review. Oncologist 24:1–8

127. Sivan A, Corrales L, Hubert N, Williams JB, Aquino-Michaels K, Earley ZM, Benyamin FW, Lei YM, Jabri B, Alegre ML, Chang EB, Gajewski TF (2015) Commensal Bifidobacterium promotes antitumor immunity and facilitates anti-PD-L1 efficacy. Science 350(6264):1084–1089. https://doi.org/10.1126/science.aac4255. Epub 2015 Nov 5. PMID: 26541606; PMCID: PMC4873287

128. Soularue E, Lepage P, Colombel JF, Coutzac C, Faleck D, Marthey L, Collins M, Chaput N, Robert C, Carbonnel F (2018) Enterocolitis due to immune checkpoint inhibitors: a systematic review. Gut 67(11):2056–2067. https://doi.org/10.1136/gutjnl-2018-316948. Epub 2018 Aug 21. PMID: 30131322

129. Spain L, Walls G, Julve M et al (2017) Neurotoxicity from immune-checkpoint inhibition in the treatment of melanoma: a single centre experience and review of the literature. Ann Oncol 28:377–385

130. Su Q, Zhang XC, Zhang CG, Hou YL, Yao YX, Cao BW (2018) Risk of immune related pancreatitis in patients with solid tumors treated with immune checkpoint inhibitors: systematic assessment with meta-analysis. J Immunol Res 2018:1027323. https://doi.org/10.1155/2018/1027323. Accessed 20 May 2020

131. Suresh K, Naidoo J (2020) Lower survival in patients who develop pneumonitis following immunotherapy for lung cancer. Clin Lung Cancer 21:e169–e170

132. Suresh K, Psoter KJ, Voong KR et al (2019) Impact of checkpoint inhibitor pneumonitis on survival in NSCLC patients receiving immune checkpoint immunotherapy. J Thorac Oncol 14:494–502

133. Sury K, Perazella MA, Shirali AC (2018) Cardiorenal complications of immune checkpoint inhibitors. Nat Rev Nephrol 14(9):571–588. https://doi.org/10.1038/s41581-018-0035-1. PMID: 30013100

134. Suzman M, Ferrucci PF, Rosenberg A, Avigan MI (2018) Hepatotoxicity of immune checkpoint inhibitors: an evolving picture of risk associated with a vital class of immunotherapy agents. Liver Int 38(6):976–987

135. Sznol M, Postow MA, Davies MJ et al (2017) Endocrine-related adverse events associated with immune checkpoint blockade and expert insights on their management. Cancer Treat Rev 58:70–76

136. Tamura T, Akimoto E (2018) Vogt-Koyanagi-Harada syndrome induced by Pembrolizumab in a patient with non-small cell lung cancer. J Thorac Oncol 13(10):1606–1607

137. Tison A, Quéré G, Misery L et al (2019) Safety and efficacy of immune checkpoint inhibitors in patients with cancer and preexisting autoimmune disease: a nationwide, multicenter cohort study. Arthritis Rheumatol 71:2100

138. Thompson JA (2018) New NCCN guidelines: recognition and management of immunotherapy-related toxicity. J Natl Compr Cancer Netw 16(5S):594–596. https://doi.org/10.6004/jnccn.2018.0047. PMID: 29784734

139. Thompson JA, Schneider BJ, Brahmer J, Andrews S, Armand P, Bhatia S, Budde LE, Costa L, Davies M et al (2020) NCCN Clinical Practice Guidelines in Oncology (NCCN Guidelines®): Management of immunotherapy-related toxicities, version 1.2020: featured updates to the NCCN guidelines. JNCCN: J Natl Compr Cancer Netw 18(3):230–241

140. Thompson JA, Schneider BJ, Brahmer J, Andrews S, Armand P, Bhatia S, Budde LE, Costa L, Davies M et al (2019) NCCN Clinical Practice Guidelines in Oncology (NCCN Guidelines®):

Management of Immunotherapy-Related Toxicities (immune checkpoint inhibitor-related toxicities). Version 1.2019. JNCCN: J Natl Compr Cancer Netw 17(3):255–289

141. U.S. Department of Health and Human Services NIH, National Cancer Institute. Common Terminology Criteria for Adverse Events (CTCAE) version 5.0. https://ctep.cancer.gov/protocoldevelopment/electronic_applications/ctc.htm#ctc_50. Published November 27, 2017. Accessed 20 Mar 2020

142. Vaddepally RK, Kharel P, Pandey R, Garje R, Chandra AB (2020) Review of indications of FDA-approved immune checkpoint inhibitors per NCCN guidelines with the level of evidence. Cancers (Basel) 12(3):738. https://doi.org/10.3390/cancers12030738. PMID: 32245016; PMCID: PMC7140028

143. Varricchi G, Marone G, Mercurio V, Galdiero MR, Bonaduce D, Tocchitti CG (2018) Immune checkpoint inhibitors and cardiac toxicity: an emerging issue. Curr Med Chem 25(11):1327–1339

144. Vétizou M, Pitt JM, Daillère R, Lepage P, Waldschmitt N, Flament C, Rusakiewicz S, Routy B, Roberti MP, Duong CP, Poirier-Colame V, Roux A, Becharef S, Formenti S, Golden E, Cording S, Eberl G, Schlitzer A, Ginhoux F, Mani S, Yamazaki T, Jacquelot N, Enot DP, Bérard M, Nigou J, Opolon P, Eggermont A, Woerther PL, Chachaty E, Chaput N, Robert C, Mateus C, Kroemer G, Raoult D, Boneca IG, Carbonnel F, Chamaillard M, Zitvogel L (2015) Anticancer immunotherapy by CTLA-4 blockade relies on the gut microbiota. Science 350(6264):1079–1084. https://doi.org/10.1126/science.aad1329. Epub 2015 Nov 5. PMID: 26541610; PMCID: PMC4721659

145. Verhaegh BPM, de Vries F, Masclee AAM et al (2016) High risk of drug-induced microscopic colitis with concomitant use of NSAIDs and proton pump inhibitors. Aliment Pharmacol Ther 43:1004–1013

146. Wanchoo R, Karam S, Uppal NN et al (2017) Adverse renal effects of immune checkpoint inhibitors: a narrative review. Am J Nephrol 45:160–169

147. Wang A, Xu Y, Fei Y, Wang M (2020) The role of immunosuppressive agents in the management of severe and refractory immune-related adverse events. Asia Pac J Clin Oncol 16(4):201–210. https://doi.org/10.1111/ajco.13332

148. Wang Y, Abu-Sbeih H, Mao E et al (2018) Endoscopic and histologic features of immune checkpoint inhibitor-related colitis. Inflamm Bowel Dis 24(8):1695–1705

149. Wang DY, Salem JE, Cohen JV et al (2018) Fatal toxic effects associated with immune checkpoint inhibitors: a systematic review and meta-analysis. JAMA Oncol 4(12):1721–1728

150. Wang W, Lie P, Guo M et al (2017) Risk of hepatotoxicity in cancer patients treated with immune checkpoint inhibitors: a systematic review and meta-analysis of published data. Int J Cancer 141:1018–1028

151. Warner BM, Baer AN, Lipson EJ et al (2019) Sicca syndrome associated with immune checkpoint inhibitor therapy. Oncologist 24:1259

152. Weber JS, Dummer R, de Pril V, Lebbie C, Hodi FS, MDX010-20 Investigators (2013) Patterns of onset and resolution of immune-related adverse events of special interest with ipilimumab: detailed safety analysis from a phase 3 trial in patients with advanced melanoma. Cancer 119(9):1675–1682

153. Weber JS, Kahler KC, Hauschild A (2012) Management of immune-mediated adverse events and kinetics of response with ipilimumab. J Clin Oncol 30(21):2691–2012

154. Wu J, Hong D, Zhang X, Lu X, Miao J (2017) PD-1 inhibitors increase the incidence and risk of pneumonitis in cancer patients in a dose-independent manner : a meta-analysis. Sci Rep 7:44173

155. Yang H, Yao Z, Zhou X, Zhang W, Zhang X, Zhang F (2020) Immune-related adverse events of checkpoint inhibitors: insights into immunological dysregulation. Clin Immunol 213:108377. https://doi.org/10.1016/j.clim.2020.108377. Epub 2020 Mar 2. PMID: 32135278

156. Zimmer L, Goldinger SM, Hofman L et al (2016) Neurological, respiratory, musculoskeletal, cardiac and ocular side effects of anti-PD-1 therapy. Eur J Cancer 60:210–225

Chapter 8
Therapeutic Advances in Small Cell Lung Cancer Management

Benjamin Newton and Anne C. Chiang

Abstract Small cell lung cancer is a recalcitrant malignancy that poses significant management challenges for the treating physician. Recent developments in our understanding of the biology of this disease have created opportunities to advance the field of small cell lung cancer treatment. Some of the most notable recent breakthroughs include immunotherapy, and novel approaches are being developed to leverage new targets for therapeutic intervention. Promising work is being done in many domains, including DNA repair, cell cycle regulation and epigenetics. With all of these discoveries, there is reason to be hopeful for further progress in the years ahead.

Keywords Lung cancer · Small cell lung cancer · Small cell lung cancer treatments

1 Introduction

Small cell lung cancer is a distinct subtype of lung cancer, comprising approximately 14% of lung cancer patients [1], with a unique biology and clinical course. Small cell lung cancer typically demonstrates aggressive behavior with rapid growth and early spread early to distant sites, and often goes undetected until the cancer has reached an advanced stage. It is also known for its sensitivity to cytotoxic chemotherapy and radiation.

Smoking is the predominant risk factor for the development of small cell lung cancer, and nearly all patients with this type of malignancy are current or former users of tobacco. Both the incidence and mortality rates of small cell lung cancer have decreased in the United States in recent decades. It has been posited that a

B. Newton, MD (✉) · A. C. Chiang, MD, PhD
Department of Medicine (Medical Oncology), Yale School of Medicine/Yale Cancer Center, New Haven, CT, USA
e-mail: Benjamin.newton@yale.edu

© Springer Nature Switzerland AG 2021
A. C. Chiang, R. S. Herbst (eds.), *Lung Cancer*, Current Cancer Research,
https://doi.org/10.1007/978-3-030-74028-3_8

potential explanation for this is a change in tobacco usage patterns, including a decrease in the percentage of smokers and a change to low tar cigarettes [1].

The biology of small cell lung cancer poses special challenges for the development of effective treatments, as it has been difficult to identify driver oncogenes amenable to targeted therapy. As a result, small cell lung cancer has been primarily viewed clinically as a single disease entity, in contrast to the increasingly personalized clinical approach used in lung adenocarcinoma. In terms of genomics, small cell lung cancer has been understood to be relatively homogeneous, with nearly universal loss-of function mutations in the tumor suppressor genes *TP53* and *RB1*. Defects in these genes tend to promote genomic instability and may increase the number of genomic alterations in the tumor. Small cell lung cancer has a very large mutation burden, as might expected in a cancer so closely associated with tobacco exposure. Nonetheless, efforts are underway to identify clinically relevant subtypes of disease, and a new model of biologically distinct small cell lung cancer subtypes has been proposed, based on the observed differential expression of four pivotal transcriptional regulators: achaete-scute homologue 1(ASCL1), neurogenic differentiation factor 1(NeuroD1), yes-associated protein (YAP1) and POU class 2 homeobox 3(POU2F3) [2]. There is evidence of a differential response to the addition of immune checkpoint inhibitors to chemotherapy among these tumor subtypes, with an inflamed, mesenchymal subtype predicting benefit from this treatment combination [3]. It is hoped that in this reconceptualization of the disease, that subtype-specific therapeutic vulnerabilities are identified, leading to more precise, effective treatments.

Despite a high tumor mutation burden observed in small cell lung cancer, immune escape mechanisms appear to be active, leading to relatively low clinical efficacy of immune checkpoint blockade as a treatment strategy, as compared to its role in non-small cell lung cancer. It has been posited that underlying causes for this could include generally low programmed death ligand 1 (PD-L1) expression, downregulation of major histocompatibility complex molecules, impairment of the host immune system through various cytokine mediated mechanisms, and through autocrine and paracrine regulation [4].

Novel approaches are being developed as therapeutic opportunities in small cell lung cancer are becoming better understood, particularly in the areas of DNA repair, cell cycle regulation and epigenetics.

At the time of diagnosis, approximately 30% of patients with small cell lung cancer will have limited stage disease, which is defined as confined to the hemithorax of origin, the mediastinum or the supraclavicular lymph nodes [5], and the ability to treat in a reasonable radiation field. Patients who have tumor that have extended beyond this are characterized as having extensive stage disease. Limited stage small cell lung cancer is potentially curable, while extensive stage small cell lung cancer is not curable, though treatment can help to improve quality of life and prolong survival.

2 Limited Stage Small Cell Lung Cancer

The International Association for the Study of Lung Cancer (IASLC) recommends using Tumor, Node, Metastasis (TNM) staging for small cell lung cancer [6]. Thorough staging for small cell lung cancer includes an MRI of the brain, as well as PET CT and CT of the chest and abdomen with contrast. For patients with limited stage small cell lung cancer, careful staging also includes pathologic mediastinal staging, which can help to discern who might benefit from surgery as part of a multimodality treatment approach, as opposed to chemoradiation, both with the intent of cure.

2.1 Surgery for Limited Stage Small Cell Lung Cancer

The majority of patients with limited stage small cell lung cancer will have evidence of mediastinal lymph node involvement. For the minority of patients that have cT1 or cT2 tumors and negative mediastinal staging, surgery is a therapeutic option. This applies to less than 5% of patients with small cell lung cancer. Patients who undergo definitive surgical resection should have a lobectomy with mediastinal node dissection. Surgery alone is not considered an adequate treatment for limited stage small cell lung cancer, as poor survival with surgery alone has been demonstrated in earlier observational studies [7–9].

In contrast, appropriate patients who undergo surgery as part of a multimodality treatment approach can derive significant clinical benefit. This was demonstrated in the International Association for the Study of Lung Cancer (IASLC) Lung Cancer Staging Project, which was a database review of over 8000 cases of small cell lung cancer, 349 of which were resected surgically. Five year survival rates were 48%, 39%, and 15% for patients with pathologic stage I, II and III disease, respectively [6]. Another review of the Surveillance, Epidemiology and End Results (SEER) database included 247 patients who underwent resection with or without radiation for stage I small cell lung cancer. Patients who underwent lobectomy without radiation had a 5 year survival rate of 50.3% and patients who underwent lobectomy with radiation had a 5 year survival rate of 57.1% [10]. In a retrospective review of the National Cancer Database of over 3000 patients with limited stage small cell lung cancer, the degree of benefit was related to degree of nodal involvement. Patients with pathologic N2 involvement had a survival benefit with the addition of postoperative radiation, while patients with N0 or N1 disease did not [11].

Observational studies suggest that outcomes are improved when surgery is followed by adjuvant chemotherapy [12], though there are no randomized trials that have compared surgery alone to surgery followed by adjuvant chemotherapy or chemoradiation. Chemotherapy typically consists of four cycles of cisplatin plus etoposide.

2.2   Chemoradiation for Limited Stage Small Cell Lung Cancer

For patients with limited stage small cell lung cancer who present with T3 or greater primary tumors, or with pathologic nodal involvement, the standard of care is concurrent chemoradiation, rather than surgery, with the start of radiation early in the chemotherapy treatment course. Patients who are treated with concurrent chemoradiation and prophylactic cranial irradiation (discussed below) have overall response rates of 80–90%, including 50–60% complete response rates. Median survival is approximately 17 months, and the five-year survival rate is approximately 20% [13, 14].

Cisplatin and etoposide are the favored agents in concurrent chemoradiation. Earlier studies of combined modality therapy in limited stage small cell lung cancer used chemotherapy regimens such as cyclophosphamide, doxorubicin, and vincristine, followed by sequential radiation therapy. Later studies showed that cisplatin and etoposide used in a sequential approach with radiation could result in favorable response and survival rates [15]. Cisplatin and etoposide was also compared to cyclophosphamide, epirubicin and vincristine, both regimens as part of concurrent chemoradiation plans for limited stage small cell lung cancer. Overall survival was significantly better with cisplatin and etoposide [16]. Two subsequent meta-analyses demonstrated a modest survival benefit in studies evaluating etoposide-based or cisplatin-based therapy for the treatment of limited stage and extensive stage small cell lung cancer [17, 18]. Cisplatin and etoposide has less associated myelotoxicity than regimens to which it has been compared and it is generally easier to combine with radiation, making it the recognized standard regimen for use in concurrent chemoradiation.

Carboplatin is often substituted for cisplatin when the toxicity profile of cisplatin precludes its use in a particular patient, and similar response rates, progression free survival and overall survival have been demonstrated in a meta-analysis comprised of four separate trials, though only two of the trials enrolled patients with limited stage small cell lung cancer [19]. Of note, toxicity profiles vary significantly, with more hematologic toxicity seen with carboplatin, and more non-hematologic toxicity seen with cisplatin. However, because the intention of treatment is cure, and because of the lack of data that directly compares these two agents in the setting of limited stage disease, cisplatin remains the drug of choice, with carboplatin as an acceptable alternative as the situation requires.

Adding radiation to chemotherapy has been shown to improve local control rates and modestly improve survival rates for patients with limited stage small cell lung cancer. This was borne out in two large meta-analyses, as well as in a more recent review of the National Cancer Data Base [13, 20, 21]. Radiation with concurrent chemotherapy is standard practice and is preferred over sequential chemotherapy and radiation. Concurrent radiotherapy has been shown to yield better survival than sequential radiotherapy, with an improvement in median overall survival of 7.5 months in a large phase III trial [22]. Radiation should start early, with cycle 1 or 2 of systemic therapy [23]. It has been demonstrated that survival improves as the time span from the start of chemotherapy to the last day of radiotherapy is minimized [24].

Limited field thoracic radiotherapy is the current standard of care. The treatment volume should contain include all gross disease present as well as all nodal regions involved at the time of diagnosis. Target volumes should be defined based on the pretreatment PET and CT imaging [25].

For limited-stage small cell lung cancer, the optimal dose and schedule of radiation have not been established [25]. Most thoracic radiation regimens that use conventional, once daily fractionation use doses of approximately 60–70 Gy, administered in 2 Gy fractions. Accelerated hyperfractionation regimens treat to 45 Gy, administered in 1.5 Gy fractions, administered twice daily over 3 weeks. The rationale for accelerated hyperfractionation is that there is less opportunity for tumor cell regeneration, as the overall treatment time is shortened, though drawbacks include increased acute toxicities, as well as a cumbersome twice daily treatment schedule. The two fractionation schedules have been compared in several randomized trials, the largest of which showed a trend toward improved median survival of 30 versus 25 months, favoring accelerated hyperfractionation, though the findings failed to achieve statistical significance [26]. As such, daily fractionation remains the standard of care.

Historically, radiographically uninvolved mediastinal nodes have been included in the radiotherapy target volume, while uninvolved supraclavicular nodes have not been included. Several small studies suggest that omission of elective nodal irradiation may result in very low rates of isolated nodal recurrence [27]. As such, elective nodal irradiation is no longer a standard part of radiation planning.

During concurrent chemoradiation, the use of myeloid growth factors is not recommended, as there is phase III evidence showing an increase in the frequency and duration of life-threatening thrombocytopenia, toxic death, non-hematologic toxicity, days spent in the hospital, antibiotic usage, and transfusions when GM-CSF is used. There was a trend towards a lower complete response rate associated with the use of GM-CSF, but the differences did not meet statistical significance [28].

Patients with limited stage small cell lung cancer who use tobacco should be encouraged to stop smoking before undergoing combined modality therapy because continued smoking may compromise survival [29].

2.3   Checkpoint Inhibitors in Limited Stage Small Cell Lung Cancer

The inhibition of programmed death ligand 1 (PD-L1) – programmed death 1 (PD-1) signaling and the resulting enhancement of tumor specific T-cell immunity represents a significant advancement in the management of small cell lung cancer. Phase 3 studies, e.g. ADRIATIC, STIMIULI, KEYLYNK-013, NRG-LU005, are underway to determine whether there is a role for checkpoint inhibitors during or following chemoradiation for limited stage small cell lung cancer, similar to studies for patients with non-small cell lung cancer [30] clinicaltrials.gov for STIMULI (NCT02046733), NRG-LU005 (NCT03811002), KEYLYNK-013 (NCT04624204). ADRIATIC and STIMULI have a design similar to the PACIFIC trial, which

Study	Phase	Treatment	Treatment Setting	# of Patients	Result
IMpower133	3	Chemotherapy + Atezolizumab	Extensive Stage First Line	403	Improved OS
CASPIAN	3	Chemotherapy + durvalumab	Extensive Stage First Line	537	Improved OS
Keynote-604	3	Chemotherapy + pembrolizumab	Extensive Stage First Line	453	Improved PFS
CheckMate451	3	Nivolumab + Ipilimumab	Maintenance following First Line Therapy	1327	No improvement in OS
CheckMate032	1/2	Nivolumab + Ipilimumab	Relapsed Disease	247 in Expansion cohort	Durable response with Nivolumab and Nivolumab +Ipilimumab
CheckMate331	3	Nivolumab	Relapsed Disease	569	No improvement in OS
Keynote158	2	Pembrolizumab	Relapsed Disease	107	Promising antitumor activity and durable responses

OS = overall survival, PFS = progression free survival

Table. 8.1 Key immunotherapy trials in small cell lung cancer

established the role of checkpoint inhibition as maintenance treatment for non-small cell lung cancer following treatment with definitive chemoradiation (Table 8.1).

2.4 Prophylactic Cranial Radiation for Limited Stage Small Cell Lung Cancer

Brain metastases are a common problem for patients with small cell lung cancer. For patients who have not developed brain metastases and have had an initial response to treatment, prophylactic cranial irradiation can help to improve outcomes. The standard dose of prophylactic cranial irradiation to the whole brain is

25 Gy in 10 daily fractions, and it is administered after the resolution of any acute toxicities of initial therapy.

In limited stage small cell lung cancer, the value of prophylactic cranial irradiation was demonstrated in a large meta-analysis which showed a significant decrease in the incidence of brain metastases (relative risk 0.46), a decrease in the 3 year cumulative incidence of brain metastases (33% vs 59%) and improved 3 year survival (20.7% vs 15.3%) [31]. The meta-analysis did include patients with extensive stage disease, with 12% of patients in the prophylactic cranial irradiation group and 17% of patients in the control group having extensive stage disease, but in general the results have been viewed to be largely representative of patients with limited stage small cell lung cancer.

2.5 Surveillance After Initial Management of Limited Stage Small Cell Lung Cancer

Because of the high relapse rate associated with limited stage small cell lung cancer, close follow up after initial treatment is essential. This should include regular oncology visits, periodic CT imaging and MRI brain surveillance, regardless of prophylactic cranial irradiation status [25]. Follow up should also include smoking cessation intervention, as indicated.

Long term survivors of small cell lung cancer are at increased risk for new primary cancers, with an estimated risk of 5–10% per year and about 30% at 5 years. New lung cancers comprise about half of these secondary malignancies, and leukemia and genitourinary malignancies are seen with increased incidence as well. As such, it is not only the risk of relapse that justifies close follow up, but also the secondary malignancy risk [32, 33].

3 Extensive Stage Small Cell Lung Cancer

Approximately 70% of patients with small cell lung cancer have extensive stage disease, for whom the main therapeutic modality is systemic therapy. For those who had a response to initial systemic therapy, subsequent thoracic radiation and prophylactic cranial irradiation may provide additional disease control. The median survival for extensive stage small cell lung cancer is about 8–13 months, with few surviving beyond 2 years. In contrast to limited stage small cell lung cancer, patients with extensive stage small cell lung cancer are treated with palliative intent.

The historical standard systemic therapy for extensive stage small cell lung cancer is platinum-based combination chemotherapy, with the most frequently used combinations consisting of cisplatin plus etoposide and carboplatin plus etoposide. Cisplatin plus etoposide replaced the older regimens of cyclophosphamide, doxorubicin and vincristine, as well as cyclophosphamide, epirubicin and vincristine, when comparable outcomes were demonstrated, along with less toxicity [16, 34, 35]. Platinum based combination chemotherapy is generally given for 4–6 cycles. Because of the palliative nature of initial systemic therapy, carboplatin is often used in place of cisplatin, due to a more favorable toxicity profile. Both drugs have been demonstrated to have similar response rates, progression free survival and overall survival in a large meta-analysis [19].

There is now a recognized role for the addition of the immune checkpoint inhibitors to platinum based chemotherapy for first line treatment of extensive stage small cell lung cancer. In a randomized trial of 403 patients with extensive stage small cell lung cancer, the addition of the anti-PD-L1 monoclonal antibody atezolizumab versus placebo to carboplatin and etoposide in the first line improved median overall survival (12.3 vs 10.3 months) and progression free survival (5.2 vs 4.3 months). Patients in the study arm received atezolizumab, carboplatin and etoposide for four cycles, followed by maintenance therapy with atezolizumab. Rates of toxicity were similar between both groups [36]. Similarly, the addition of the anti-PD-L1 monoclonal antibody durvalumab to etoposide and either carboplatin or cisplatin showed improved overall survival (13 vs 10.3 months) in the CASPIAN trial [37]. In this study, the addition of a second of the CTLA-4 monoclonal antibody, tremelimumab, did not meet its primary endpoint of overall survival. Nonetheless, these findings led to the FDA approval of both atezolizumab and durvalumab for treatment of extensive stage small cell lung cancer together with chemotherapy. Another trial, Keynote-604, was designed to evaluate the addition of the PD-1 monoclonal antibody pembrolizumab to etoposide and either carboplatin or cisplatin. Progression free survival benefit was demonstrated, but while the coprimary endpoint of overall survival trended favorably at 10.8 vs 9.7 months, it narrowly missed the threshold for statistical significance [38].

It has been proposed that the function of first line checkpoint inhibitor therapy combined with chemotherapy in small cell lung cancer is primarily that of a maintenance agent. Notably, a phase 3 trial, CheckMate-451, which looked at the PD-1 monoclonal antibody nivolumab and the cytotoxic T-lymphocyte associated protein 4 (CTLA-4) monoclonal antibody ipilimumab in the maintenance setting for patients with extensive stage small cell lung cancer without disease progression following first line platinum based chemotherapy, failed to meet its primary endpoint of overall survival [39]. Future studies may lead to clarity on this point.

3.1   Thoracic Irradiation as Consolidation Therapy

For patients who have had a favorable response to initial systemic therapy, thoracic radiation therapy after initial systemic therapy can provide additional benefit. This was demonstrated in a large phase 3 study wherein patients who were initially treated with four to six cycles of platinum-based chemotherapy and had at least partial response to treatment were randomized to receive either thoracic radiation in addition to standard prophylactic cranial radiation or prophylactic cranial radiation alone. Overall survival was improved at the 2 year mark (12% vs 3%, respectively). Progression free survival was also significantly improved [40]. Further analysis revealed that the benefit was limited to patients who had residual disease in the thorax based on imaging following systemic therapy, and not in those who had a complete response [41]. As such, this approach is generally restricted to those who have residual thoracic disease following systemic therapy. Thoracic radiotherapy should be considered for all patients with extensive stage small cell lung cancer who meet this criteria, however, this has not been tested in patients who have received frontline immunotherapy.

3.2 Prophylactic Cranial Radiation in Extensive Stage Small Cell Lung Cancer

Historically, patients with extensive stage small cell lung cancer would receive prophylactic cranial irradiation following initial systemic therapy. This practice was based on a phase 3 trial conducted by the European Organization for Research and Treatment of Cancer (EORTC) which studied patients who initially received chemotherapy and had an initial response, and were then randomized to prophylactic cranial irradiation or no further treatment. Those patients treated with prophylactic cranial irradiation had a lower incidence of symptomatic brain metastases (15% vs 40%), modestly improved median overall survival (6.7 vs 5.4 months) and a significantly improved 1 year overall survival rate (27% vs 13%) [42]. In a more recent phase 3 trial by Takahashi and colleagues [43], patients who had responded to initial therapy and had no brain metastases on subsequent MRI were randomized to prophylactic cranial irradiation or no further treatment. In this study, the primary endpoint was overall survival, but the trial was stopped early due to futility, and overall survival was shown to be worse with prophylactic cranial irradiation (11.6 vs 13.7 months), though there was a decrease in the incidence of brain metastases with prophylactic cranial irradiation, a secondary endpoint of the study. As for the seemingly contradictory outcomes regarding overall survival, it has been posited that the absence of brain imaging prior to trial enrollment and substantial variations in radiation doses and fractions in the earlier EORTC study may account for these differences. The latter study suggests that prophylactic cranial irradiation should be omitted for extensive stage disease, provided that periodic MRI brain surveillance is done instead [25].

4   Brain Metastasis

Patients who present with brain metastases, in contrast, are treated with whole brain radiotherapy, for which the recommended dose is 30 Gy in 10 daily fractions, because of the proclivity for the development of multiple central nervous system metastases among these patients. More neurotoxicity is observed at this higher dose, than what is typically seen with prophylactic cranial irradiation. Patients who develop brain metastasis after prophylactic cranial irradiation may be able to receive whole brain radiotherapy in select circumstances, though there is controversy surrounding its safety and efficacy, and experience is largely limited to single center observational studies. These studies, while not limited to small cell lung cancer, potentially suggest a role for re-treatment in patients with good performance status and stable extracranial disease [44, 45]. Stereotactic radiosurgery has also been successfully used in selected cases to avoid repeat whole brain irradiation as a salvage therapy for patients with brain metastases following prophylactic cranial irradiation, and is preferred over whole brain radiotherapy when feasible [46]. For salvage stereotactic radiosurgery, having stable extracranial disease is an important factor predicting overall survival.

Toxicities associated with prophylactic cranial irradiation are a more relevant consideration as overall treatment for small cell lung cancer advances. The most significant toxicity concern is delayed neurocognitive impairment, and age is an important predictor of this problem. In a phase 2 Radiation Therapy Oncology Group (RTOG) study, 83% of patients older than 60 years experienced chronic neurotoxicity 12 months after prophylactic cranial irradiation compared to 56% of patients under age 60 [47]. The administration of memantine during and after prophylactic cranial irradiation can be considered, as it has been shown to decrease neurocognitive impairment for those receiving whole brain radiotherapy [25, 48].

In an ongoing effort to minimize treatment related toxicity, there is also growing interest in hippocampus sparing whole brain radiotherapy. Cranial irradiation can lead to a loss of hippocampal neurogenesis, which in effect can suppress new memory formation. Conformally avoiding the hippocampus during cranial irradiation using intensity modulated radiotherapy is being tested in the phase III setting; initial results point to less neurocognitive toxicity, without affecting intracranial progression free survival and overall survival [49].

5   Treatment of Refractory and Relapsed Small Cell Lung Cancer

For patients with small cell lung cancer, the development of resistance to treatment is a major problem. Relapse following initial response to treatment occurs in approximately 80% of patients with limited stage disease, and almost all patients with extensive stage disease. Second-line treatment is always given with palliative intent.

The likelihood of response to second line systemic therapy is highly dependent on the time from initial therapy to relapse [50]. In characterizing relapse, a distinction is often made between resistant relapse and sensitive relapse (relapse less than or more than 90 days from initial therapy, respectively). Patients with resistant relapse generally have a poor response rate of less than 10% to most agents, while patients with sensitive relapse have an expected response rate of approximately 25%.

For patients who develop relapse greater than 6 months after initial treatment, consideration should be given to retreatment with the original regimen [25]. This paradigm was established when the earlier regimen of cyclophosphamide, doxorubicin and etoposide was repeated at the time of relapse, yielding response rates of 62% [51]. Retreatment after 6 months of remission has been adapted to platinum based chemotherapy combinations currently in use. This strategy is likely to receive increasing attention as the use of chemotherapy combined with immune checkpoint inhibitor therapy in the first line becomes more common and time to relapse increases.

The approach to second line treatment also depends on the patient's initial treatment, as there is an established role both for immune checkpoint inhibitor therapy as well as cytotoxic therapy for relapsed small cell lung cancer. For individuals that received an immune checkpoint inhibitor as part of first line therapy, the optimal therapy at the time of relapse is not yet known. For those that have not received an immune checkpoint inhibitor in the first line and have no contraindications, it is reasonable to select immune checkpoint inhibitor based therapy at the time of relapse.

5.1   Checkpoint Inhibitor Therapy for Relapsed Disease

Checkpoint inhibitors improve survival in combination with first line chemotherapy followed by checkpoint inhibitor maintenance, as was demonstrated in the CASPIAN and IMpower133 trials [36, 37]. Notably, the role of checkpoint inhibitors purely in the maintenance setting following first line chemotherapy, specifically nivolumab and ipilimumab, was not established in the CheckMate-451 study, which did not meet the primary endpoint of overall survival [39]. Nonetheless, nivolumab and ipilimumab were both studied in patients with relapsed disease in the pivotal phase 1/2 trial, CheckMate 032 [52]. This study, initially comprised of a nonrandomized cohort, and subsequently followed by a randomized expansion cohort [53], suggests that while nivolumab monotherapy and nivolumab plus ipilimumab are both active with durable responses and manageable safety profiles, the combination of nivolumab plus ipilimumab can improve disease outcomes more than nivolumab monotherapy, though the frequency of adverse events is higher. In the preliminary analysis of the randomized portion of the study, an objective response was achieved in 21% of patients receiving nivolumab plus ipilimumab, compared to 12% in patients receiving nivolumab alone. Overall survival at 1 year was 42% for patients receiving nivolumab plus ipilimumab, compared to 30% in patients receiving nivolumab alone. It is worth noting that a phase 3 trial, CheckMate-331, which compared nivolumab to second line chemotherapy for patients with relapsed small cell lung cancer following exposure to platinum based chemotherapy did not meet its endpoint of overall survival [54]. Nonetheless, findings from CheckMate 032 led to the inclusion of nivolumab in the National Comprehensive Cancer Network (NCCN) guidelines as therapeutic options for patients with recurrent small cell lung cancer, although category 3.

There is a need to define biomarkers that can identify patients who will benefit from immune checkpoint inhibitor therapy. In Checkmate 032, there was no association with PD-L1 expression and benefit from treatment with nivolumab, but there was a subsequent exploratory analysis which demonstrated that tumor mutational burden (TMB) could serve as a predictive biomarker for response to nivolumab plus ipilimumab [55]. In this retrospective analysis, whole exome sequencing was done, and TMB was calculated as the total number of missense mutations in the tumor. Based on TMB, patients were divided into tertiles, and the response rates in the highest tertile was 46% with nivolumab plus ipilimumab and 21% with nivolumab alone, whereas in the lowest tertile the response rates were 22% with the combination and 5% with nivolumab alone. A prospective trial is needed to confirm this finding before TMB can be used as a biomarker to predict for responsiveness to checkpoint inhibitor therapy.

The IgG4 PD-1 monoclonal antibody pembrolizumab has also been studied for activity in the setting of relapse in the advanced small cell lung cancer cohort of KEYNOTE-158, a phase 2 basket study of 10 tumor types as well as microsatellite instability-high (MSI-H) tumors [56]. In this study, results were stratified by PD-L1 Combined Positive Score (CPS), which is the number of PD-L1 staining cells (tumor cells, lymphocytes, macrophages) divided by the total viable tumor cells, multiplied by 100. With pembrolizumab, there was a 35.7% overall response rate in patients with a CPS greater than or equal to 1, and a 6.6% overall response rate in patients with a CPS less than 1. Among treatment responders, the response was often noted to be durable. Pembrolizumab was also shown to have activity in previously treated small cell lung cancer in the phase Ib study, KEYNOTE-28, in which a 33% objective response rate was observed among 24 patients with PD-L1 positive small cell lung cancer [57]. A recent analysis of the pooled data from these two studies found that pembrolizumab had antitumor activity with durable responses, with over half of the responders having a response lasting at least 18 months [58]. KEYNOTE -604 [38], a randomized phase 3 trial adding pembrolizumab to chemotherapy compared to placebo did not show significant different in overall survival, although there was a significant difference in PFS.

It is important to be aware of the spectrum of possible immune mediated adverse events that can be seen with immune checkpoint inhibitors. For patients with immune mediated adverse events, high-dose corticosteroids are recommended based on the severity of the toxicity. Nivolumab and ipilimumab should be discontinued for severe or life-threatening immune mediated adverse events.

5.2 Chemotherapy for Relapsed Disease

For patients who already received immune checkpoint inhibitor therapy in the first line or who are not eligible for such therapy, single agent chemotherapy can be used. Multiple cytotoxic agents have modest activity in this setting, including lurbinectidin, topotecan, irinotecan, paclitaxel, temozolomide, vinorelbine, oral etoposide, gemcitabine, bendamustine, and cyclophosphamide, doxorubicin and vincristine [25].

Lurbinectidin is a selective inhibitor of oncogenic transcription, as it covalently binds to residues lying in the minor groove of DNA, which can result in cell cycle arrest. This agent has demonstrated activity as a second line treatment based on a single arm phase 2 basket trial which showed a 35% overall response rate [59]. This drug was approved by the FDA for use as second-line therapy in 2020, and it is now listed as a preferred regimen for second line therapy by the National Comprehensive Cancer Network. A phase 3 study for this drug in combination with doxorubicin is ongoing.

Topotecan is also approved by the FDA as second-line therapy in small cell lung cancer. It has been shown to increase survival compared to supportive care, and was demonstrated to be more effective in controlling cancer related symptoms than cyclophosphamide, doxorubicin, and vincristine [60, 61]. Oral and parenteral forms of this drug have been shown to be equally effective.

Among the available second line cytotoxic agents, temozolomide also deserves mention, as data suggests it may have activity against brain metastases [62] which could make it a preferential consideration for patients who have already received whole brain irradiation and have limited options for further radiation therapy. The DNA repair protein, methylated O^6-methylguanine-DNA methyltransferase (MGMT), is often aberrantly expressed in small cell lung cancer, and temozolomide has been associated with improved outcomes in the presence of *MGMT* promoter hypermethylation.

During palliative systemic therapy for relapsed disease, response assessment by CT should occur after every 2–3 cycles of therapy. Treatment should continue until 2 cycles beyond best response, progression of disease, or unacceptable toxicity [25].

5.3 Beyond the Second Line

While nivolumab is the only drug approved by the US FDA as a third line therapy for small cell lung cancer, immune checkpoint therapy is now being used in the first and second lines, and as a result there is currently no established third line regimen for extensive stage small cell lung cancer. Under these circumstances, participation in a clinical trial is preferred. Proper patient selection for treatment beyond the second line is essential, as performance status can often be significantly compromised by this time. In the scenario where continued treatment is elected, most oncologists select a non-cross resistant regimen from the commonly used second line agents outlined above.

6 Novel Treatments

New treatment approaches are critically needed in small cell lung cancer, and as the biology of small cell lung cancer is better understood, there is hope for the identification and leveraging of new targets and the development of improved therapeutic approaches in the future.

6.1 DNA Repair

Poly (ADP-ribose) polymerase enzymes are involved in DNA damage repair, and proteomic profiling has found PARP-1 overexpression in small cell lung cancer [63].

PARP inhibitors have been demonstrated to have activity in this disease, both as single agents, as well as in combination with cytotoxic chemotherapy. In a phase 2 study evaluating the addition of velaparib to cisplatin and etoposide as first line therapy for extensive stage small cell lung cancer, improved progression free survival was demonstrated but not overall survival [64]. Another phase 2 trial evaluated addition of velaparib to temozolomide in patients with recurrent small cell lung cancer and demonstrated a higher response rate (39% vs 14%) but no difference in 4 month progression free survival or overall survival [65].

The protein Schlafen-11 (SLFN-11) regulates response to DNA damage and may have a role as a biomarker of responsiveness to PARP inhibitors in small cell lung cancer [66]. Biomarkers are needed to identify a potential subset of patients who might derive benefit from the use of PARP inhibitors.

Wee-1 is a nuclear kinase belonging to the Ser/Thr family of protein kinases, and is an important regulator of cell cycle progression. In p53 defective tumors, the inhibition of Wee-1 results in the abrogation of DNA damage checkpoint G2, sensitizing malignant cells to DNA damaging agents [67]. Wee-1 inhibitors are currently being studied in combination with olaparib for activity in small cell lung cancer.

6.2 MYC Gene Family

The MYC family genes are amplified in approximately 20% of small cell lung cancers [68], often in a mutually exclusive manner with other commonly affected genes including *TP53* and *RB1*. There are inherent difficulties in the rational design of inhibitors of MYC and other transcription factors. MYC is a transcriptional regulator of aurora kinases A and B, and when MYC is amplified and P53 mutations are absent, a growth advantage is seen, such that MYC amplification can predict sensitivity to aurora kinase inhibitors [69]. Alisertib, a selective aurora kinase A inhibitor, was evaluated in a phase 2 study of patients with relapsed or progressive small cell lung cancer and was demonstrated to have a response rate of 21% [70]. Alisertib was subsequently combined with paclitaxel in a phase 2 trial and compared with paclitaxel alone, with the rationale that the two drugs could work synergistically to interfere with the assembly of the mitotic spindle [71]. Favorable progression free survival was demonstrated with the combination, but not overall response rate or overall survival, and there was a higher rate of treatment discontinuation due to adverse effects.

6.3   Epigenetics

Promoter methylation and histone acetylation becomes dysregulated in small cell lung cancer, and these conditions affect gene transcription. Histone deacetylases regulate histone acetylation, leading to increased accessibility of promoter regions and increased transcription of genes. The histone deacetylase inhibitor belinostat has been shown to have synergistic activity when administered simultaneously with cisplatin and etoposide [72], leading to the development of a phase I first line trial for advanced small cell lung cancer [73].

6.4   Other Approaches

The Notch pathway is important for early lung development as it regulates stem cell renewal self-renewal, and this pathway can become dysregulated in small cell lung cancer. Notch signaling can have oncogenic or tumor suppressive effects depending on the cellular environment but in small cell lung cancer, Notch pathway inhibition promotes tumor growth and metastasis [74]. Delta-like protein 3 (DLL3) is an inhibitory Notch ligand, which is upregulated in 80% of patients with small cell lung cancer [75].

   Tarextumab, a fully human IgG2 antibody which selectively inhibits Notch2 and 3 receptor function, has been studied in the phase II setting together with etoposide plus either cisplatin or carboplatin chemotherapy, but no benefit over placebo was demonstrated. The antibody-drug conjugate rovalpituzumab teserine (ROVA-T) links a humanized monoclonal antibody targeting DLL3 and the cytotoxic payload agent pyrrolobenzodiazepine and was studied in the phase 2 TRINITY trial, which yielded lackluster results in patients whose tumors were positive for DLL3 and who had received at least two prior regimens for small cell lung cancer [76]. This drug is now being studied in combination with other therapeutic agents in the phase 1 setting.

   Recently, a bispecific T-cell engager (BiTE) antibody, AMG 757, composed of two single chain variable fragments has been developed, one end directed against DLL3 and the other end directed against the CD3 antigen found on cytotoxic T lymphocytes (CTL). This bispecific antibody is intended to bind the DLL3 antigen on DLL3 expressing tumor cells, and also to bind to the CTL, and in so doing redirect the CTL to the tumor cell, resulting in CTL mediated cell death. This drug is being explored in a Phase 1 study following front line platinum based therapy, both as a maintenance agent, as well as for progressive disease following initial treatment [77].

7 Conclusion

Small cell lung cancer is an aggressive and deadly disease that poses an enormous challenge to clinicians and investigators alike. While there have been advances in the management of this disease, limited tissue availability for translational research has been a substantial limitation to progress. Nonetheless, as knowledge grows regarding tumor immunology and genomic alterations, there is reason to be optimistic about substantial progress in the years ahead.

References

1. Govindan R, Page N, Morgensztern D et al (2006) Changing epidemiology of small cell lung cancer in the United States over the last 30 years: analysis of the surveillance, epidemiologic and end results database. J Clin Oncol 24(28):4349–4544
2. Rudin CM, Poirier JT, Byers LA, Dive C, Dowlati A, George J, Heymach JV, Johnson JE, Lehman JM, MacPherson D, Massion PP (2019) Molecular subtypes of small cell lung cancer: a synthesis of human and mouse model data. Nat Rev Cancer 19(5):289–297
3. Gay CM, Stewart CA, Park EM et al (2021) Patterns of transcription factor programs and immune pathway activation define four major subtypes of SCLC with distinct therapeutic vulnerabilities. Cancer Cell 39(3): 346–360
4. Tian Y, Zhai X, Han A, Zhu H, Yu J (2019) Potential immune escape mechanisms underlying the distinct clinical outcome of immune checkpoint blockades in small cell lung cancer. J Hematol Oncol 12(67):1–12
5. Murray N, Coy P, Pater JL (1993) Importance of timing for thoracic irradiation in the combined modality treatment of limited-stage small-cell lung cancer. The National Cancer Institute of Canada Clinical Trials Group. J Clin Oncol 11(2):336–344
6. Vallieres E, Shepherd FA, Crowley J et al (2009) The IASLC Lung Cancer Staging Project: proposals regarding the relevance of TNM in the pathologic staging of small cell lung cancer in the forthcoming(seventh) edition of the TNM classification for lung cancer. J Thorac Oncol 4(9):1049–1059
7. Fox W, Miller AB, Tall R (1966) Comparative trial of surgery and radiotherapy for the primary treatment of small-celled or oat celled carcinoma of the bronchus. First report to the Medical Research Council by the working-party on the evaluation of different methods of therapy in carcinoma of the bronchus. Lancet 2(7471):979–986
8. Fox W, Scadding JG (1973) Medical Research Council comparative trial of surgery and radiotherapy for the primary treatment of small-celled or oat-celled carcinoma of the bronchus. Ten-year follow-up. Lancet 2(7820):63–65
9. Martini N, Wittes RE, Hilaris BS et al (1975) Oat cell carcinoma of the lung. Clin Bull 5(4):144–148

10. Yu JB, Decker RH, Detterbeck FC, Wilson LD (2010) Surveillance epidemiology and end results evaluation of the role of surgery for stage I small cell lung cancer. J Thorac Oncol 5(2):215–219

11. Wong AT, Rineer J, Schwartz D, Schreiber D (2016) Assessing the impact of postoperative radiation therapy for completely resected limited-stage small cell lung cancer using database. J Clin Oncol 11(2):242–248

12. Yang CF, Chan DY, Speicher PJ, Gulack BC, Wang X, Hartwig MG, Onatis MW, Tong BC, D'Amico TA, Berry MF, Marpole DH (2016) Role of adjuvant therapy in a population-based cohort of patients with early-stage small-cell lung cancer. J Clin Oncol 34(10):1057

13. Gaspar LE, Gay GE, Crawford J et al (2005) Limited -stage small cell lung cancer (stages I-III): observations from the National Cancer Database. Clin Lung Cancer 6:355–360

14. Janne PA, Freidlin B, Saxman S et al (2002) Twenty-five years of clinical research for patients with limited-stage small cell lung carcinoma in North America. Cancer 95(7):1528–1538

15. Evans WK, Shepherd FA, Feld R et al (1985) VP-16 and cisplatin as first line therapy for small-cell lung cancer. J Clin Oncol 3(11):1471–1477

16. Sundstrum S, Bremnes RM, Kaasa S, Aasebo U, Hatlevoll R, Dahle R, Boye N, Wang M, Vigander T, Vilsvik J, Skovlund E, Hannisdal E, Aamdal S, Norwegian Lung Cancer Study Group (2002) Cisplatin and etoposide regimen is superior to cyclophosphamide, epirubicin and vincristine regimen in small-cell lung cancer: results from a randomized phase III trial with 5 year's follow up. J Clin Oncol 20(24):4665–4672

17. Pujol JL, Carestia L, Daures JP (2000) Is there a case for cisplatin in the treatment of small-cell lung cancer? A meta-analysis of randomized trial of a cisplatin-containing regimen versus a regimen without this alkylating agent. Br J Cancer 83(1):8–15

18. Mascaux C, Paesmans M, Berghmans T, Branle F, Lafitte JJ, Lemaitre F, Meert AP, Vermylen P, Sculier JP, European Lung Cancer Working Party (ELCWP) (2000) A systemic review of the role of etoposide and cisplatin in the chemotherapy of small cell lung cancer with methodology assessment and meta-analysis. Lung Cancer 30(1):23–36

19. Rossi A, Di Maio M, Chiodini P et al (2012) Carboplatin- or cisplatin-based chemotherapy in the first-line treatment of small-cell lung cancer: the COCIS meta-analysis of individual patient data. J Clin Oncol 30(14):1692–1698

20. Warde P, Payne D (1992) Does thoracic irradiation improve survival and local control in limited-stage small-cell carcinoma of the lung? A meta-analysis. J Clin Oncol 10(6):890–895

21. Pignon JP, Arriagada R, Ihde DC et al (1992) A meta-analysis of thoracic radiotherapy for small-cell lung cancer. N Engl J Med 327(23):1618–1624

22. Takada M, Fukuoka M, Kawahara M et al (2002) Phase III study of concurrent versus sequential thoracic radiotherapy in combination with cosplatin and etoposide for limited-stage small-cell lung cancer: results of the Japan Clinical Oncology Group Study 9104. J Clin Oncol 20(14):3054–3060

23. Fried DB, Morris DE, Poole C et al (2004) Systematic review evaluating the timing of thoracic radiation therapy in combined modality therapy for limited-stage small-cell lung cancer. J Clin Oncol 22(23):4837–4845

24. De Ruysscher D, Pijls-Johannesma M, Bentzen SM et al (2006) Time between the first day of chemotherapy and the last day of chest radiation is the most important predictor of survival in limited-disease small-cell lung cancer. J Clin Oncol 24(7):1057–1063

25. NCCN guidelines, version 1.2019, 10/10/18. 12/29/18

26. Faivre-Finn C, Snee M, Ashcroft L, Appel W, Barlesi F, Bhatnagar A, Bezjak A, Cardenal F, Fournel P, Harden S, Le Pechoux C, McMenemin R, Mohammed N, O'Brien M, Pantrotto J, Surmonth V, Van Meerbeeck JP, Woll PJ, Lorigan P, Blackhall F, CONVERT Study Team (2017) Concurrent once-daily versus twice daily chemoradiotherapy in patients with limited-stage small-cell lung cancer (CONVERT): an open-label, phase 3, randomized, superiority trial. Lancet Oncol 18(8):1116–1125

27. Gregory MM, Belderbos JS, Kepka L, Martel MK, Jeremic B (2008) Report from the International Atomic Energy Agency (IAEA) consultant,s meeting on elective nodal irradiation in lung cancer: small-cell lung cancer (SCLC). Int J Radiat Oncol Biol Phys 72(2):327–334

28. Bunn PA, Crowley J, Kelly K, Hazuka MB, Beasley K, Upchurch C, Livinsgston R, Weiss GR, Hicks WJ, Gandara DR et al (1995) Chemoradiotherapy with or without granulocyte-macrophage colony-stimulating factor in the treatment of limited-stage small-cell lung cancer: a prospective phase III randomized study of the Southwest Oncology Group. J Clin Oncol 13(7):1632–1641

29. Videtic GM, Stitt LW, Dar AR et al (2003) Continued cigarette smoking by patient receiving concurrent chemoradiotherapy for limited-stage small-cell lung cancer is associated with decreased survival. J Clin Oncol 21(8):1544–1549

30. clinicaltrials.gov. 2019 [cited 2019 January 13, 2019]; a phase III, randomized, double-blind, placeo-controlled, multi-center, International Study of Durvalumab or Durvalumab and Tremelimumab as consolidation treatment for patients with Stage I-III Limited Disease small-cell lung cancer who have not progressed following concurrent chemoradiation therapy (ADRIATIC) clinicaltrials.gov for STIMULI (NCT02046733), NRG-LU005 (NCT03811002), KEYLYNK-013 (NCT04624204)

31. Auperin A, Arriagada R, Pignon JP et al (1999) Prophylactic cranial irradiation for patient with small-cell lung cancer in complete remission. Prophylactic Cranial Irradiation Overview Collaborative Group. N Engl J Med 341(7):476–484

32. Sagman U, Lishner M, Maki E, Sheperd FA, Haddad R, Evans WK (1992) Secondary malignancies following diagnosis of small-cell lung cancer. J Clin Oncol 10:1525–1533

33. Tucker MA, Murray N, Shaw EG, Ettinger DS, Mabry M, Hubber MH (1997) Second primary cancer related to smoking and treatment of small-cell lung cancer. J Natl Cancer Inst 279(10):726G

34. Roth BJ, Johnson DH, Einhorn LH, Schacter LP, Cherng NC, Cohen HJ, Crawford J, Randolph JA, Goodlow JL, Broun GO (1992) Randomized study of cyclophosphamide, doxorubicin and vincristine versus etoposde and cisplatin versus alternation of these two regimens in extensive small-cell lung cancer: a phase III trial of the Southeastern Cancer Study Group. J Clin Oncol 10(2):282–291

35. Fukuoka M, Furuse K, Saijo N et al (1991) Randomized trial of cyclophosphamide, doxorubicin and vincristine versus cisplatin and etoposide versus alternations of these regimens in small-cell lung cancer. J Natl Cancer Inst 83(12):855–861

36. Horn L, Mansfield AS, Szczesna A et al (2018) First-line atezolizumab plus chemotherapy in extensive- stage small-cell lung cancer. N Engl J Med 379(23):2220–2229

37. Paz-Ares L, Dvorkin M, Chen Y, Reinmuth N, Hotta K, Trukhin D, Statsenko G, Hochmair M, Ozguroglu M, Ji J, Voitko O, Poltoratskiy A, Ponce S, Verderame F, Havel L, Bondarenko I, Kazarnowicz A, Losonczy G, Conev N, Armostrong J, Byrne N, Shire N, Jiang H, Goldman J (2019) Durvalumab plus platinum-etoposide versus platinum etoposide in first-line treatment of extensive-stage small cell lung cancer (CASPIAN): a randomized, controlled, open-label, phase 3 trial. Lancet 394(10212):1929–1939

38. Rudin CM, Awad MM, Navarro A et al (2020) KEYNOTE-604: pembrolizumab (pembro) or placebo plus etoposide and platinum (EP) as first-line therapy for extensive-stage small-cell lung cancer (SCLC). J Clin Oncol 38(suppl):abstr 9001

39. Bristol-Myers Squibb Announces CheckMate −451 Study did not meet primary endpoint of overall survival with opdivo plus yervoy vs. placebo as a maintenance therapy in patients with extensive-stage small cell lung cancer after completion of first-line... (2018) https://news.bms.com/press-release/corporatefinancial-news/bristol-myers-squibb-announces-checkmate-451-study-did-not-meet

40. Slotman BJ, van Tinteren H, Praag JO et al (2015) Use of thoracic radiotherapy for extensive stage small-cell lung cancer: a phase 3 randomised controlled trial. Lancet 385(9962):36–42

41. Slotman BJ, van Tinteren H, Praag JO, Knegjens JL, El Sharouni SY, Hatton M, Keijser A, Faivre-Finn C, Senan S (2015) Radiotherapy for extensive stage small-cell lung cancer – Author's reply. Lancet 385(9975):1292–1293

42. Slotman B, Faivre-Finn C, Kramer G et al (2007) Prophylactic cranial irradiation in extensive small-cell lung cancer, prophylactic cranial irradiation in extensive small-cell lung cancer. N Engl J Med 357(7):664–672
43. Takahashi T, Yamanaka T, Seto T et al (2017) Prophylactic cranial irradiation versus observation in patients with extensive-disease small-cell lung cancer: a multicentre, randomised, open-Label, phase 3 trial. Lancet 18(5):663–671
44. Son CH, Jimenez R, Niemierko A, Loeffler JS, Oh KS, Shih HA (2012) Outcomes after whole brain reirradiation in patients with brain metastases. Int J Radiat Oncol Biol Phys 82(2):e167–e172
45. Sadikov E, Bezjak A, Yi QL, Wells W, Dawson L, Millar BA, Laperriere N (2007) Value of whole brain re-irradiation for brain metastases- single centre experience. Clin Oncol (R Coll Radiol) 19(7):532–538
46. Harris S, Chan MD, Lovato JF, Ellis TL, Tatter SB, Bourland JD, Munley M, deGuzman AF, Shaw EG, Urbanic JJ, McMullen KP (2012) Gamma knife stereotactic radiosurgery as salvage therapy after failure of whole-brain radiotherapy in patients with small-cell lung cancer. Int J Radiat Oncol Biol Phys 82(1):e53–e59
47. Wolfson AH, Bae K, Komaki R, Meyers C, Movsas B, Le Pechoux C, Werner-Wasik M, Videtic GM, Garces YI, Choy H (2011) Primary analysis of a phase II randomized trial Radiation Therapy Oncology Group (RTOG) 0212: impact of different total doses and schedules of prophylactic cranial irradiation on chronic neurotoxicity and quality of life for patients with limited disease small cell lung cancer. Int J Radiat Oncol Biol Phys 81(1):77–84
48. Brown PD, Pugh S, Laack NN et al (2013) Memantine for the prevention of cognitive dysfunction in patients receiving whole brain radiotherapy: a randomized, double-blind, placebo-controlled trial. Neuro Oncol 10(15):1429–1437
49. Gondi V, Deshmukh S, Brown PD et al (2018) Preservation of neurocognitive finction with conformal avoidance of the hippocampus during whole-brain radiotherapy for brain metastases: Preliminary result of phsae III trial NRG Oncology CC001. 2018 annual meeting of ASTRO. Abstract LBA9
50. Owonikoko TK, Behera M, Chen Z et al (2012) A systematic analysis of efficacy of second line chemotherapy in sensitive and refractory small cell lung cancer. J Thorac Oncol 7(5):866–872
51. Postmus PE, Berendsen HH, van Zandwijk N, Splinter TA, Burghouts JT, Bakker W (1987) Retreatment with the induction regimen in small cell lung cancer relapsing after an initial response to short term chemotherapy. Eur J Cancer Clin Oncol 23(9):1409–1411
52. Antonia SJ, López-Martin JA, Bendell J, Ott PA, Taylor M, Eder JP, Jager D, Pietanza MC, Le DT, de Braud F, Morse MA, Ascierto PA, Horn L, Amin A, Pillai RN, Evans J, Chau I, Bono P, Atmaca A, Sharms P, Harbison CT, Lin CS, Christensen O, Calvo E (2016) Nivolumab alone and nivolumab plus ipilimumab in recurrent small-cell lung cancer (CheckMate 032): a multicentre, open-label, phase 1/2 trial. Lancet Oncol 17(7):883–895
53. Hellman MD, Ott PA, Zugazagoitia J et al (2018) Nivolumab (nivo) +/– ipilulumab (ipi) in advanced small-cell lung cancer (SCLC): first report of a randomized expansion cohort from CheckMate 032. J Clin Oncol 35(suppl):abstr 8503
54. Bristol-myers squibb announces phase 3 CheckMate-331 study does not meet primary endpoint of overall survival with opdivo versus chemotherapy in patients with previously treated relapsed small cell lung cancer (2018) https://news.bms.com/press-release/corporatefinancial-news/bristol-myers-squibb-announces-phase-3-checkmate-331-study-doe
55. Hellman MD, Callahan MK, Awad MM, Calvo E, Ascierto PA, Atamca A, Rizvi NA, Hirsch FR, Selvaggi G, Szustakowski JD, Sasson A, Golhar R, Chang H, Geese WJ, Antonia SJ (2018) Tumor mutational burden and efficacy of nivolumab monotherapy and in combination with ipilimumab in small-cell lung cancer. Cancer Cell 33(5):853–861
56. Cheol Chung H, Lopez-Martin JA, Kao SC, Miller WH, Ros W, Gao B, Marabelle A, Gottfried M, Zer A, Delord JP, Penel N (2018) Phase 2 study of pembrolizumab in advanced small-cell lung cancer (SCLC): KEYNOTE-158. J Clin Oncol 36(15_suppl):8506

57. Ott PA, Elez E, Hiret S, Kim DW, Morosky A, Saraf S, Piperdi B, Mehnert JM (2017) Pembrolizumab in patients with extensive stage small cell lung cancer: results from the phase Ib KEYNOTE-028 study. J Clin Oncol 35(34):3823–3829
58. Cavallo J (2019) AACR 2019: data analysis shows activity of pembrolizumab in pretreated patients with advanced small cell lung cancer. Available from: http://www.ascopost.com
59. Trigo J, Subbiah V, Besse B, Moreno V, López R, Sala MA, Peters S, Ponce S, Fernández C, Alfaro V, Gómez J (2020) Lurbinectidin as second-line threatment for patient with small-cell lung cancer: a single-arm, open-label, phase 2 basket trial. Lancet Oncol 21(5):645–654
60. O'Brien ME, Ciuleanu TE, Tsekov H, Shparyk Y, Cucevia B, Juhasz G, Thatcher N, Ross GA, Dane GC, Crofts T (2006) Phase III trial comparing supportive care alone with supportive care with oral topotecan in patients with relapsed small-cell lung cancer. J Clin Oncol 24(34):5441–5447
61. von Pawel J, Schiller JH, Shepherd FA et al (1999) Topotecan versus cyclophosphamide, doxorubicin and vincristine for the treatment of recurrent small-cell lung cancer. J Clin Oncol 17(2):658
62. Pietanza MC, Kadota K, Huberman K et al (2012) Phase II trial of temozolomide in patients with relapsed sensitive or refractory small cell lung cancer, with assessment of methylguanine-DNA methyltransferase as a potential biomarker. Clin Cancer Res 18(4):1138–1145
63. Byers LA, Wang J, Nilsson MB, Fujimoto J, Saintigny P, Yordy J et al (2012) Proetomic profiling identifies dysregulated pathways in small cell lung cancer and novel therapeutic targets including PARP1. Cancer Discov 2:798–811
64. Owonikoko T, Dahlberg S, Sica G et al (2017) Randomized trial of cisplatin and etoposide in combination with velaparib or placebo for extensive stage small cell lung cancer: ECOG-ACRIN 2511 study. J Clin Oncol 35(15_suppl):8505
65. Pietanza CM, Waqar S, Krug LM et al (2018) Randomized, double blind, phase II study of temozolomide in combination with either velaparib or placebo in patients with relapsed-sensitive or refractory small-cell lung cancer. J Clin Oncol 36(23):2386–2394
66. Lok BH, Gardner E, Scheenberger VE et al (2017) PARP inhibitor activity correlates with SLFN-11 expression and demonstrates synergy with temozolomide in small-cell lung cancer. Clin Cancer Res 23:523–525
67. Syljuasen RG, Hasvold G, Hauge S et al (2015) Targeting lung cancer through inhibition of checkpoint kinases. Front Genet 6:70
68. Hwang DH, Sun H, Rodig SJ et al (2015) Myc protein expression correlates with MYC amplification in small-cell lung carcinoma. Histopathology 67:81–89
69. Sos ML, Dietlein F, Peifer M et al (2012) A framework for the identification of actionable cancer genome dependencies in small cell lung cancer. Proc Natl Acad Sci USA 109:17034–17039
70. Melichar B, Adenis A, Lockhart AC et al (2015) Safety and activity of alisertib, an investigational aurora kinase A inhibitor, in patients with breast cancer, small-cell lung cancer, non-small cell lung cancer, head and neck squamous cell carcinoma, and gastro-oesophageal adenocarcinoma, a five arm phase 2 study. Lancet Oncol 16:395–405
71. Owonikoko T, Nackaerts K, Csozi T, Ostoros G, Baik C, Ullmann CD, Zagadailov E, Sheldon-Waniga E, Huebner D, Leonard EJ, Spigel D (2017) OA05.05 randomized phase 32 study: alisertib (MLN8237) of placebo + paclitaxel as second-line therapy for small-cell lung cancer (SCLC). J Thorac Oncol 12(1 supplement):S261–S262
72. Luchenko VL, Salcido CD, Zhang Y et al (2011) Schedule-dependent synergy of histone deacetylase inhibitors with DNA damaging agents in small-cell lung cancer. Cell Cycle 10:3119–3128
73. Balasubramaniam S, Redon CE, Peer CJ, Bryla C, Lee MJ, Trepel JB, Tomita Y, Rajan A, Giaccone G, Bonner WM, Figg WD (2018) Phase I trial of belinostat with cisplatin and etoposide in advanced solid tumors, with a focus on neuroendocrine and small cell cancers of the lung. Anti-Cancer Drugs 29(5):457–465
74. Kunnimalayaan M, Chen H (2007) Tumor suppressor role of Notch-1 signaling in neuroendocrine tumors. Oncologist 12(5):535–542

75. Saunders LR, Bankovich AJ, Anderson WC et al (2015) A DLL3-targeted antibody-drug conjugate eradicates high grade pulmonary neuroendocrine tumor-initiating cells in vivo. Sci Transl Med 7:302ra136
76. Carbone DP, Morgensztern D, Moulec SL et al (2018) Efficacy and safety of rovalpituzumab teserine in patients with DLL3-expressing, >3rd line small cell lung cancer: results from the phase 2 TRINITY trial. J Clin Oncol 36:abstract 8507
77. Study evaluating safety, tolerability and PK of AMG757 in adults with small cell lung cancer (2019). Available from: www.cancer.gov

Chapter 9
Small Cell Lung Cancer: Biology Advances

Christine L. Hann

Abstract Small-cell lung cancer (SCLC) represents about 13% of all lung cancers and is hallmarked by early metastatic behavior and poor prognosis. Recently immune checkpoint inhibitors have been approved for use in combination with etoposide plus a platinum agent as initial therapy for patients extensive stage SCLC; with the triplet regimen, the median overall survival is approximately 12 months. Over the past 4 years, several agents, including immune checkpoint inhibitors, have also received FDA-approval for SCLC in the relapsed setting, based primarily on objective response rates or duration of response, but not improvement in survival. Analyses of SCLC models have identified molecular subtypes based on the relative expression of key transcriptional regulators. These analyses are leading to a better understanding of SCLC biology and may help identify distinct therapeutic vulnerabilities among subsets of this disease. Ideally, these investigations will lead to more personalized therapeutic approaches and better outcomes for patients diagnosed with this aggressive cancer.

Keywords Immune checkpont inhibitor · Trascriptional program · Genomics

1 Introduction

Small cell lung cancer (SCLC) is a poorly-differentiated neuroendocrine carcinoma that accounts for approximately 13% of all lung cancer cases [1]. SCLC is initially responsive chemotherapy and radiation treatment, however, in the majority of cases, patients develop and succumb to treatment-refractory recurrence. As a result SCLC has one of the highest case-fatality rates among cancers. In the US, approximately 30,000 deaths annually are attributable to SCLC.

C. L. Hann (✉)
Johns Hopkins University School of Medicine, Baltimore, MD, USA
e-mail: chann1@jhmi.edu

© Springer Nature Switzerland AG 2021
A. C. Chiang, R. S. Herbst (eds.), *Lung Cancer*, Current Cancer Research,
https://doi.org/10.1007/978-3-030-74028-3_9

197

Due to the early metastatic behavior of SCLC, patients with any stage of disease are recommended to receive systemic chemotherapy. From the 1980s through 2018, etoposide plus a platinum agent (EP) was the standard of care for 1st line systemic therapy in the U.S. in extensive stage disease. Starting in 2016, promising results of immune checkpoint inhibitor (ICI) studies were reported in the relapsed SCLC setting resulting in FDA approvals of the PD-1 inhibitors, nivolumab and pembrolizumab [2–4]. In 2019, based on a statistically significant, though modest, improvement in overall survival when combined with carboplatin plus etoposide, the PD-L1 inhibitor, atezolizumab received FDA-approval in the first-line setting for ES SCLC [5]. A similar improvement in OS was reported when durvalumab was added to etoposide plus either cisplatin or carboplatin in therapy-naïve ES SCLC patients leading to the approval of durvalumab in this setting as well [6]. In 2020, the transcriptional inhibitor, lurbinectedin, received FDA-approval for patients with relapsed SCLC based on results from a large phase 2 study [7].

Advances in genomic, proteomic and epigenomic profiling have enabled a better understanding of SCLC biology as has the development of more biologically relevant preclinical SCLC models. In 2012 SCLC was included in the Recalcitrant Cancer Research Act which called on the National Cancer Institute to develop a scientific framework to assist in making progress against this deadly disease. This initiative highlighted the ongoing unmet need in SCLC therapeutic development and has contributed to a groundswell of interest in SCLC research. Results of this research has added to the work of prior decades and are bringing new insights to our:understanding of SCLC biology as summarized in the next sections.

2   Identifying Therapeutic Targets in SCLC

SCLC tumors are hallmarked by near universal inactivation of *TP53* and *RB1*. Underscoring the fundamental role of these two tumor suppressor genes in SCLC, loss of *TP53* and *RB1* in pulmonary cells results in the development of SCLC-like tumors in genetically engineered mouse models (GEMMs) [8]. More recent genomic analyses of SCLC tumors have confirmed frequent loss of *TP53* and *RB1* and amplification of MYC family members and further identified frequent mutations of chromatin remodeling proteins (EP300, CREBBP and MLL2) and Notch family members [9, 10]. Proteomic and epigenetic studies have reported high expression of PARP1, BCL2 and EZH2 [11]. Although many of these alterations are considered major contributors to SCLC pathogenesis, thus far clinical studies have not yielded successful targeted approaches in this disease. SCLC is still treated as a single entity where all patients are offered the same treatment options and the final decisions are based primarily on clinical attributes such as major organ function, performance status, prior toxicities or trial availability. Recently researchers have proposed a new nomenclature for biologic subsets of SCLC based on dominant transcriptional profiles [12]. Ideally this approach will lead to a better understanding of therapeutic vulnerabilities of SCLC and a more personalized approach to care of patients afflicted with this cancer.

2.1 DNA Damage Response (DDR) Proteins

Poly (ADP-ribose) polymerase (PARP) family proteins have multiple activities, most notably in DNA repair [13]. PARP is highly expressed at the mRNA and protein levels in SCLC and in preclinical studies, PARP inhibitors were able to synergize with chemotherapy and radiation in SCLC models [11, 14–16]. These findings have led to clinical evaluation of PARP inhibitors in various disease settings. ECOG 2511, a phase 1/2 study of cisplatin plus etoposide with or without veliparib in chemotherapy-naïve patients with SCLC, reported that the addition of veliparib to EP was associated with an improvement of PFS, the study's primary endpoint [17]. A similar study, using carboplatin in this setting instead of cisplatin, has been completed and results are pending (NCT02289690). In the relapsed setting, a randomized phase 2 study of temozolomide (TMZ) plus veliparib or placebo in patients with recurrent SCLC (NCI 9026) reported an increased ORR for the combination arm, however, the primary endpoint of improvement in PFS at 4 months was not met [18]. A phase 1/2 study of the PARP inhibitor, olaparib, in combination with TMZ in patients with relapsed SCLC reported a ORR of 41.7% and mOS of 8.5 months [19]. Talazoparib, a PARP inhibitor with the most potent PARP-DNA trapping activity among agents currently in trials, demonstrated modest single agent activity with a ORR of 9% in relapsed SCLC in a phase 1 study [20].

Ongoing PARP inhibitor trials in SCLC include: nanoparticle camptothecin (CRLX101) plus olaparib in relapsed SCLC (NCT02769962), liposomal irinotecan (MM398) plus veliparib (NCT02631733) and talazoparib in combination with low-dose TMZ (NCT03672773). In the first-line setting. Preclinically the addition of talazoparib was able to potentiate the effects of ionizing radiation in a panel of SCLC cell lines and SCLC PDXs [16]. A study of olaparib and low dose radiotherapy in SCLC is ongoing (NCT03532880).

The DNA/RNA helicase, Schlafen 11 (SLFN11), regulates responses to DNA damage and replication stress, and has been identified as a candidate biomarker of sensitivity to PARP inhibitors [14, 16, 21]. In correlative studies from the NCI9026 study of TMZ with or without veliparib, SLFN11 expression was associated with improved PFS and OS in patients who received TMZ plus veliparib compared with those who received TMZ only [18]. Data from a PDX co-clinical trial for the phase 2 study of olaparib plus TMZ, however, did not find an correlation between SLFN11 expression and response to olaparib/TMZ. In these models resistance to olaparib/TMZ was associated with low basal expression of inflammatory-response genes [19].

WEE1 is a serine/threonine kinase that regulates the G2/M checkpoint by phosphorylating CDC2 and inactivating CDC2/Cyclin B complexes. Defects in the G1/S checkpoint due to loss of *TP53* and *RB1* renders SCLC reliant on the G2/M checkpoint; thus inhibition of WEE1 can increase sensitivity to DNA-damaging agents. In preclinical studies, the WEE1 inhibitor, AZD1775, enhanced the antitumor activity of the PARP inhibitor, olaparib in *TP53* deficient cells [22]. In the SUKES phase 2 umbrella trial AZD1775 did not show significant single agent activity in patients with relapsed SCLC [23]. AZD1775 is also being evaluated in combination with carboplatin a phase 2 multi-drug, multi-arm study in patients with relapsed SCLC (BALTIC study; NCT02937818).

Checkpoint kinase 1 (CHK1) mediates cell cycle arrest at G2/M. CHK1 inhibition in the context of *TP53* loss, can render cells vulnerable to DNA damaging agents [24]. CHK1 is highly expressed in SCLC and in preclinical studies the CHK1 inhibitor, prexasertib (LY2606368) displayed significant activity, alone or in combination with cisplatin or olaparib. In this work, MYC overexpression was found to be predictive of prexasertib sensitivity [25]. A phase 2 study of prexasertib in relapsed SCLC is has completed enrollment and results are pending (NCT02735980).

2.2 DDR Inhibition and Immunotherapy

In breast, colorectal and ovarian preclinical models, PARP inhibition was shown to enhance immune checkpoint blockade by inducing an interferon-mediated immune response (STING signaling) by increasing cytosolic DNA [26]. The combination of PARP inhibitor, olaparib, and PD-L1 blockade was also synergistic in a transplantable GEMM of SCLC. The CHK1 inhibitor, prexasertib, similarly improved responses to PD-L1 antibodies in SCLC GEMMs [27]. In each case, the combinatorial activity of these DDR inhibitors with PD-L1 agents was dependent on the activation of the cGAS–STING pathway [27]. A basket study of durvalumab plus olaparib (MEDIOLA) included a cohort of patients with relapsed SCLC. While the SCLC cohort failed to meet its primary endpoint of ORR [28], additional studies combining DDR inhibitors and ICI are under development exploring different scheduling and incorporating additional correlative studies. SWOG S1929 is a biomarker-based randomized phase 2 study of maintenance atezolizumab vs atezolizumab plus talazoparib in patients with SFLN11 (+) ES SCLC (NCT04334941).

2.3 MYC

MYC family of proto-oncogenes are transcription factors that control a multitude of intracellular processes including growth and cell cycle entry. MYC paralogs, MYC, MYCL and MYCN are amplified or overexpressed in approximately 20% of SCLC cases [9, 10]. MYC expression, in the context of *RB1* and *TP53* loss (the RPM model), promotes rapid development of non-neuroendocrine SCLC in GEMMs [29]. MYC, more than MYCN or MYCL, represses *BCL2* transcription [30]. In preclinical models, expression of MYC or MYCN is associated with chemotherapy resistance [31, 32]. In a large study of SCLC PDXs, resistance to platinum plus etoposide correlated to increased expression of a MYC gene signature [31]. MYCN overexpression in treatment-naïve GEMMs accelerated SCLC development and diminished responses to EP [32]. Using a CRISPER-screen in this context, the deubiquitinase, USP7, could restore chemotherapy-sensitivity [32].

While direct inhibition of MYC remains a challenge, targeting its downstream effectors may prove more efficacious [33]. MYC-driven SCLC cell lines and GEMMs are sensitized to chemotherapy when treated with Aurora kinase inhibitors [29, 34]. Consistent with these findings, a phase 1/2 study patients with relapsed SCLC reported a 21% ORR to the aurora kinase A (AURKA) inhibitor, alisertib [35]. Clinical activity has also been reported for the combination of paclitaxel with alisertib, with benefit particularly in the MYC-high subset of patients [36]. In a CRISPR activation model, MYC was found to repress BCL2 expression and renders cells sensitized to DDR inhibitors. The combination of a CHK1 inhibitor, prexasertib, and alisertib, prolonged survival of RPM GEMMs when compared with chemotherapy [30]. A Phase 1 clinical trial of the AURKB inhibitor, AZD2811, in patients with relapsed or refractory SCLC is ongoing (NCT02579226).

Metabolomic studies of SCLC cell lines have identified two groups of SCLC delineated by expression of the Achaete-scute homolog-1 (ASCL1) transcription factor [37]. ASCL1^{Low} cells express high levels of guanosine biosynthetic enzymes, IMPDH1 and IMPDH2, both of which are transcriptional targets of MYC. IMPDH inhibition resulted in growth suppression of ASCL1^{Low} cells and improved survival in RPM mice suggesting an potentially exploitable dependency in MYC-driven tumors [37]. MYC-driven SCLC cell are dependent on arginine and depletion of arginine was able to promote survival of RPM mice [38]. A phase 2 study of single agent pegylated arginine deiminase (ADI-PEG20; NCT01266018), however, reported lack of efficacy in a cohort of patients with refractory SCLC. Future directions for this therapeutic approach may require biomarker selection to identify patients who are most likely to benefit.

2.4   Targets in Developmental Pathways

The Notch signaling pathway regulates cell-fate decisions, renewal and homeostasis. NOTCH proteins can be oncogenic or tumor suppressive, depending on their cellular context. In a large genomic study loss of function alterations of Notch family members were reported in 25% of cases, suggesting that Notch functions in a tumor suppressive manner in SCLC [9]. Additional studies, however, have demonstrated that Notch blockade suppresses tumor growth [39]. The ability to directly target Notch signaling for clinical benefit will likely require careful patient selection based on tumor dependency on activated Notch.

Delta-like Ligand 3 (DLL3) is a Notch ligand highly expressed in SCLC and other neuroendocrine tumors and sparingly expressed in normal tissue, making it an attractive target for therapies. The DLL3-targeted antibody-drug conjugate, Rovalpituzumab tesirine (Rova-T), demonstrated significant activity in preclinical models of SCLC and in early phase clinical studies [40, 41]. Follow-up studies including a single-arm phase 2 study in the 3rd line and beyond setting (TRINITY), and randomized phase 3 studies in second-line (TAHOE) and maintenance setting after induction chemotherapy (MERU) failed to meet their primary endpoints and treatment emergent adverse events were substantial. A pilot study of Rova-T in combination with 1st-line chemotherapy was completed and reported a safe dosing combination but did not show any benefit when of Rova-T was added to EP [42]. The Rova-T program was discontinued in 2019 [43].

Selective expression of DLL3 allows for additional targeted approaches including T-cell redirecting therapy, imaging and delivery of radionuclides. DLL3-targeted T-cell redirecting therapeutic strategies include a bispecific T cell engager (BiTE; AMG-757) that binds to DLL3 and CD3, and AMG-119, a chimeric antigen receptor (CAR) T cell therapy targeting DLL3. Each have each demonstrated preclinical activity in SCLC models [44, 45]. AMG-757 and AMG-119 are currently being evaluated in phase I clinical trials for subjects with relapsed SCLC (NCT03319940 and NCT03392064, respectively), ushering in a novel immunotherapeutic approach for SCLC and potentially other DLL3-expressing tumors. The SC16 DLL3 antibody is also being used to develop novel imaging and therapeutic approaches in SCLC. A ^{89}Zr-labelled anti-DLL3 antibody (^{89}Zr-SC16) is under development as a PET-radiotracer and was able to delineate SCLC tumors from normal tissue in mouse models [46]. An observational clinical trial is currently underway to assess biodistribution, safety and correlate tumor uptake of the PET radiotracer to tissue expression of DLL3 (NCT04199741).

2.5 BCL2

BCL2, a central regulator of the intrinsic apoptotic pathway, is overexpressed in the majority of SCLC cases [47, 48]. Preclinical strategies targeting BCL2 have demonstrated potent efficacy in various preclinical models of SCLC [49–52]. Clinical trials of BCL2-directed therapy including antisense strategies or the dual BCL-2/BCL-xL inhibitor, navitoclax, however, have not demonstrated benefit as monotherapy in relapsed SCLC or in the first-line setting when combined with EP [53–55]. A major limitation of navitoclax is an on-target thrombocytopenia due to BCL-xL inhibition in circulating platelets; this activity limited the use of navitoclax with chemotherapy. Preclinical data using SCLC cell lines, PDXs and GEMMs have demonstrated combinatorial efficacy when PI3K/mTOR inhibitor were added to navitoclax, a strategy which ideally could avoid the dose-limiting thrombocytopenia that has limited clinical evaluation of navitoclax. Based on these findings, a phase 1/2 study of navitoclax plus the TORC1/2 inhibitor, vistusertib, in recurrent SCLC is ongoing (NCT03366103). APG-1252, a more potent BCL2 inhibitor with strong binding affinities to BCL2, BCL-xL and BCL-W, is being evaluated in combination with paclitaxel in relapsed SCLC (NCT04210037, NCT03387332). The BCL-2 specific inhibitor, venetoclax, is effective at reducing tumor size in high

BCL-2 expressing PDXs and would allow for concomitant treatment with cytotoxic agents [56]. Venetoclax is currently under evaluation in the front-line setting, either as maintenance with atezolizumab after carboplatin, etoposide and atezolizumab induction (NCT04422210). A study of venetoclax in combination with irinotecan is ongoing (NCT04543916).

2.6 Epigenetic Inhibitors

Frequent mutations in chromatin remodeling genes including CREBBP, EP300 and MLL2 have been reported in genomic studies of SCLC, suggesting that perturbation of epigenetic programming may play a role in SCLC pathogenesis [9, 10, 57]. Enhancer of zeste homolog 2 (EZH2), a histone-lysine N-methyltransferase of the polycomb repressor complex 2, regulates gene expression by catalyzing the methylation of H3K27 [21, 58, 59]. EZH2 expression is under the control of the E2F family of transcription factors which are, in turn negatively regulated by Rb. Thus *RB* loss is associated with high expression of EZH2 and, consistent with this, EZH2 is highly expressed in SCLC [11, 59, 60]. A preclinical study of acquired chemotherapy resistance in SCLC PDXs reported that EZH2 could silence SLFN11 expression resulting in chemotherapy resistance [61]. Inhibition of EZH2 was able to maintain chemotherapy sensitivity. The EZH2 inhibitor, DS-3201b, is currently in clinical evaluation in combination with irinotecan in relapsed SCLC (NCT03879798).

Lysine specific histone demethylase 1A (LSD1) demethylates H3K4me1 and H3K4me2 to control target gene transcription and is highly expressed in SCLC [62]. In preclinical studies, the LSD1 inhibitor, GSK2879552, was able to suppress tumor growth in SCLC cell lines and PDX models and sensitivity to the drug correlated with a hypomethylation signature [63]. A Phase 1 clinical trial of GSK2879552 did not demonstrate a favorable benefit:risk ratio and the study was terminated (NCT02034123). Treatment of SCLC preclinical models with the LSD1 inhibitor, ORY-1001, suppresses tumorigenesis in SCLC PDXs via activation of the NOTCH pathway and resultant inhibition of ASCL1 [64]. A phase 2 study of ORY-1001 in combination with EP in patients with relapsed SCLC is currently enrolling patients (the CLEPSIDRA study).

3 Immunotherapy: Recent Approvals, Biomarkers and Novel Combinations

Two randomized phase III studies, IMpower133 and CASPIAN, have shown that the addition of an anti-PD-L1 antibody to EP improves survival in patients with chemotherapy-naïve ES SCLC [5, 6]. The 2–3 month survival benefit in each study was modest but represented the first improvement over EP since the doublet was established as the standard of care 1st line regimen in the 1980s. Based on this improvement in mOS, atezolizumab and durvalumab have each received FDA-approval in the first-line setting. In the relapsed setting, nivolumab and pembrolizumab had initially received FDA-approval for the treatment of relapsed SCLC after two lines of therapy based on results from CheckMate-032 and pooled analysis from KEYNOTE-028 and -158 [2, 65, 66]. For each nivolumab and pembrolizumab, approval was based on ORR and durability of response and the indications for each have been withdrawn due to failure to meet post-marketing requirements. Combined ICI therapy with nivolumab plus ipilimumab was studied as a part of the CHECKMATE-032 trial and reported higher response rates than nivolumab monotherapy but at the cost of significant toxicities. This combination has not received FDA-approval for SCLC [3]. Notably, these studies of ICI in relapsed SCLC were conducted prior to the use of PD-L1 blockade in the front-line setting. Thus the benefit of anti-PD-1 antibodies for relapsed SCLC after prior exposure to ICI therapy is unknown. Future development in this area is focused on identifying biomarkers of response to immunotherapy and novel immunotherapy combinations.

PD-L1 expression is a predictive biomarker for ICI in several contexts; notably in the use pembrolizumab monotherapy in the 1st line setting for non-small cell lung cancer (NSCLC) [67]. A correlation of PD-L1 expression and responses to ICI therapy in SCLC, however, has been less clear. In CheckMate-032, PD-L1 tumor proportion score of $\geq 1\%$ did not correlate with responses to either nivolumab monotherapy or nivolumab plus ipilimumab [3, 68]. In contrast, in the SCLC cohort of KEYNOTE-158, a combined proportion score (CPS) of $\geq 1\%$ was associated with a significantly higher ORR with pembrolizumab monotherapy [4].

In a retrospective biomarker analysis of CheckMate-032, high tissue tumor mutation burden (tTMB) was associated with improved ORR, PFS and OS for nivolumab monotherapy or nivolumab plus ipilimumab [68]. In contrast, high blood TMB was not associated with benefit when atezolizumab was added to EP in IMpower133 [5]. The multi-cohort KEYNOTE-158 study included prospective tTMB analysis and reported that tTMB-high status identified solid tumor patients with a high response rate to pembrolizumab monotherapy compared with those with tTMB-low tumors. This association appeared to hold for subset of SCLC patients in this study as well [69].

Approaches to augmenting ICI responses in SCLC include combinatorial strategies with DDR targeting agents such as PARP and CHK1 inhibitors. The preclinical data supporting these approaches are described in more detail in the DDR section. Another area of active research involves engaging macrophages and natural killers cells within the tumor microenvironment. CD47, a cell-surface molecule highly expressed in SCLC acts as a ligand for SIRPα, a regulatory protein expressed on macrophages and dendritic cells. Binding of CD47 to SIRPα inhibits activation and phagocytic activity of macrophages and may contribute to immune escape [70, 71]. Inhibition of CD47/SIRPα by either anti-CD47 antibodies or direct inactivation of CD47 suppressed growth of SCLC in preclinical models [71]. Phase 1 studies using anti-CD47 antibodies are currently underway.

4 A New Classification System: SCLC Subtypes Based on Dominant Gene Expression Profile

In 2018, a framework to define SCLC subsets based on differential gene expression of four key transcriptional regulators was proposed [12]. Analysis of the gene expression profiling of SCLC patient tumors, cell lines, and murine models of SCLC revealed that discrete subtypes of SCLC can be distinguished by their relative expression of ASCL1 (~70% of cases), neurogenic differentiation factor 1 (NEUROD1; ~11%), POU class 2 homeobox 3 (POU2F3; ~16%), and yes-associated protein 1 (YAP1; ~2%) [12]. While the majority of SCLC cases have a neuroendocrine (NE) phenotype, preclinical modeling has identified a subset of SCLC that has non-neuroendocrine phenotype (non-NE) and is hallmarked by a more mesenchymal profile [72]. The 4 transcriptional subsets also align to histologic subtypes: NE SCLC include ASCL1 ("classic") and NeuroD1 ("variant") predominant subsets, while non-NE SCLC include the YAP1 and POU2F3 subsets [12].

ASCL1 and *NEUROD1* are each critical in normal neuroendocrine development [73, 74]. In SCLC GEMMs, ASCL1, but not NeuroD1, is required for initiation of tumors; NeuroD1 high tumors, however, may derive from ASCL1-high precursors [75, 76]. ASCL1 and NeuroD1 bind to distinct super-enhancers leading to different downstream gene expression profiles. Target genes of *ASCL1* include *RET, BCL2, MYCL1, SOX2, FOX2A* and *DLL3* [40]. In contrast, NeuroD1 target genes include *MYC, INSM1* and *HES6* [75]. Consistent with this, MYC overexpression in the *Trp53/Rb1* conditional knockout mouse results in the development of NeuroD1-high subtype of SCLC [29]. In contrast to distinct expression of ASCL1 and NeuroD1 in preclinical models, a tissue-based study of SCLC subtype staining reports frequent co-expression of ASCL1 and NeuroD1 [77].

POU2F3-positive SCLC (SCLC-P) lacks neuroendocrine characteristics and does not express high levels of ASCL1 or NeuroD1 [77, 78]. SCLC-P cells maintain a distinct transcriptional signature similar to tuft cells implicating a different cell of origin than other SCLC subsets [78]. CRISPR studies identified a vulnerability of POU2F3-expressing cells to IGF-1R inhibitors [78]. While ASCL1, NeuroD1 and POU2F3 are considered drivers of their respective subsets, it is unclear if this is the case of YAP1.

YAP1 is a key component of the HIPPO pathway and is expressed in small fraction of SCLC tumors [77, 79]. The paucity of YAP1 expressing tumors makes it a challenging SCLC subset to study. Insights from preclinical data supports that *RB1* wild-type SCLC may co-segregate with a YAP1 expression profile [79]. The CDK4/6 cyclin dependent kinases phosphorylate and inactivate Rb, preventing cell cycle arrest. In preclinical work, YAP1 (+) SCLC cell lines were sensitive to several CDK4/6 inhibitors [79]. Currently a clinical trial of the CDK4/6 inhibitor, abemaciclib, is open to patients with *RB* wild-type relapsed SCLC (NCT04010357).

ASCL1, NeuroD1, POU2F3 and YAP1 expression can be assessed by immunohistochemistry (IHC), ideally allowing this classification to be broadly accessible [77]. A recent tissue-based analysis of 174 SCLC samples reported that

ASCL1-dominant expression was present in 69% of samples, NeuroD1 in 17%, POU2F3 in 7% and YAP1 was rare [77]. Based on the known downstream targets of each of these transcriptional programs, SCLC subtypes may harbor unique therapeutic vulnerabilities. Agents hypothesized to target therapeutic vulnerabilities of these SCLC subsets have been or are currently under clinical investigation including BCL2 inhibitors, AURKi, and IGF-1R inhibitors. These studies do not have biomarker selection. Correlation of outcomes of patients, either on study or receiving standard of care therapy, with these SCLC subtypes may enable a better understanding of the predictive or prognostic value of subtype classification. This in turn may pave the way for prospective subset-specific clinical trials and more effective therapeutic development.

5   Conclusions

Recent clinical studies of immune checkpoint inhibitors led to the first FDA-approvals of novel therapies in SCLC in the last 20 years. The addition of an anti-PD-L1 antibody, atezolizumab or durvalumab, to first-line chemotherapy in ES SCLC results in a survival improvement and both of these agents are now approved for therapy-naïve patients. The transcriptional inhibitor, lurbinectedin, has also received FDA-approval in relapsed SCLC. These approvals mark a historic time for SCLC therapeutic development with multiple agents receiving FDA-approval within 2 years. These new treatment options, however, provide only a modest benefit and lack biomarker selection; SCLC is still treated as a singular disease and remains an area of unmet need. To improve the long-term outcome of SCLC patients, ongoing research efforts continue to focus on developing a deeper understanding of SCLC biology and identifying vulnerabilities which can be exploited for therapeutic benefit. SCLC has not been amenable to the personalized approaches enabled by targetable tumor-specific genomic alterations found in other tumor types. Recent insights into the biology SCLC point to a potential classification SCLC subtypes based dominant transcriptional programs and provide a new framework for efforts to develop biomarker-based approaches to this deadly disease.

References

1. Siegel RL, Miller KD, Jemal A (2020) Cancer statistics, 2020. CA Cancer J Clin 70(1):7–30. https://doi.org/10.3322/caac.21590
2. Ready N, Farago AF, de Braud F, Atmaca A, Hellmann MD, Schneider JG et al (2019) Third-line nivolumab monotherapy in recurrent SCLC: CheckMate 032. J Thorac Oncol 14(2):237–244. https://doi.org/10.1016/j.jtho.2018.10.003
3. Antonia SJ, Lopez-Martin JA, Bendell J, Ott PA, Taylor M, Eder JP et al (2016) Nivolumab alone and nivolumab plus ipilimumab in recurrent small-cell lung cancer (CheckMate 032): a

multicentre, open-label, phase 1/2 trial. Lancet Oncol 17(7):883–895. https://doi.org/10.1016/S1470-2045(16)30098-5

4. Chung HC, Lopez-Martin JA, Kao SC-H, Miller WH, Ros W, Gao B et al (2018) Phase 2 study of pembrolizumab in advanced small-cell lung cancer (SCLC): KEYNOTE-158. J Clin Oncol 36(15_suppl):8506. https://doi.org/10.1200/JCO.2018.36.15_suppl.8506

5. Horn L, Mansfield AS, Szczesna A, Havel L, Krzakowski M, Hochmair MJ et al (2018) First-line atezolizumab plus chemotherapy in extensive-stage small-cell lung Cancer. N Engl J Med 379(23):2220–2229. https://doi.org/10.1056/NEJMoa1809064

6. Paz-Ares L, Dvorkin M, Chen Y, Reinmuth N, Hotta K, Trukhin D et al (2019) Durvalumab plus platinum-etoposide versus platinum-etoposide in first-line treatment of extensive-stage small-cell lung cancer (CASPIAN): a randomised, controlled, open-label, phase 3 trial. Lancet 394(10212):1929–1939. https://doi.org/10.1016/S0140-6736(19)32222-6

7. Trigo J, Subbiah V, Besse B, Moreno V, Lopez R, Sala MA et al (2020) Lurbinectedin as second-line treatment for patients with small-cell lung cancer: a single-arm, open-label, phase 2 basket trial. Lancet Oncol 21(5):645–654. https://doi.org/10.1016/S1470-2045(20)30068-1

8. Meuwissen R, Linn SC, Linnoila RI, Zevenhoven J, Mooi WJ, Berns A (2003) Induction of small cell lung cancer by somatic inactivation of both Trp53 and Rb1 in a conditional mouse model. Cancer Cell 4(3):181–189

9. George J, Lim JS, Jang SJ, Cun Y, Ozretic L, Kong G et al (2015) Comprehensive genomic profiles of small cell lung cancer. Nature 524(7563):47–53. https://doi.org/10.1038/nature14664

10. Rudin CM, Durinck S, Stawiski EW, Poirier JT, Modrusan Z, Shames DS et al (2012) Comprehensive genomic analysis identifies SOX2 as a frequently amplified gene in small-cell lung cancer. Nat Genet 44(10):1111–1116. https://doi.org/10.1038/ng.2405

11. Byers LA, Wang J, Nilsson MB, Fujimoto J, Saintigny P, Yordy J et al (2012) Proteomic profiling identifies dysregulated pathways in small cell lung cancer and novel therapeutic targets including PARP1. Cancer Discov 2(9):798–811. https://doi.org/10.1158/2159-8290.CD-12-0112

12. Rudin CM, Poirier JT, Byers LA, Dive C, Dowlati A, George J et al (2019) Molecular subtypes of small cell lung cancer: a synthesis of human and mouse model data. Nat Rev Cancer 19(5):289–297. https://doi.org/10.1038/s41568-019-0133-9

13. Simbulan-Rosenthal CM, Rosenthal DS, Boulares AH, Hickey RJ, Malkas LH, Coll JM et al (1998) Regulation of the expression or recruitment of components of the DNA synthesome by poly(ADP-ribose) polymerase. Biochemistry 37(26):9363–9370. https://doi.org/10.1021/bi9731089

14. Murai J, Huang S-YN, Das BB, Renaud A, Zhang Y, Doroshow JH et al (2012) Trapping of PARP1 and PARP2 by clinical PARP inhibitors. Cancer Res 72(21):5588–5599. https://doi.org/10.1158/0008-5472.CAN-12-2753

15. Cardnell RJ, Byers LA (2014) Proteomic markers of DNA repair and PI3K pathway activation predict response to the PARP inhibitor BMN 673 in small cell lung cancer--response. Clin Cancer Res 20(8):2237. https://doi.org/10.1158/1078-0432.CCR-13-3391

16. Laird JH, Lok BH, Ma J, Bell A, de Stanchina E, Poirier JT et al (2018) Talazoparib is a potent radiosensitizer in small cell lung cancer cell lines and xenografts. Clin Cancer Res 24(20):5143–5152. https://doi.org/10.1158/1078-0432.CCR-18-0401

17. Owonikoko TK, Dahlberg SE, Sica GL, Wagner LI, Wade JL, Srkalovic G et al (2018) Randomized phase II trial of cisplatin and etoposide in combination with veliparib or placebo for extensive-stage small-cell lung cancer: ECOG-ACRIN 2511 study. J Clin Oncol 37(3):222–229. https://doi.org/10.1200/JCO.18.00264

18. Pietanza MC, Waqar SN, Krug LM, Dowlati A, Hann CL, Chiappori A et al (2018) Randomized, double-blind, phase II study of temozolomide in combination with either veliparib or placebo in patients with relapsed-sensitive or refractory small-cell lung cancer. J Clin Oncol 36(23):2386–2394. https://doi.org/10.1200/JCO.2017.77.7672

19. Farago AF, Yeap BY, Stanzione M, Hung YP, Heist RS, Marcoux JP et al (2019) Combination olaparib and temozolomide in relapsed small-cell lung cancer. Cancer Discov 9(10):1372–1387. https://doi.org/10.1158/2159-8290.CD-19-0582
20. de Bono J, Ramanathan RK, Mina L, Chugh R, Glaspy J, Rafii S et al (2017) Phase I, dose-escalation, two-part trial of the PARP inhibitor talazoparib in patients with advanced germ-line BRCA1/2 mutations and selected sporadic cancers. Cancer Discov 7(6):620. https://doi.org/10.1158/2159-8290.CD-16-1250
21. Allison Stewart C, Tong P, Cardnell RJ, Sen T, Li L, Gay CM et al (2017) Dynamic variations in epithelial-to-mesenchymal transition (EMT), ATM, and SLFN11 govern response to PARP inhibitors and cisplatin in small cell lung cancer. Oncotarget 8(17):28575–28587. https://doi.org/10.18632/oncotarget.15338
22. Lallo A, Frese KK, Morrow C, Szczepaniak Sloane R, Gulati S, Schenk MW et al (2018) The combination of the PARP inhibitor olaparib and the Wee1 inhibitor AZD1775 as a new therapeutic option for small cell lung cancer. Clin Cancer Res 24(20):5153–5164. https://doi.org/10.1158/1078-0432.CCR-17-2805
23. Park S, Shim J, Jung HA, Sun J-M, Lee S-H, Park W-Y et al (2019) Biomarker driven phase II umbrella trial study of AZD1775, AZD2014, AZD2811 monotherapy in relapsed small cell lung cancer. J Clin Oncol 37(15_suppl):8514. https://doi.org/10.1200/JCO.2019.37.15_suppl.8514
24. Ma CX, Janetka JW, Piwnica-Worms H (2011) Death by releasing the breaks: CHK1 inhibitors as cancer therapeutics. Trends Mol Med 17(2):88–96. https://doi.org/10.1016/j.molmed.2010.10.009
25. Sen T, Tong P, Stewart CA, Cristea S, Valliani A, Shames DS et al (2017) CHK1 inhibition in small-cell lung cancer produces single-agent activity in biomarker-defined disease subsets and combination activity with cisplatin or olaparib. Cancer Res 77(14):3870–3884. https://doi.org/10.1158/0008-5472.CAN-16-3409
26. Shen J, Zhao W, Ju Z, Wang L, Peng Y, Labrie M et al (2019) PARPi triggers the STING-dependent immune response and enhances the therapeutic efficacy of immune checkpoint blockade independent of BRCAness. Cancer Res 79(2):311–319. https://doi.org/10.1158/0008-5472.CAN-18-1003
27. Sen T, Rodriguez BL, Chen L, Corte CMD, Morikawa N, Fujimoto J et al (2019) Targeting DNA damage response promotes antitumor immunity through STING-mediated T-cell activation in small cell lung cancer. Cancer Discov 9(5):646–661. https://doi.org/10.1158/2159-8290.CD-18-1020
28. Thomas A, Vilimas R, Trindade C, Erwin-Cohen R, Roper N, Xi L et al (2019) Durvalumab in combination with olaparib in patients with relapsed SCLC: results from a phase II study. J Thorac Oncol 14(8):1447–1457. https://doi.org/10.1016/j.jtho.2019.04.026
29. Mollaoglu G, Guthrie MR, Bohm S, Bragelmann J, Can I, Ballieu PM et al (2017) MYC drives progression of small cell lung cancer to a variant neuroendocrine subtype with vulnerability to aurora kinase inhibition. Cancer Cell 31(2):270–285. https://doi.org/10.1016/j.ccell.2016.12.005
30. Dammert MA, Bragelmann J, Olsen RR, Bohm S, Monhasery N, Whitney CP et al (2019) MYC paralog-dependent apoptotic priming orchestrates a spectrum of vulnerabilities in small cell lung cancer. Nat Commun 10(1):3485. https://doi.org/10.1038/s41467-019-11371-x
31. Drapkin BJ, George J, Christensen CL, Mino-Kenudson M, Dries R, Sundaresan T et al (2018) Genomic and functional fidelity of small cell lung cancer patient-derived xenografts. Cancer Discov 8(5):600–615. https://doi.org/10.1158/2159-8290.CD-17-0935
32. Grunblatt E, Wu N, Zhang H, Liu X, Norton JP, Ohol Y et al (2020) MYCN drives chemoresistance in small cell lung cancer while USP7 inhibition can restore chemosensitivity. Genes Dev 34(17–18):1210–1226. https://doi.org/10.1101/gad.340133.120
33. McKeown MR, Bradner JE (2014) Therapeutic strategies to inhibit MYC. Cold Spring Harb Perspect Med 4(10):a014266. https://doi.org/10.1101/cshperspect.a014266

34. Sos ML, Dietlein F, Peifer M, Schöttle J, Balke-Want H, Müller C et al (2012) A framework for identification of actionable cancer genome dependencies in small cell lung cancer. Proc Natl Acad Sci U S A 109(42):17034–17039. https://doi.org/10.1073/pnas.1207310109

35. Melichar B, Adenis A, Lockhart AC, Bennouna J, Dees EC, Kayaleh O et al (2015) Safety and activity of alisertib, an investigational aurora kinase A inhibitor, in patients with breast cancer, small-cell lung cancer, non-small-cell lung cancer, head and neck squamous-cell carcinoma, and gastro-oesophageal adenocarcinoma: a five-arm phase 2 study. Lancet Oncol 16(4):395–405. https://doi.org/10.1016/S1470-2045(15)70051-3

36. Owonikoko TK, Niu H, Nackaerts K, Csoszi T, Ostoros G, Mark Z et al (2020) Randomized phase II study of paclitaxel plus alisertib versus paclitaxel plus placebo as second-line therapy for SCLC: primary and correlative biomarker analyses. J Thorac Oncol 15(2):274–287. https://doi.org/10.1016/j.jtho.2019.10.013

37. Huang F, Ni M, Chalishazar MD, Huffman KE, Kim J, Cai L et al (2018) Inosine monophosphate dehydrogenase dependence in a subset of small cell lung cancers. Cell Metab 28(3):369–382.e365. https://doi.org/10.1016/j.cmet.2018.06.005

38. Chalishazar MD, Wait SJ, Huang F, Ireland AS, Mukhopadhyay A, Lee Y et al (2019) MYC-driven small-cell lung cancer is metabolically distinct and vulnerable to arginine depletion. Clin Cancer Res 25(16):5107. https://doi.org/10.1158/1078-0432.CCR-18-4140

39. Lim JS, Ibaseta A, Fischer MM, Cancilla B, O'Young G, Cristea S et al (2017) Intratumoural heterogeneity generated by Notch signalling promotes small-cell lung cancer. Nature 545(7654):360–364. https://doi.org/10.1038/nature22323

40. Saunders LR, Bankovich AJ, Anderson WC, Aujay MA, Bheddah S, Black K et al (2015) A DLL3-targeted antibody-drug conjugate eradicates high-grade pulmonary neuroendocrine tumor-initiating cells in vivo. Sci Transl Med 7(302):302ra136. https://doi.org/10.1126/scitranslmed.aac9459

41. Rudin CM, Pietanza MC, Bauer TM, Ready N, Morgensztern D, Glisson BS et al (2017) Rovalpituzumab tesirine, a DLL3-targeted antibody-drug conjugate, in recurrent small-cell lung cancer: a first-in-human, first-in-class, open-label, phase 1 study. Lancet Oncol 18(1):42–51. https://doi.org/10.1016/S1470-2045(16)30565-4

42. Hann C, Burns T, Dowlati A, Morgensztern D, Koch M, Chang Y et al (2019) A phase 1 study evaluating rovalpituzumab tesirine (ROVA-T) in frontline treatment of patients (pts) with extensive stage small cell lung cancer (ES SCLC). Ann Oncol 30(suppl_5):v710–v717. https://doi.org/10.1093/annonc/mdz264

43. AbbVie Rova-T Press Release, 8/29/19

44. Baeuerle PA, Kufer P, Bargou R (2009) BiTE: teaching antibodies to engage T-cells for cancer therapy. Curr Opin Mol Ther 11(1):22–30

45. Giffin M, Cooke K, Lobenhofer E, Friedrich M, Raum T, Coxon A (2018) P3.12–03 targeting DLL3 with AMG 757, a BiTE® antibody construct, and AMG 119, a CAR-T, for the treatment of SCLC. J Thorac Oncol 13(10):S971. https://doi.org/10.1016/j.jtho.2018.08.1826

46. Sharma SK, Pourat J, Abdel-Atti D, Carlin SD, Piersigilli A, Bankovich AJ et al (2017) Noninvasive interrogation of DLL3 expression in metastatic small cell lung cancer. Cancer Res 77(14):3931–3941. https://doi.org/10.1158/0008-5472.CAN-17-0299

47. Ben-Ezra JM, Kornstein MJ, Grimes MM, Krystal G (1994) Small cell carcinomas of the lung express the Bcl-2 protein. Am J Pathol 145(5):1036–1040

48. Jiang SX, Kameya T, Sato Y, Yanase N, Yoshimura H, Kodama T (1996) Bcl-2 protein expression in lung cancer and close correlation with neuroendocrine differentiation. Am J Pathol 148(3):837–846

49. Zangemeister-Wittke U, Schenker T, Luedke GH, Stahel RA (1998) Synergistic cytotoxicity of bcl-2 antisense oligodeoxynucleotides and etoposide, doxorubicin and cisplatin on small-cell lung cancer cell lines. Br J Cancer 78(8):1035–1042

50. Oltersdorf T, Elmore SW, Shoemaker AR, Armstrong RC, Augeri DJ, Belli BA et al (2005) An inhibitor of Bcl-2 family proteins induces regression of solid tumours. Nature 435(7042):677–681. nature03579 [pii]. https://doi.org/10.1038/nature03579

51. Tahir SK, Yang X, Anderson MG, Morgan-Lappe SE, Sarthy AV, Chen J et al (2007) Influence of Bcl-2 family members on the cellular response of small-cell lung cancer cell lines to ABT-737. Cancer Res 67(3):1176–1183. https://doi.org/10.1158/0008-5472.CAN-06-2203

52. Hann CL, Daniel VC, Sugar EA, Dobromilskaya I, Murphy SC, Cope L et al (2008) Therapeutic efficacy of ABT-737, a selective inhibitor of BCL-2, in small cell lung cancer. Cancer Res 68(7):2321–2328. https://doi.org/10.1158/0008-5472.CAN-07-5031

53. Rudin CM, Otterson GA, Mauer AM, Villalona-Calero MA, Tomek R, Prange B et al (2002) A pilot trial of G3139, a bcl-2 antisense oligonucleotide, and paclitaxel in patients with chemo-refractory small-cell lung cancer. Ann Oncol 13(4):539–545

54. Gandhi L, Camidge DR, Ribeiro de Oliveira M, Bonomi P, Gandara D, Khaira D et al (2011) Phase I study of Navitoclax (ABT-263), a novel Bcl-2 family inhibitor, in patients with small-cell lung cancer and other solid tumors. J Clin Oncol 29(7):909–916. https://doi.org/10.1200/JCO.2010.31.6208

55. Rudin CM, Hann CL, Garon EB, Ribeiro de Oliveira M, Bonomi PD, Camidge DR et al (2012) Phase II study of single-agent navitoclax (ABT-263) and biomarker correlates in patients with relapsed small cell lung cancer. Clin Cancer Res 18(11):3163–3169. https://doi.org/10.1158/1078-0432.CCR-11-3090

56. Lochmann TL, Floros KV, Naseri M, Powell KM, Cook W, March RJ et al (2018) Venetoclax is effective in small-cell lung cancers with high BCL-2 expression. Clin Cancer Res 24(2):360–369. https://doi.org/10.1158/1078-0432.CCR-17-1606

57. Augert A, Zhang Q, Bates B, Cui M, Wang X, Wildey G et al (2017) Small cell lung cancer exhibits frequent inactivating mutations in the histone methyltransferase KMT2D/MLL2: CALGB 151111 (alliance). J Thorac Oncol 12(4):704–713. https://doi.org/10.1016/j.jtho.2016.12.011

58. Margueron R, Li G, Sarma K, Blais A, Zavadil J, Woodcock CL et al (2008) Ezh1 and Ezh2 maintain repressive chromatin through different mechanisms. Mol Cell 32(4):503–518. https://doi.org/10.1016/j.molcel.2008.11.004

59. Poirier JT, Gardner EE, Connis N, Moreira AL, de Stanchina E, Hann CL et al (2015) DNA methylation in small cell lung cancer defines distinct disease subtypes and correlates with high expression of EZH2. Oncogene 34(48):5869–5878. https://doi.org/10.1038/onc.2015.38

60. Hubaux R, Thu KL, Coe BP, MacAulay C, Lam S, Lam WL (2013) EZH2 promotes E2F-driven SCLC tumorigenesis through modulation of apoptosis and cell-cycle regulation. J Thorac Oncol 8(8):1102–1106. https://doi.org/10.1097/JTO.0b013e318298762f

61. Gardner EE, Lok BH, Schneeberger VE, Desmeules P, Miles LA, Arnold PK et al (2017) Chemosensitive relapse in small cell lung cancer proceeds through an EZH2-SLFN11 axis. Cancer Cell 31(2):286–299. https://doi.org/10.1016/j.ccell.2017.01.006

62. Shi Y, Lan F, Matson C, Mulligan P, Whetstine JR, Cole PA et al (2004) Histone demethyl-ation mediated by the nuclear amine oxidase homolog LSD1. Cell 119(7):941–953. https://doi.org/10.1016/j.cell.2004.12.012

63. Mohammad HP, Smitheman KN, Kamat CD, Soong D, Federowicz KE, Van Aller GS et al (2015) A DNA hypomethylation signature predicts antitumor activity of LSD1 inhibitors in SCLC. Cancer Cell 28(1):57–69. https://doi.org/10.1016/j.ccell.2015.06.002

64. Augert A, Eastwood E, Ibrahim AH, Wu N, Grunblatt E, Basom R et al (2019) Targeting NOTCH activation in small cell lung cancer through LSD1 inhibition. Sci Signal 12(567):eaau2922. https://doi.org/10.1126/scisignal.aau2922

65. Ott PA, Elez E, Hiret S, Kim D-W, Morosky A, Saraf S et al (2017) Pembrolizumab in patients with extensive-stage small-cell lung cancer: results from the phase Ib KEYNOTE-028 study. J Clin Oncol 35(34):3823–3829. https://doi.org/10.1200/JCO.2017.72.5069

66. Chung HC, Piha-Paul SA, Lopez-Martin J, Schellens JHM, Kao S, Miller WH et al (2020) Pembrolizumab after two or more lines of previous therapy in patients with recurrent or meta-static SCLC: results from the KEYNOTE-028 and KEYNOTE-158 studies. J Thorac Oncol 15(4):618–627. https://doi.org/10.1016/j.jtho.2019.12.109

67. Reck M, Rodríguez-Abreu D, Robinson AG, Hui R, Csőszi T, Fülöp A et al (2019) Updated analysis of KEYNOTE-024: pembrolizumab versus platinum-based chemotherapy for advanced non–small-cell lung cancer with PD-L1 tumor proportion score of 50% or greater. J Clin Oncol 37(7):537–546. https://doi.org/10.1200/JCO.18.00149

68. Hellmann MD, Rizvi NA, Goldman JW, Gettinger SN, Borghaei H, Brahmer JR et al (2017) Nivolumab plus ipilimumab as first-line treatment for advanced non-small-cell lung cancer (CheckMate 012): results of an open-label, phase 1, multicohort study. Lancet Oncol 18(1):31–41. https://doi.org/10.1016/S1470-2045(16)30624-6

69. Marabelle A, Fakih M, Lopez J, Shah M, Shapira-Frommer R, Nakagawa K et al (2020) Association of tumour mutational burden with outcomes in patients with advanced solid tumours treated with pembrolizumab: prospective biomarker analysis of the multicohort, open-label, phase 2 KEYNOTE-158 study. Lancet Oncol 21(10):1353–1365. https://doi.org/10.1016/S1470-2045(20)30445-9

70. Matozaki T, Murata Y, Okazawa H, Ohnishi H (2009) Functions and molecular mechanisms of the CD47-SIRPalpha signalling pathway. Trends Cell Biol 19(2):72–80. https://doi.org/10.1016/j.tcb.2008.12.001

71. Weiskopf K, Jahchan NS, Schnorr PJ, Cristea S, Ring AM, Maute RL et al (2016) CD47-blocking immunotherapies stimulate macrophage-mediated destruction of small-cell lung cancer. J Clin Invest 126(7):2610–2620. https://doi.org/10.1172/jci81603

72. Gazdar AF, Carney DN, Nau MM, Minna JD (1985) Characterization of variant subclasses of cell lines derived from small cell lung cancer having distinctive biochemical, morphological, and growth properties. Cancer Res 45(6):2924–2930

73. Borges M, Linnoila RI, van de Velde HJ, Chen H, Nelkin BD, Mabry M et al (1997) An achaete-scute homologue essential for neuroendocrine differentiation in the lung. Nature 386(6627):852–855. https://doi.org/10.1038/386852a0

74. Neptune ER, Podowski M, Calvi C, Cho JH, Garcia JG, Tuder R et al (2008) Targeted disruption of NeuroD, a proneural basic helix-loop-helix factor, impairs distal lung formation and neuroendocrine morphology in the neonatal lung. J Biol Chem 283(30):21160–21169. https://doi.org/10.1074/jbc.M708692200

75. Borromeo MD, Savage TK, Kollipara RK, He M, Augustyn A, Osborne JK et al (2016) ASCL1 and NEUROD1 reveal heterogeneity in pulmonary neuroendocrine tumors and regulate distinct genetic programs. Cell Rep 16(5):1259–1272. https://doi.org/10.1016/j.celrep.2016.06.081

76. Schaffer BE, Park KS, Yiu G, Conklin JF, Lin C, Burkhart DL et al (2010) Loss of p130 accelerates tumor development in a mouse model for human small-cell lung carcinoma. Cancer Res 70(10):3877–3883

77. Baine MK, Hsieh MS, Lai WV, Egger JV, Jungbluth A, Daneshbod Y et al (2020) Small cell lung carcinoma subtypes defined by ASCL1, NEUROD1, POU2F3 and YAP1: comprehensive immunohistochemical and histopathologic characterization. J Thorac Oncol 15(12):1823–1835. https://doi.org/10.1016/j.jtho.2020.09.009

78. Huang Y-H, Klingbeil O, He X-Y, Wu XS, Arun G, Lu B et al (2018) POU2F3 is a master regulator of a tuft cell-like variant of small cell lung cancer. Genes Dev 32(13–14):915–928. https://doi.org/10.1101/gad.314815.118

79. McColl K, Wildey G, Sakre N, Lipka MB, Behtaj M, Kresak A et al (2017) Reciprocal expression of INSM1 and YAP1 defines subgroups in small cell lung cancer. Oncotarget 8(43):73745–73756. https://doi.org/10.18632/oncotarget.20572

Chapter 10
Immunotherapy and Radiotherapy: New Strategies

Allison M. Campbell and Roy H. Decker

Abstract Ionizing radiation is a local therapeutic intervention that plays a role in the multipronged approach to the treatment of non-small cell lung cancer. Case reports of excellent clinical responses in patients treated with both checkpoint inhibition and radiation point to a synergy between these two modalities that may extend the reach of radiotherapy from a local to a systemic treatment. Radiotherapy has been referred to as an *in situ* vaccine, given that its application has the potential to liberate tumor antigen in the context of pro-inflammatory cell death. This chapter describes interactions between radiotherapy and the immune system, with a particular focus on an emerging mechanistic understanding of how radiation can materially contribute to an anti-tumor immune response.

Keywords Immunotherapy · Radiotherapy · Abscopal responses · Innate immunity · Adaptive immunity

1 Introduction

Radiotherapy (RT) is a major component of the therapeutic arsenal deployed against non-small cell lung cancer (NSCLC). RT is often conceptualized as a purely local treatment, meaning it acts where it's directed without causing a systemic anti-cancer response. RT exerts its effects by damaging the DNA of cancer cells, leading to tumor killing. The immunological milieu around and within the tumor has an important role to play in the clinical response to radiation and other therapeutic modalities. RT is capable of eliciting an immune response, which is systemic by nature. Synergy between the immune system and RT has allowed radiation to impact overall disease burden in a way that was previously underappreciated.

A. M. Campbell (✉) · R. H. Decker
Department of Therapeutic Radiology, Yale School of Medicine/Yale Cancer Center, New Haven, CT, USA
e-mail: allison.campbell@yale.edu; roy.decker@yale.edu

© Springer Nature Switzerland AG 2021
A. C. Chiang, R. S. Herbst (eds.), *Lung Cancer*, Current Cancer Research,
https://doi.org/10.1007/978-3-030-74028-3_10

The combination of immunotherapy and RT is conceptually grounded in the ability of the immune system to handle cell death caused by radiation damage to the DNA of tumor cells. The subsequent cell death liberates tumor antigen that is processed by the immune system, potentially in such a way to facilitate the development of an anti-tumor immune response. When immunologic conditions are favorable, the anti-tumor response may have off-target or "abscopal" effects that occur at a distance from the irradiated site, turning a local therapy into one with systemic properties. Clinical case reports and pre-clinical studies have demonstrated synergistic benefit in using both immunotherapy and radiotherapy, but further studies are required to determine how these two modalities are best combined. This chapter will discuss the concept of radiotherapy as an *in situ* vaccine and detail the ways in which it has been shown to activate the innate and adaptive immune systems. These mechanistic insights directly translate into critical areas for future research and highlight unanswered questions within the field.

2 Radiotherapy as In Situ Vaccine

2.1 Principles of Vaccination as Applied to NSCLC

Classically, the idea of vaccination referred to the development of a protective immunity against pathogens that would effectively defend against subsequent encounters, but the concept has expanded to include therapeutic vaccines that are employed to treat established disease [5]. There are two components of a vaccine: (1) an antigen that serves as the target for the adaptive immune system and (2) an adjuvant that serves to engage the innate immune system and provide the required costimulatory signals to trigger a response. The term "antigen" derives directly from its effect on the host immune system, namely, the generation of an adaptive immune response against itself. An "adjuvant" enhances the immune response to the antigen. While there have been outstanding vaccination successes in the realm of infectious disease, in cancer significant barriers to success remain.

The rationale for cancer vaccination comes from the observation that immune activation can lead to tumor regression. Tumor infiltrating lymphocytes (TILs) have been identified as a prognostic features in multiple cancer subtypes [25, 33, 56, 77], and there has been significant interest in the creation and maintenance of an anti-tumor response through cancer vaccination [15]. Cancer vaccination encompasses a variety of methodologic approaches aimed at providing the immune system with antigen coupled with various adjuvants, with the goal being the activation of cytotoxic T cells—the primary effector of the anti-tumor response.

Peptide vaccines deliver antigen in a form that can bind MHC class I and be presented to cytotoxic T cells. Cellular vaccines are composed of cancer cell lines. Using intact cancer cell lines provides immunological access to a broad array of possible antigens that are taken up by dendritic cells and cross presented to T cells.

Viral-based strategies consist of using a viral carrier to deliver the antigen of interest, with the virus itself serving as adjuvant. The overall efficacy of the different vaccination methods has been thus far disappointing in NSCLC. But the basic principles of vaccination—the coupling of antigen and adjuvant to achieve an effective immunological response—still holds as a sound guiding principle. The generation of an immune response to altered self will always be more challenging than a response against a foreign agent. The margin for success is narrower because of the immunosuppressive environment of the tumor and the inherent controls built into the immune system itself to prevent harmful immunopathology. To this end, there has recently been an expansion of the concept of vaccination within the oncologic context: the triggering of *in situ*, proinflammatory cell death of the tumor itself.

2.2 Radiotherapy as Both Antigen and Adjuvant

Natural selection exerts pressure on proliferating tumor cells. Clones that escape immunological containment go on to survive and divide further. The ideal vaccine would therefore be personalized to a patient's particular tumor at the time of therapeutic intervention. The ideal vaccine would be delivered with an adjuvant capable of activating the innate immune system that allowed for the optimal engagement of adaptive immunity. In a perfect world, RT is capable of killing tumor cells *in situ* providing an array of antigen for the adaptive immune system to peruse. When tumor cells die, they are potentially capable of releasing danger-associated molecular patterns (DAMPs) that serve the role of adjuvant by activating the innate immune system [20].

The "abscopal effect" refers to regression of tumors outside a radiation field. The phenomenon was described initially in 1953 [66] but has gained prominence in recent years after a series of case reports describing dramatic systemic tumor responses in the setting of checkpoint inhibition and radiotherapy. The phenomenon has been observed in multiple tumor types, with a systematic review identifying 46 reported cases in the literature as of 2016 [1].

The drama of such responses point to what might be clinically possible for more patients in broader circumstances as our understanding of basic biology increases. That several of these high profile abscopal cases occurred in the setting of checkpoint inhibition implied a special synergy between radiation and immunotherapy. Support for this idea can also be found in a secondary analysis of the KEYNOTE-001 trial, which demonstrated that median overall survival doubled from 5.3 months to 10.7 months in patients with NSCLC who received radiotherapy prior to pembrolizumab [81]. Such observations suggest that there may be ways to alter the immunologic milieu to favor the successful engagement of the adaptive immune system in a larger number of patients.

In addition to checkpoint inhibitors, other adjuvant agents have been delivered in conjunction with radiation to help ensure that the innate immune system is adequately engaged. A proof-of-principle phase I trial introduced the combination of granulocyte macrophage-colony stimulating factor (GM-CSF) with radiotherapy in patients with metastatic cancer. 11 of 29 patients demonstrated an abscopal response, defined as a ≥30% decrease in the longest diameter of the best responding lesion [34]. An ongoing clinical trial in breast cancer is combining topical imiquimod with RT in patients with skin metastases. Imiquimod functions as an adjuvant by activating Toll-like Receptor 7 (TLR7), a receptor of the innate immune system [21].

The synergy of radiotherapy and immunotherapy represents an emerging approach toward improved outcomes in NSCLC. The sections that follow discuss pre-clinical studies that explore and characterize the influence of RT on innate and adaptive immune systems.

3 Radiotherapy and the Innate Immune System

3.1 Immunogenic Cell Death

The innate immune system is the first line of defense against invading pathogens. It recognizes pathogens by their evolutionary signatures, also known as their pathogen associated molecular patterns (PAMPs). The receptors of the innate immune system are called pattern recognition receptors (PRRs). The innate immune system also detects danger signals, or danger associated molecular patterns (DAMPs) associated with threats to genomic integrity [53]. DAMPs that occur in conjunction with PAMPs indicate the need for a robust defense of the self. Cell death alone is insufficient to prompt an immune response. Cellular turnover in the human body is estimated to be on the order of tens of billions of cells per day [38]. Most of these cells die by apoptosis, a process that promotes tolerance and prevents autoimmunity [37]. Cell death associated with the release of DAMPs elicits the engagement of the innate immune system. There are an array of ways in which cells can die that trigger the innate immune system. These include necrosis to necroptosis, pyroptosis, and autophagic cell death [6, 31, 32].

Radiation is known to induce cellular senescence and mitotic catastrophe, but these terms refer to the loss of proliferative capacity—not the rupture of the plasma membrane and cessation of cellular function. From an immunologic standpoint, these forms of death are "invisible" until such a time that the cellular corpse is engulfed by a macrophage and the immune system must discriminate between self and non-self. Self/non-self discrimination is one of the cardinal features of the immune system. Inability to tolerate self-derived antigen leads to autoimmunity.

While in vitro studies have demonstrated the many ways tumor cells *can* die, the data regarding the *in vivo* behavior of tumor cells in response to radiation are insufficient to determine how irradiated tumor cells *do* die. The manner of cellular demise may change based on RT dose and fractionation. Cell death within a living organism is a complex process that can range from tolerogenic and sedate to wildly immunologically provocative. Pre-clinical studies of RT-induced immunological responses have shed light on the importance of achieving inflammatory cell death to engage the innate immune system and set the stage for an adaptive anti-tumoral immunity. Involved pathways will be discussed in the following sections.

3.2 DNA Damage Machinery and Pattern Recognition Receptors: An Emerging Overlap

When viewed from the perspective of the preservation genomic integrity, it makes intuitive sense that proteins that detect damage in the DNA Damage Response (DDR) pathway double as Pattern Recognition Receptors (PRRs) in the innate immune system, given that both systems serve to detect nucleic acid damage. This idea is supported by the observation that DNA damaging agents, including RT, induce inflammatory responses [55]. These responses are mediated by the expression of type I interferon (IFN), which is also one of the key cytokines induced by viral infection [44]. Consistent with this, it has been observed that cells that have sustained DNA damage subsequently attain a degree of anti-viral resistance [59].

There are several points of contact between the innate immune system and the DDR machinery that have already been identified. Ku70, a protein involved in non-homologous end joining (NHEJ), also serves as a DNA sensor that induces type III interferon [100]. The NHEJ protein known as DNA-PK also acts as a pattern recognition receptor for cytoplasmic DNA, leading to activation of the transcription factor IRF3 [28]. Rad50 is also involved in NHEJ but has been shown to be capable inducing interleukin-1 (IL-1) and activating nuclear factor-kB (NF-kB) [76].

PRRs of the innate immune system recognize an array of molecules, one of which is cytosolic nucleic acid. In this context, discrimination between self and non-self is based upon the availability, localization, and structure of the sensed DNA [79]. Availability for sensing is determined by concentration, which considers both degradation rate and "shielding" by associated protein. Localization refers to the cellular compartment in which the nucleic acid is detected. Structure includes information about conformation and any chemical modifications to the nucleic acid [79]. Both DNA and RNA are recognized by the innate immune system. This chapter discusses innate immune recognition of RT induced damage, focusing on four emerging pathways, detailed in Fig. 10.1 and described in the following sections.

3.3 Recognition of DNA Damage with cGAS/STING

Cyclic adenosine monophosphate synthase (cGAS) is a PRR that detects DNA in the cytosol [85]. Detection occurs in a sequence independent manner and results in a conformational change that allows for the conversion of guanosine triphosphate (GTP) into cyclic GMP-AMP (cGAMP) [51]. cGAMP in turn binds the adaptor

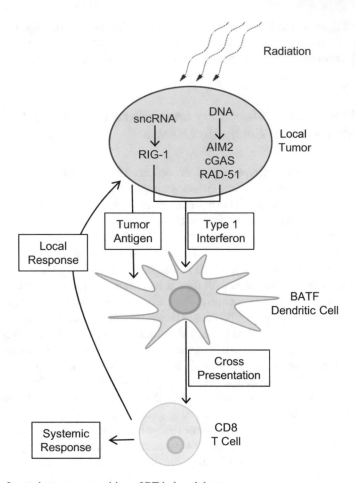

Fig. 10.1 Innate immune recognition of RT-induced damage

protein stimulator of IFN gene (STING) [45, 86]. STING subsequently forms a homodimer and recruits TANK-binding kinase (TBK1) and interferon regulatory factor 3 (IRF3) [58, 88]. Activation of this pathway leads to the production of type I IFN. Interestingly, STING is also capable of interacting with the IκB kinase (IKK) to activate NF-κB [27], which is another innate immune transcription factor with multiple pro-inflammatory downstream targets [89].

Radiotherapy has been shown to be capable of activating the cGAS/STING axis in pre-clinical mouse models. In the presence of checkpoint inhibition and following an RT regimen of 8 Gy × 3, cGAS has been shown to recognize damaged DNA and activate STING. Downstream of this activation dendritic cells successfully recruited cytotoxic T cells and subsequent tumor regression was observed [91]. It has also been demonstrated that STING is required for IFNβ production after irradiation. In the absence of STING, there is a failure of dendritic cell cross presentation and engagement of adaptive immunity [23].

3.4 Recognition of DNA Damage with AIM2

Absent in melanoma 2 (AIM2) is a cytosolic DNA sensor that binds directly to double stranded DNA (dsDNA) with its C-terminal domain [16, 29, 42, 75]. Its N-terminal pyrin domain interacts with the inflammasome adaptor known as apoptosis-associated speck-like protein (ASC) which then recruits pro-caspase-1 to create the macromolecular complex known as the inflammasome [62]. When the inflammasome assembles, pro-caspase-1 is cleaved into its active form. This results in the release of proinflammatory cytokines, such as IL-1β and IL-18. It is also capable of triggering a form of immunogenic cell death known as pyroptosis, which results from caspase-1 forming pores in the plasma membrane. This in turn effects cellular lysis, allowing undegraded nucleic acid to be released into the extracellular space [6].

RT is capable of inducing DNA damage that is sensed by AIM2. In a murine model of radiation-induced gastrointestinal and hematologic syndromes, AIM2 deficient mice were shown to be protected from the death of intestinal epithelial cells and bone marrow cells respectively. AIM2 was found to sense radiation-induced DNA damage and to mediate pyroptotic cell death and proinflammatory cytokine secretion [43]. Intriguingly, AIM2 has a role in the regulation of tumorigenesis itself, independent of inflammasome activation [62, 63]. In a mouse model of colitis AIM2 has been shown to prevent colorectal cancer in an inflammasome-independent fashion. AIM2 deficient mice developed severe colitis and a higher tumor burden upon exposure to mutagenic agents [96]. Overexpression of AIM2 in colon cancer cell lines results in cell cycle arrest at the G2/M checkpoint [70].

3.5 RAD51 at the Intersection of the DNA Damage Response and Innate Immunity

RAD51 is a multifunctional protein, involved in DNA replication and repair. Under normal physiologic conditions it plays multiple roles in managing replication forks, including replication restart when a fork encounters DNA damage [7]. After cellular irradiation, RAD51 assists in double strand break (DSB) repair via homologous recombination (HR). It is capable of binding both single-strand DNA (ssDNA) and double-strand DNA (dsDNA). The overlapping role RAD51 plays in innate immunity and the DDR pathway after radiotherapy has emerged only recently. *In vitro*, shRNA-mediated depletion of RAD51 results in induction of innate immune response pathway genes after irradiation, which corresponded with an increase in the levels of nuclear-derived ssDNA and dsDNA in the cytosol. This increased level of DNA in the cytosol results in STING activation and TBK1 phosphorylation [8]. At baseline, RAD51 blocks degradation of newly replicated DNA by MRE11, a nuclease that destroys DNA in response to replication stress [39]. Inhibition of MRE11 attenuates cytosolic self-DNA accumulation in cells with depleted RAD51 [8].

RAD51 overexpression is observed in many cancer subtypes, which correlates with an increased efficiency of repair and subsequent resistance to therapy that relies on DNA damage, such as chemotherapy and RT [52]. RAD51 expression, phosphorylation, and nuclear translocation can be affected by signaling through innate immune pathways. Urokinase-type plasminogen activator receptor (PLAUR) is a molecule expressed in most solid cancers and is associated with a poor prognosis [36]. It has no transmembrane domains, but signals in association with other surface receptors [10]. PLAUR, in combination with TLR4 mediates activation of CHK1 and RAD51 as part of an autocrine/paracrine signaling pathway, which leads to improved DNA repair [68]. This pathway indicates that not only can the innate immune system be activated by disruptions in genomic integrity, but that the reverse is also true—repair pathways can be influenced downstream of innate immune signaling.

3.6   Radiotherapy and RNA Sensing: RIG-I

The three routes of engaging the innate immune system described above all rely on recognition of DNA damage. RNA sensing is also a critical component of anti-viral detection. The retinoic acid inducible gene I (RIG-I) is part of a class of like receptors known as the RIG-I-like receptor (RLR) family. RIG-I is an RNA helicase that recognizes viral RNA and signals through the mitochondrial anti-viral signaling protein (MAVS). It is a critical component of the cellular defense against viral infection and its activation leads to production of type I IFN [99]. RIG-I itself is an IFN-stimulated gene (ISG), meaning type I IFN signaling is capable of upregulating its expression.

In an *in vivo*, pre-clinical study using a murine model, the deletion of RIG-I protected mice from death following total body irradiation. Depletion of RIG-I conferred radioresistance upon cell lines derived from human tumors. RT was found to result in the binding of RIG-I with small non-coding RNAs (sncRNA) U1 and U2, which translocated from the nucleus to the cytoplasm after radiotherapy. This subsequently resulted in the production of IFN-β [72]. The upregulation of sncRNAs by radiotherapy and the translocation of these molecules to the cytosol is a process that requires further investigation, but may yield clinical dividends. Interestingly, a regulatory mechanism for RIG-I signaling has been identified in the form of an IFN-inducible long noncoding RNA (lncRNA) known Lsm3b, which competes with viral RNA for RIG-I binding [47]. This type I IFN inducible regulatory pathway illustrates the principle that the induction of a proinflammatory response and its negative feedback mechanism often occur in short succession, if not simultaneously.

3.7 Type I IFN in Acute and Chronic Settings

The final common pathway of innate recognition of cytosolic DNA and RNA is the activation of type I IFN. This cytokine family consists of IFNα and IFNβ. IFNβ can be produced by nearly all cell types, and is thus a key mediator of antiviral defense, while IFNα serves a more specialized role and is produced only by cells from the hematopoietic lineage. Type I IFN induces a cell-intrinsic viral defense, called the "antiviral state" leading to the promotion of antigen presentation to T cells and natural killer cells on MHC-I molecules, which results in the killing of infected cells. Type I IFN is also capable of activating the adaptive immune system, which results in a tailored defense against non-self antigen [46].

Type I IFNs bind to the transmembrane interferon α receptor (IFNAR) and activate transcription factors from the IFN-regulatory factor family. Downstream of this transcription factor, several hundred ISGs are induced. Their collective activation creates and characterizes the antiviral state [61, 80], which impairs the ability of a virus to replicate its genome and infect additional cells: viral transcripts are degraded; mRNA translation is blocked; IFNAR signaling sensitizes cells to apoptosis, cells become more sensitive to NK cell and cytotoxic T cell-mediated killing [84].

In the acute setting, signaling by type I IFN establishes a foundation for the coming adaptive, T cell mediated response. In the chronic setting, however, type I IFN can suppress the production of proinflammatory cytokines and promote the release of IL-10, which results in inhibition of adaptive immunity. It can also lead to the upregulation of the programmed death-ligand 1 (PD-L1), which promotes T cell exhaustion. In these settings, blockade of type I IFN signaling or deficiency in IFNAR results in decreased expression of PD-L1 and IL-10 [46]. From an evolutionary perspective, this immunosuppressive property of chronic type I IFN signaling can be understood as a means to limit excessive immunopathology in the setting of an infection that fails to clear. Given that cancer represents a chronic threat from altered-self, and it is therefore no surprise that in this setting type I IFN can have both immunostimulatory and immunosuppressive effects.

3.8 Immunostimulatory Effects of Acute Type I IFN in Cancer

Both RT and chemotherapy are capable of inducing type I IFN, which is, in turn required for regression of tumors in response to therapy. In the pre-clinical setting, it has been demonstrated that B16 melanoma tumors implanted into IFNAR knockout mice fail to regress after radiotherapy, but this phenotype can be rescued by adenovirus-mediated delivery of IFNβ [14]. Conditional knockout of the IFNAR receptor has also been demonstrated to block dendritic cell mediated priming of T cells after RT [23], indicating the importance of type I IFNs for the engagements of adaptive immunity. These observations also hold in setting of chemotherapy where it has been demonstrated that tumor cells lacking IFNAR failed to respond to anthra-cyclines [82]. In the clinical setting, it has been observed that in breast cancer patients a complete response to neoadjuvant chemotherapy was associated with the ISG known as MX1, which is induced by anthracycline treatment [82].

3.9   Immunosuppressive Effects of Chronic Type I IFN in Cancer

Type I IFN has been demonstrated to upregulate PD-L1 in the tumor microenviron-ment [97], and that upregulation co-localizes with the presence of an inflammatory response [90]. In addition to PD-L1, there are other IFN-stimulated genes (ISGs) ISGs that play inhibitory roles. Melanoma metastases have been shown to have a type I IFN transcriptional profile, and when analyzed for negative regulators of T cell function, elevated indolamine 2,3 dioxygenase (IDO) expression correlated with a subset of tumors with an inflamed signature [83]. IDO is an inhibitory enzyme involved in tryptophan catabolism. It is induced in a STING-dependent manner and acts to inhibit inflammation [67]. Interestingly, not only does IDO control inflam-mation, but it also actively promotes self-tolerance. IDO-deficient mice suffer from an autoimmune phenotype with broad defects in tolerance to dead cell debris [73].

Chronic type I IFN signaling in tumor cells is known to be capable of conferring resistance to both RT and chemotherapy via the induction of a collection of genes known as the interferon-related DNA damage resistance signature (IRDS) [94]. This gene signature has also been observed in tumors exposed to exosomes pro-duced by stromal cells. These exosomes contained non-coding RNA capable of acti-vating RIG-I and inducing downstream type I IFN. The downstream induction of the signal transducer and activator of transcription 1 (STAT1) leads to cooperation with the neurogenic locus notch homolog protein 3 (NOTCH3) signaling pathway, the ultimate effect of which is to increase therapeutic resistance [11].

The innate immune system is a profoundly powerful tool and must regulate itself to ensure that it does not cause lethal immunopathology in its own host. These regulatory mechanisms that protect the host from autoimmunity also come into play in cancer, tipping the balance of response in favor of an immunosup-pressed tumor microenvironment (Fig. 10.2). Like many components of the immune system, the type I IFN pathway, when chronically activated, triggers its own inhibition. The emerging picture of type I IFN suggests that an acute burst of this signaling pathway is important for engaging the adaptive immune system. Its regulatory role under conditions of chronic inflammation suggests that, in an onco-logic setting, attempts to stimulate these pathways over a prolonged period may not have the desired effect.

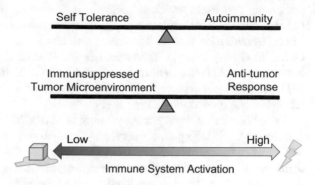

Fig. 10.2 Relationship between immune system activation and self/non-self discriminatory function

4 Radiotherapy and the Adaptive Immune System

4.1 Priming of the Adaptive Immune System

Adaptive immunity is conferred by B and T cells and differs from innate immunity in several key features. Adaptive immunity is slow to develop, but highly specific to particular non-self antigens. Once the pathogen has been cleared, the resultant immunologic memory protects the host upon a second exposure to an offending agent. A comprehensive discussion of all features of adaptive immunity is beyond the scope of this chapter, which will focus specifically on the interaction between the innate immune system and the development of the T cell repertoire.

Given their destructive potential, cytotoxic (CD8) T cells require multiple signals for activation: (1) signaling through the T cell receptor (TCR) (2) engagement of costimulatory receptors during direct cell-to-cell contact, and (3) the presence of pro-inflammatory innate signals. Helper (CD4) T cells and dendritic cells work together to generate an effector CD8 population that is licensed to kill infected cells [74]. CD4 T cells and CD8 T cells interact with the same dendritic cell, which displays their cognate antigen [26, 41]. The presence of CD4 T cell help improves the capabilities of CD8 effectors, including inhibitory receptor downregulation and the capacity to infiltrate into peripheral tissues [2].

4.2 The Importance of Cross-Presentation in the Anti-tumoral Response

Cytotoxic T cell responses in the oncologic setting rely on a phenomenon known as cross presentation. Cross presentation refers to the process by which professional antigen presenting cells, specifically dendritic cells, process and present extracellular antigen for the express purpose of priming CD8 T cells [48]. This allows for CD8 T cell responses to be generated against antigens that aren't expressed by the presenting cell itself, which is particularly important in the setting of cancer. In order for this process complete, dendritic cells must capture foreign antigen in the setting of activation signals. There are particular subsets of dendritic cells that specialize in cross-priming. Conventional dendritic cells (cDC) that express the basic leucine zipper ATF-like transcription factor 3 (BATF3) are efficient cross-presenters [87]. Plasmacytoid dendritic cells (pDCs) have a particular facility for cross presentation and the production of Type I IFN.

Type I IFN can stimulate cross-priming in both viral and oncologic settings [54], and the cGAS/STING pathway serves as a critical source of this innate signal. In the setting of radiotherapy-induced DNA damage, the cGAS/STING pathway in dendritic cells is required for the cross priming of CD8 T cells [23]. In pre-clinical models, cGAS has been shown to be required for effective checkpoint blockade in mice, and cGAMP explicitly enhanced cross-presentation of tumor associated antigen to T cells [92]. Treatment with cGAMP or STING agonists enhances immunity and promotes CD8 T cell mediated tumor regression [19]. These studies illustrate the critical connection between innate immune signals and the initiation of an adaptive response.

In the absence of innate signaling, cross-presentation leads to an outcome called cross-tolerance. This process is critical to the maintenance of self-tolerance and avoiding autoimmunity. Just as an activated dendritic cell is in the position of subsequently activating T cells, cross-presentation by an inactivated dendritic cell results in T cell deletion or tolerance [64]. In the setting of cancer, immature dendritic cells have been found in the tumor microenvironment, and any cross-priming performed in the absence of innate engagement is likely to contribute to the overall immunosuppression within this setting.

4.3   Radiotherapy and Immunological Memory

Though there have been several studies in the pre-clinical setting documenting the importance of CD8 T cells to tumor rejection and systemic responses, there have been few studies to date that explicitly interrogating the creation of a persistent memory CD8 population. A recent study in a murine model examined RT in combination with intra-tumoral CD40. The formation of immunologic memory was assessed by rechallenging mice with a higher dose of tumor cells. All mice were protected from rechallenge in a T cell-dependent manner [98]. Memory T cells are likely to play a role in tumor immunosurveillance; their quick response rates to antigen exposure and high level of cytotoxic cytokines make them ideal candidates to control tumor growth [9], but additional studies are needed to define their role in the context of radiotherapy.

4.4 T Cell Exhaustion within the Tumor Microenvironment

The tumor microenvironment, by its very nature, serves as a constant source of antigenic stimulation, which contributes to the development of immunological tolerance. As tumor cells proliferate, natural selection favors the survival of those cells that are able to evade immunological detection. These cells in turn modify their local environment to further promote immunosuppression [3]. An additional barrier to the creation and maintenance of an effective response is the similarity between tumor antigen and self; tumor antigen is better described as altered self than nonself, and, as discussed in previous sections, there are strong, evolutionarily conserved mechanisms in place to prevent anti-self responses. Even if antigen is successfully recognized as non-self, unless it rapidly cleared, the chronic nature of the exposure will lead to downstream immunosuppression.

T cell exhaustion is a state that occurs upon exposure to persistent antigen, and is characterized by loss of effector function and memory capabilities [95]. Exhausted T cells upregulate many inhibitory receptors. Two of the most clinically relevant are PD-1 and cytotoxic T-lymphocyte-associated protein 4 (CTLA-4). Signaling through these pathways results in the suppression of a previously active effector T cell response. It has been demonstrated that upregulation of PD-L1 on neoplastic cells is an important mechanism of immunological evasion [49]. Monoclonal antibodies targeting CTLA-4 and PD-1/PD-L1 have been approved for treatment in multiple cancer types, including NSCLC.

In the clinical setting, checkpoint inhibition has proven to be one of the most important and promising immunotherapeutic interventions in NSCLC. In the clinical setting, multiple randomized controlled trials have demonstrated increased overall survival when checkpoint inhibitors are combined with chemotherapy and radiation [12, 13, 60]. Of particular note is the PACIFIC trial, which demonstrated that the addition of durvalumab (an anti-PD-L1 antibody) to definitive chemoradiotherapy in patients with locally advanced NSCLC significantly improved progression free survival [4].

4.5 Checkpoint Inhibition and Radiotherapy

In addition to its role in the reversal of T cell exhaustion, checkpoint inhibition may also improve priming of an initial response to newly liberated antigen by facilitating a more permissive environment for T cell activation. Given that RT is capable of liberating antigen via cell death and activating the innate immune system, the opportunity exists to harness synergy between RT and checkpoint inhibition. As discussed in the early portion of this chapter, harnessing of the abscopal effect represents a particularly valuable new strategy for improving therapeutic responses in NSCLC.

In the pre-clinical setting, it has been demonstrated that immunological responses to radiotherapy are improved in the setting of checkpoint inhibition. Radiotherapy administered in conjunction with anti-CTLA-4 immunotherapy stimulated CD8 T cell production of tumor-specific IFNγ on restimulation with tumor antigen [24]. In the pre-clinical setting RT has been demonstrated to be capable of overcoming resistance to checkpoint inhibition in a murine model of lung cancer. Tumors resistant to anti-PD-1 therapy were radiated, resulting in the production of type I IFN, which restored the responsiveness of tumors to checkpoint inhibition [93].

Whether RT is exerting its effects by reversal of T cell exhaustion versus more permissive priming is a question that it still incompletely understood. A recent study in the pre-clinical setting created a state of immunosuppression in mice at the time of tumor implantation, which prevented to the formation of an initial anti-tumor response. When the mice were then treated with a regimen of anti-CTLA-4 and RT, there was failure of tumor regression, indicating that the initial response was required, and combined RT and anti-CTLA-4 failed to effectively prime a new response in an immunosuppressive context [18]. Now that checkpoint inhibitors are approved for use in a front-line context, before the host immune system has been profoundly suppressed by cytotoxic chemotherapy, it may be that systemic immunological responses to RT will become more common.

5 Maximizing the Clinical Utility of Radiotherapy in an Era of Checkpoint Inhibition: New Strategies

5.1 Rational Treatment Design

At present, insufficient evidence exists to recommend a particular combination of RT dose and fractionation in the setting of checkpoint inhibition. The ultimate goal of such a combination is a systemic or abscopal response following the joint administration of immunotherapy and RT. Many questions remain to be answered before such a strategy can be optimized, regarding factors such as target, timing, dose, and fractionation. When considering the potential interactions between RT-induced DNA damage and the immune system, there is a fine balance between inducing an anti-tumor response and inducing tolerance.

5.2 Choice of Target

Not all sites are immunologically equivalent within the body, and some sites, such as the brain, the testes, the eye, and the placenta are protected by anatomic barriers that make establishment of an inflammatory infiltrate technically difficult. Independent of anatomical barriers, there are also cellular and metabolic mechanisms capable of controlling inflammation at these sites [65], and when these are considered, locations of immune privilege expand to include other organs, such as the hair follicle, the colon, and the bone marrow [30]. In the reports of the abscopal effect in the clinical literature, there appears to be a trend favoring visceral organs over bone [50]. Though the propensity of different anatomical sites to be more or less immunogenic has not been examined in a systematic, prospective way, this raises the possibility that delivery of RT to privileged sites is less likely to induce a productive immune response.

A related consideration is the cost/benefit analysis of elective nodal irradiation (ENI). On one hand, elective nodal radiation is attractive due to the potential for RT to address microscopic disease in draining lymph nodes and for this reason it is performed in multiple oncologic contexts. However, radiation on lymph nodes also has the potential to result in increased immunosuppression, leading to a compromised adaptive response. The utility of targeting versus avoiding draining lymph nodes in the setting of metastatic disease when the therapeutic aim is to elicit an abscopal response is unknown, and requires dedicated investigation in both pre-clinical and clinical contexts.

5.3   Timing

No consensus exists as to whether RT and immunotherapy are best administered simultaneously or sequentially. Nor is there a consensus regarding whether RT should precede or follow immunotherapy given sequential administration. In principle, the combination of RT and immunotherapy can serve as either a priming event or an immunological booster.

RT administered prior to or concurrent with checkpoint inhibition may allow for more effective immunological priming as tumor antigen is liberated after RT-induced cell death. There have been no prospective studies specifically designed to answer whether RT is best positioned before or after immunotherapy, however there is pertinent indirect evidence in the form of the KEYNOTE-001 and PACIFIC trials. A secondary analysis the of KEYNOTE-001 trial demonstrated that patients with prior radiotherapy had improved overall survival after receiving pembrolizumab [81]. The PACIFIC trial also administered RT prior to immunotherapy and demonstrated an overall survival benefit [4].

The use of RT after administration of checkpoint inhibition is also a potentially viable strategy. High profile case reports exist describing the abscopal effect resulted after radiotherapy was added to checkpoint inhibition [71]. Though there have yet to be any prospective studies explicitly interrogating this strategy, a potential parallel can be drawn from the pre-clinical surgical literature, given that surgical intervention also has the capacity to liberate tumor antigen. In a murine model of metastatic breast cancer, checkpoint inhibition prior to resection improved survival when compared to concomitant administration of immunotherapy [57].

5.4 Dose and Fractionation

In the preclinical setting there is a wide array of results comparing the immunological responses to variations in dose and fractionation. Given the delicate nuance of immunological response and its profound dependency on in vivo context, this should not be surprising. *Ex vivo* studies and studies carried out in immortalized cell lines have shown a broad range of immunological responses, but the degree to which these can be meaningfully extrapolated to the clinical setting is unclear. When considering the generation of systemic responses in the setting of combined immunotherapy and RT, in this section, in vivo studies are likely to be the most valuable indicators in the absence of prospective clinical trials.

Case reports describing the abscopal effect range widely in dose and fractionation strategy. When the 47 cases described in the literature between 1969 and 2014 are considered, the median total dose was found to be 31 Gy and with a median dose per fraction of 3 Gy. Doses ranged from 0.45 to 60.75 Gy [1]. In the modern setting, hypofractionated regimens paired with checkpoint inhibition are commonly reported. Regimens that have been described in case reports include 9.5 Gy × 3 fractions [71], 17 Gy × 3 fraction [40], and 6 Gy × 5 fractions [35]. In murine models of the abscopal effect, there has also been a general convergence upon hypofractionated regimens, though to some degree this reflects the observations from the clinical setting. Across multiple studies, regiments that elicit systemic responses include of 24 Gy in 3 fractions [24], 30 Gy in 5 fractions [24], 15 Gy in 2 fractions [78], and 12 Gy in a single fraction [22].

The convergence upon hypofractionated regimens also reflects the conceptual shift in understanding toward the importance of generating an immunogenic form of cell death. Cellular demise occurs on a spectrum from tolerogenic (apoptosis) to immunogenic (necrosis). Ablative doses of radiotherapy seem more likely to elicit the latter than the former, but this has not been directly assessed. Our knowledge of cellular death pathways is hampered by the difficulty of visualizing and assessing such death in vivo. Further complicating matters, a binary conception of cell death—immunogenic versus tolerogenic—is unlikely to reflect reality. Cell death is more appropriately rendered as a spectrum, determined by the quality and quantity of antigen made available to the immune system [17].

6 Conclusions

Dramatic clinical outcomes in the setting of immunotherapy and radiotherapy illustrate what is possible when these two modalities are used in combination. The power of the immune system lies in its systemic nature; priming or recall responses in one location can translate to responses throughout the entire organism. In clinical oncology, the idea of tipping the immunological balance in the tumor microenvironment away from immunosuppression and toward immune activation now undergirds a host of in-progress clinical trials [69]. In addition to checkpoint inhibitors that block either the CTLA-4 pathway or the PD-1 pathway, other agents that influence immune checkpoints are under investigation. As strategies evolve, both innate and adaptive immunity are being targeted. When it comes to the use of these therapies in conjunction with RT, many questions still remain. It is worth noting that there may be more than one answer, depending on the state of the host and the context in which an immunological response is generated.

The optimal strategy for sequencing RT and immunotherapy has yet to be determined. The optimal dose and fractionation strategy to provide the best chance of inducing proinflammatory cell death has yet to be determined, and all RT targets may not be equally likely to induce a robust immunological response. When designing these therapeutic strategies, it is easy to forget that cell death occurs in a spectrum from tolerogenic to immunogenic and that the immune system is calibrated to attack non-self while preserving the body of its host. A myriad of genetic pathways intersect to determine the propensity of any individual organism to respond robustly or apathetically to any given antigenic stimulus. Those pathways are perturbed by the pillars of modern cancer therapy. Surgery, chemotherapy, radiation, and immunotherapy all influence the final outcome.

A common theme in this chapter is that chronic immune activation engages negative feedback mechanisms to regulate the scope and destructiveness of the immune response.. This principle holds in the innate immune system as well as the adaptive immune system, and has been evolutionarily conserved to limit self-inflicted damage. It is useful to think of the immune system as regulating itself like a thermostat, responding to environmental stimuli with a burst of heat (immunological activation) or cold (immunological suppression) as appropriate. In order to generate an effective anti-tumor response the self-correcting nature of the system must be accounted for, and the set point must be either perturbed, or the balance tipped in favor of immunological activation for a long enough period of time to eradicate the tumor without significant injury to the self. It may be that personalized combinations of radiotherapeutic and immunotherapeutic regimens, tailored to an individual's immunological baseline as it changes with time and with therapy will be required to successfully educate and engage the body's own defense system in the attack against altered self.

References

1. Abuodeh Y, Venkat P, Kim S (2016) Systematic review of case reports on the abscopal effect. Curr Probl Cancer 40:25–37
2. Ahrends T, Spanjaard A, Pilzecker B, Bąbała N, Bovens A, Xiao Y, Jacobs H, Borst J (2017) CD4. Immunity 47:848–861.e5
3. Anderson KG, Stromnes IM, Greenberg PD (2017) Obstacles posed by the tumor microenvironment to T cell activity: A case for synergistic therapies. Cancer Cell 31:311–325
4. Antonia SJ, Villegas A, Daniel D, Vicente D, Murakami S, Hui R, Yokoi T, Chiappori A, Lee KH, DE Wit M, Cho BC, Bourhaba M, Quantin X, Tokito T, Mekhail T, Planchard

D, Kim YC, Karapetis CS, Hiret S, Ostoros G, Kubota K, Gray JE, Paz-Ares L, De Castro Carpeño J, Wadsworth C, Melillo G, Jiang H, Huang Y, Dennis PA, Özgüroğlu M, PACIFIC Investigators (2017) Durvalumab after chemoradiotherapy in stage III non-small-cell lung cancer. N Engl J Med 377:1919–1929

5. Banchereau J, Palucka K (2018) Immunotherapy: Cancer vaccines on the move. Nat Rev Clin Oncol 15:9–10
6. Bergsbaken t, Fink SL, Cookson b T (2009) Pyroptosis: host cell death and inflammation. Nat Rev Microbiol 7:99–109
7. Bhat KP, Cortez D (2018) RPA and RAD51: fork reversal, fork protection, and genome stability. Nat Struct Mol Biol 25:446–453
8. Bhattacharya S, Srinivasan K, Abdisalaam S, Su F, Raj P, Dozmorov I, Mishra R, Wakeland EK, Ghose S, Mukherjee S, Asaithamby A (2017) RAD51 interconnects between DNA replication, DNA repair and immunity. Nucleic Acids Res 45:4590–4605
9. Blanc C, Hans S, Tran T, Granier C, Saldman A, Anson M, Oudard S, Tartour E (2018) Targeting resident memory T cells for cancer immunotherapy. Front Immunol 9:1722
10. Blasi F, Sidenius N (2010) The urokinase receptor: focused cell surface proteolysis, cell adhesion and signaling. FEBS Lett 584:1923–1930
11. Boelens MC, Wu TJ, Nabet BY, Xu B, Qiu Y, Yoon T, Azzam DJ, Twyman-Saint Victor C, Wiemann BZ, Ishwaran H, Ter Brugge PJ, Jonkers J, Slingerland J, Minn AJ (2014) Exosome transfer from stromal to breast cancer cells regulates therapy resistance pathways. Cell 159:499–513
12. Borghaei H, Paz-Ares L, Horn L, Spigel DR, Steins M, Ready NE, Chow LQ, Vokes EE, Felip E, Holgado E, Barlesi F, Kohlhäufl M, Arrieta O, Burgio MA, Fayette J, Lena H, Poddubskaya E, Gerber DE, Gettinger SN, Rudin CM, Rizvi N, Crinò L, Blumenschein GR, Antonia SJ, Dorange C, Harbison CT, Graf Finckenstein, F. & Brahmer, J. R. (2015) Nivolumab versus docetaxel in advanced nonsquamous non-small-cell lung cancer. N Engl J Med 373:1627–1639
13. Brahmer J, Reckamp KL, Baas P, Crinò L, Eberhardt WE, Poddubskaya E, Antonia S, Pluzanski A, Vokes EE, Holgado E, Waterhouse D, Ready N, Gainor J, Arén Frontera O, Havel L, Steins M, Garassino MC, Aerts JG, Domine M, Paz-Ares L, Reck M, Baudelet C, Harbison CT, Lestini B, Spigel DR (2015) Nivolumab versus docetaxel in advanced squamous-cell non-small-cell lung Cancer. N Engl J Med 373:123–135
14. Burnette BC, Liang H, Lee Y, Chlewicki L, Khodarev NN, Weichselbaum RR, Fu YX, Auh SL (2011) The efficacy of radiotherapy relies upon induction of type i interferon-dependent innate and adaptive immunity. Cancer Res 71:2488–2496
15. Butterfield LH (2015) Cancer vaccines. BMJ 350:h988
16. Bürckstümmer T, Baumann C, Blüml S, Dixit E, Dürnberger G, Jahn H, Planyavsky M, Bilban M, Colinge J, Bennett KL, Superti-Furga G (2009) An orthogonal proteomic-genomic screen identifies AIM2 as a cytoplasmic DNA sensor for the inflammasome. Nat Immunol 10:266–272
17. Campbell AM, Decker RH (2017) Mini-review of conventional and hypofractionated radiation therapy combined with immunotherapy for non-small cell lung cancer. Transl Lung Cancer Res 6:220–229
18. Crittenden MR, Zebertavage L, Kramer G, Bambina S, Friedman D, Troesch V, Blair T, Baird JR, Alice A, Gough MJ (2018) Tumor cure by radiation therapy and checkpoint inhibitors depends on pre-existing immunity. Sci Rep 8:7012
19. Demaria O, De Gassart A, Coso S, Gestermann N, Di Domizio J, Flatz L, Gaide O, Michielin O, Hwu P, Petrova TV, Martinon F, Modlin RL, Speiser DE, Gilliet M (2015) STING activation of tumor endothelial cells initiates spontaneous and therapeutic antitumor immunity. Proc Natl Acad Sci U S A 112:15408–15413
20. Demaria S, Formenti SC (2012) Radiation as an immunological adjuvant: current evidence on dose and fractionation. Front Oncol 2:153

21. Demaria S, Vanpouille-Box C, Formenti SC, Adams S (2013) The TLR7 agonist imiqui-mod as an adjuvant for radiotherapy-elicited in situ vaccination against breast cancer. Onco Targets Ther 2:e25997

22. Deng L, Liang H, Burnette B, Beckett M, Darga T, Weichselbaum RR, Fu YX (2014) Irradiation and anti-PD-L1 treatment synergistically promote antitumor immunity in mice. J Clin Invest 124:687–695

23. Deng L, Liang H, Xu M, Yang X, Burnette B, Arina A, Li XD, Mauceri H, Beckett M, Darga T, Huang X, Gajewski TF, Chen ZJ, Fu YX, Weichselbaum RR (2014) STING-dependent cytosolic DNA sensing promotes radiation-induced type I interferon-dependent antitumor immunity in immunogenic tumors. Immunity 41:843–852

24. Dewan MZ, Galloway AE, Kawashima N, Dewyngaert JK, Babb JS, Formenti SC, Demaria S (2009) Fractionated but not single-dose radiotherapy induces an immune-mediated abscopal effect when combined with anti-CTLA-4 antibody. Clin Cancer Res 15:5379–5388

25. Dieci MV, Mathieu MC, Guarneri V, Conte P, Delaloge S, Andre F, Goubar A (2015) Prognostic and predictive value of tumor-infiltrating lymphocytes in two phase III random-ized adjuvant breast cancer trials. Ann Oncol 26:1698–1704

26. Eickhoff S, Brewitz A, Gerner MY, Klauschen F, Komander K, Hemmi H, Garbi N, Kaisho T, Germain RN, Kastenmüller W (2015) Robust anti-viral immunity requires multiple distinct T cell-dendritic cell interactions. Cell 162:1322–1337

27. Fang R, Wang C, Jiang Q, Lv M, Gao P, Yu X, Mu P, Zhang R, Bi S, Feng JM, Jiang Z (2017) NEMO-IKKβ are essential for IRF3 and NF-κB activation in the cGAS-STING pathway. J Immunol 199:3222–3233

28. Ferguson BJ, Mansur DS, Peters NE, Ren H, Smith GL (2012) DNA-PK is a DNA sensor for IRF-3-dependent innate immunity. elife 1:e00047

29. Fernandes-Alnemri T, Yu J, Datta P, Wu J, Alnemri E (2009) AIM2 activates the inflamma-some and cell death in response to cytoplasmic DNA. Nature 458:509–513

30. Fujisaki J, Wu J, Carlson AL, Silberstein L, Putheti P, Larocca R, Gao W, Saito TI, Lo Celso C, Tsuyuzaki H, Sato T, Côté D, Sykes M, Strom TB, Scadden DT, Lin CP (2011) In vivo imaging of Treg cells providing immune privilege to the haematopoietic stem-cell niche. Nature 474:216–219

31. Galluzzi L, Buqué A, Kepp O, Zitvogel L, Kroemer G (2017) Immunogenic cell death in cancer and infectious disease. Nat Rev Immunol 17:97–111

32. Galluzzi L, Kepp O, Chan FK, Kroemer G (2017) Necroptosis: mechanisms and relevance to disease. Annu Rev Pathol 12:103–130

33. Geng Y, Shao Y, He W, Hu W, Xu Y, Chen J, Wu C, Jiang J (2015) Prognostic role of tumor-infiltrating lymphocytes in lung cancer: a meta-analysis. Cell Physiol Biochem 37:1560–1571

34. Golden EB, Chhabra A, Chachoua A, Adams S, Donach M, Fenton-Kerimian M, Friedman K, Ponzo F, Babb JS, Goldberg J, Demaria S, Formenti SC (2015) Local radiotherapy and granulocyte-macrophage colony-stimulating factor to generate abscopal responses in patients with metastatic solid tumours: a proof-of-principle trial. Lancet Oncol 16:795–803

35. Golden EB, Demaria S, Schiff PB, Chachoua A, Formenti SC (2013) An abscopal response to radiation and ipilimumab in a patient with metastatic non-small cell lung cancer. Cancer Immunol Res 1:365–372

36. Gonias SL, Hu J (2015) Urokinase receptor and resistance to targeted anticancer agents. Front Pharmacol 6:154

37. Green DR, Ferguson T, Zitvogel L, Kroemer G (2009) Immunogenic and tolerogenic cell death. Nat Rev Immunol 9:353–363

38. Hancock J (2010) Cell signaling: life, death, and apoptosis. Oxford University Press, Lavis

39. Hashimoto Y, Ray Chaudhuri A, Lopes M, Costanzo V (2010) Rad51 protects nascent DNA from Mre11-dependent degradation and promotes continuous DNA synthesis. Nat Struct Mol Biol 17:1305–1311

40. Hiniker SM, Chen DS, Reddy S, Chang DT, Jones JC, Mollick JA, Swetter SM, Knox SJ (2012) A systemic complete response of metastatic melanoma to local radiation and immu-notherapy. Transl Oncol 5:404–407

41. Hor JL, Whitney PG, Zaid A, Brooks AG, Heath WR, Mueller SN (2015) Spatiotemporally distinct interactions with dendritic cell subsets facilitates CD4+ and CD8+ T cell activation to localized viral infection. Immunity 43:554–565

42. Hornung V, Ablasser A, Charrel-Dennis M, Bauernfeind F, Horvath G, Caffrey D, Latz E, Fitzgerald K (2009) AIM2 recognizes cytosolic dsDNA and forms a caspase-1-activating inflammasome with ASC. Nature 458:514–518

43. Hu B, Jin C, Li HB, Tong J, Ouyang X, Cetinbas NM, Zhu S, Strowig T, Lam FC, Zhao C, Henao-Mejia J, Yilmaz O, Fitzgerald KA, Eisenbarth SC, Elinav E, Flavell RA (2016) The DNA-sensing AIM2 inflammasome controls radiation-induced cell death and tissue injury. Science 354:765–768

44. Härtlova A, Erttmann SF, Raffi FA, Schmalz AM, Resch U, Anugula S, Lienenklaus S, Nilsson LM, Kröger A, Nilsson JA, Ek T, Weiss S, Gekara NO (2015) DNA damage primes the type I interferon system via the cytosolic DNA sensor STING to promote anti-microbial innate immunity. Immunity 42:332–343

45. Ishikawa H, Ma Z, Barber GN (2009) STING regulates intracellular DNA-mediated, type I interferon-dependent innate immunity. Nature 461:788–792

46. Ivashkiv LB, Donlin LT (2014) Regulation of type I interferon responses. Nat Rev Immunol 14:36–49

47. Jiang M, Zhang S, Yang Z, Lin H, Zhu J, Liu L, Wang W, Liu S, Liu W, Ma Y, Zhang L, Cao X (2018) Self-recognition of an inducible host lncRNA by RIG-I feedback restricts innate immune response. Cell 173:906–919.e13

48. Joffre OP, Segura E, Savina A, Amigorena S (2012) Cross-presentation by dendritic cells. Nat Rev Immunol 12:557–569

49. Juneja VR, Mcguire KA, Manguso RT, Lafleur MW, Collins N, Haining WN, Freeman GJ, Sharpe AH (2017) PD-L1 on tumor cells is sufficient for immune evasion in immunogenic tumors and inhibits CD8 T cell cytotoxicity. J Exp Med 214:895–904

50. Kang J, Demaria S, Formenti S (2016) Current clinical trials testing the combination of immunotherapy with radiotherapy. J Immunother Cancer 4:51

51. Kato K, Omura H, Ishitani R, Nureki O (2017) Cyclic GMP-AMP as an endogenous second messenger in innate immune signaling by cytosolic DNA. Annu Rev Biochem 86:541–566

52. Klein HL (2008) The consequences of Rad51 overexpression for normal and tumor cells. DNA Repair (Amst) 7:686–693

53. Krysko DV, Garg AD, Kaczmarek A, Krysko O, Agostinis P, Vandenabeele P (2012) Immunogenic cell death and DAMPs in cancer therapy. Nat Rev Cancer 12:860–875

54. Le Bon A, Etchart N, Rossmann C, Ashton M, Hou S, Gewert D, Borrow P, Tough DF (2003) Cross-priming of CD8+ T cells stimulated by virus-induced type I interferon. Nat Immunol 4:1009–1015

55. Li T, Chen ZJ (2018) The cGAS-cGAMP-STING pathway connects DNA damage to inflammation, senescence, and cancer. J Exp Med 215:1287–1299

56. Lianyuan T, Dianrong X, Chunhui Y, Zhaolai M, Bin J (2018) The predictive value and role of stromal tumor-infiltrating lymphocytes in pancreatic ductal adenocarcinoma (PDAC). Cancer Biol Ther 19:296–305

57. Liu J, Blake SJ, Yong MC, Harjunpää H, Ngiow SF, Takeda K, Young A, O'donnell JS, Allen S, Smyth MJ, Teng MW (2016) Improved efficacy of neoadjuvant compared to adjuvant immunotherapy to eradicate metastatic disease. Cancer Discov 6:1382–1399

58. Liu S, Cai X, Wu J, Cong Q, Chen X, Li T, Du F, Ren J, Wu YT, Grishin NV, Chen ZJ (2015) Phosphorylation of innate immune adaptor proteins MAVS, STING, and TRIF induces IRF3 activation. Science 347:aaa2630

59. Luthra P, Aguirre S, Yen BC, Pietzsch CA, Sanchez-Aparicio MT, Tigabu B, Morlock LK, García-Sastre A, Leung DW, Williams NS, Fernandez-Sesma A, Bukreyev A, Basler CF (2017) Topoisomerase II inhibitors induce DNA damage-dependent interferon responses circumventing Ebola virus immune evasion. MBio 8:e00368-17

60. Lynch TJ, Bondarenko I, Luft A, Serwatowski P, Barlesi F, Chacko R, Sebastian M, Neal J, Lu H, Cuillerot JM, Reck M (2012) Ipilimumab in combination with paclitaxel and carboplatin as first-line treatment in stage IIIB/IV non-small-cell lung cancer: results from a randomized, double-blind, multicenter phase II study. J Clin Oncol 30:2046–2054

61. Macmicking JD (2012) Interferon-inducible effector mechanisms in cell-autonomous immunity. Nat Rev Immunol 12:367–382

62. Man SM, Karki R, Kanneganti TD (2016) AIM2 inflammasome in infection, cancer, and autoimmunity: role in DNA sensing, inflammation, and innate immunity. Eur J Immunol 46:269–280

63. Man SM, Zhu Q, Zhu L, Liu Z, Karki R, Malik A, Sharma D, Li L, Malireddi RK, Gurung P, Neale G, Olsen SR, Carter RA, Mcgoldrick DJ, Wu G, Finkelstein D, Vogel P, Gilbertson RJ, Kanneganti TD (2015) Critical role for the DNA sensor AIM2 in stem cell proliferation and cancer. Cell 162:45–58

64. Mcdonnell AM, Robinson BW, Currie AJ (2010) Tumor antigen cross-presentation and the dendritic cell: where it all begins? Clin Dev Immunol 2010:539519

65. Mellor AL, Munn DH (2008) Creating immune privilege: active local suppression that benefits friends, but protects foes. Nat Rev Immunol 8:74–80

66. Mole RH (1953) Whole body irradiation; radiobiology or medicine? Br J Radiol 26:234–241

67. Munn DH, Mellor AL (2016) IDO in the tumor microenvironment: inflammation, counter-regulation, and tolerance. Trends Immunol 37:193–207

68. Narayanaswamy PB, Tkachuk S, Haller H, Dumler I, Kiyan Y (2016) CHK1 and RAD51 activation after DNA damage is regulated via urokinase receptor/TLR4 signaling. Cell Death Dis 7:e2383

69. Patel SA, Minn AJ (2018) Combination cancer therapy with immune checkpoint blockade: mechanisms and strategies. Immunity 48:417–433

70. Patsos G, Germann A, Gebert J, Dihlmann S (2010) Restoration of absent in melanoma 2 (AIM2) induces G2/M cell cycle arrest and promotes invasion of colorectal cancer cells. Int J Cancer 126:1838–1849

71. Postow MA, Callahan MK, Barker CA, Yamada Y, Yuan J, Kitano S, Mu Z, Rasalan T, Adamow M, Ritter E, Sedrak C, Jungbluth AA, Chua R, Yang AS, Roman RA, Rosner S, Benson B, Allison JP, Lesokhin AM, Gnjatic S, Wolchok JD (2012) Immunologic correlates of the abscopal effect in a patient with melanoma. N Engl J Med 366:925–931

72. Ranoa DR, Parekh AD, Pitroda SP, Huang X, Darga T, Wong AC, Huang L, Andrade J, Staley JP, Satoh T, Akira S, Weichselbaum RR, Khodarev NN (2016) Cancer therapies activate RIG-I-like receptor pathway through endogenous non-coding RNAs. Oncotarget 7:26496–26515

73. Ravishankar B, Liu H, Shinde R, Chandler P, Baban B, Tanaka M, Munn DH, Mellor AL, Karlsson MC, Mcgaha TL (2012) Tolerance to apoptotic cells is regulated by indoleamine 2,3-dioxygenase. Proc Natl Acad Sci U S A 109:3909–3914

74. Ridge JP, Di Rosa F, Matzinger P (1998) A conditioned dendritic cell can be a temporal bridge between a CD4+ T-helper and a T-killer cell. Nature 393:474–478

75. Roberts T, Idris A, Dunn J, Kelly G, Burnton C, Hodgson S, Hardy L, Garceau V, Sweet M, Ross I, Hume D, Stacey K (2009) HIN-200 proteins regulate caspase activation in response to foreign cytoplasmic DNA. Science 323:1057–1060

76. Roth S, Rottach A, Lotz-Havla AS, Laux V, Muschaweckh A, Gersting SW, Muntau AC, Hopfner KP, Jin L, Vanness K, Petrini JH, Drexler I, Leonhardt H, Ruland J (2014) Rad50-CARD9 interactions link cytosolic DNA sensing to IL-1β production. Nat Immunol 15:538–545

77. Rozek LS, Schmit SL, Greenson JK, Tomsho LP, Rennert HS, Rennert G, Gruber SB (2016) Tumor-infiltrating lymphocytes, Crohn's-like lymphoid reaction, and survival from colorectal cancer. J Natl Cancer Inst 108:djw027

78. Schaue D, Ratikan JA, Iwamoto KS, Mcbride WH (2012) Maximizing tumor immunity with fractionated radiation. Int J Radiat Oncol Biol Phys 83:1306–1310

79. Schlee M, Hartmann G (2016) Discriminating self from non-self in nucleic acid sensing. Nat Rev Immunol 16:566–580
80. Schoggins JW, Wilson SJ, Panis M, Murphy MY, Jones CT, Bieniasz P, Rice CM (2011) A diverse range of gene products are effectors of the type I interferon antiviral response. Nature 472:481–485
81. Shaverdian N, Lisberg AE, Bornazyan K, Veruttipong D, Goldman JW, Formenti SC, Garon EB, Lee P (2017) Previous radiotherapy and the clinical activity and toxicity of pembrolizumab in the treatment of non-small-cell lung cancer: a secondary analysis of the KEYNOTE-001 phase 1 trial. Lancet Oncol 18:895–903
82. Sistigu A, Yamazaki T, Vacchelli E, Chaba K, Enot DP, Adam J, Vitale I, Goubar A, Baracco EE, Remédios C, Fend L, Hannani D, Aymeric L, Ma Y, Niso-Santano M, Kepp O, Schultze JL, Tüting T, Belardelli F, Bracci L, La Sorsa V, Ziccheddu G, Sestili P, Urbani F, Delorenzi M, Lacroix-Triki M, Quidville V, Conforti R, Spano JP, Pusztai L, Poirier-Colame V, Delaloge S, Penault-Llorca F, Ladoire S, Arnould L, Cyrta J, Dessoliers MC, Eggermont A, Bianchi ME, Pittet M, Engblom C, Pfirschke C, Préville X, Uzè G, Schreiber RD, Chow MT, Smyth MJ, Proietti E, André F, Kroemer G, Zitvogel L (2014) Cancer cell-autonomous contribution of type I interferon signaling to the efficacy of chemotherapy. Nat Med 20:1301–1309
83. Spranger S, Spaapen RM, Zha Y, Williams J, Meng Y, Ha TT, Gajewski TF (2013) Up-regulation of PD-L1, IDO, and T(regs) in the melanoma tumor microenvironment is driven by CD8(+) T cells. Sci Transl Med 5:200ra116
84. Stetson DB, Medzhitov R (2006) Type I interferons in host defense. Immunity 25:373–381
85. Sun L, Wu J, Du F, Chen X, Chen ZJ (2013) Cyclic GMP-AMP synthase is a cytosolic DNA sensor that activates the type I interferon pathway. Science 339:786–791
86. Sun W, Li Y, Chen L, Chen H, You F, Zhou X, Zhou Y, Zhai Z, Chen D, Jiang Z (2009) ERIS, an endoplasmic reticulum IFN stimulator, activates innate immune signaling through dimerization. Proc Natl Acad Sci U S A 106:8653–8658
87. Sánchez-Paulete AR, Teijeira A, Cueto FJ, Garasa S, Pérez-Gracia JL, Sánchez-Arráez A, Sancho D, Melero I (2017) Antigen cross-presentation and T-cell cross-priming in cancer immunology and immunotherapy. Ann Oncol 28:xii74
88. Tanaka Y, Chen ZJ (2012) STING specifies IRF3 phosphorylation by TBK1 in the cytosolic DNA signaling pathway. Sci Signal 5:ra20
89. Taniguchi K, Karin M (2018) NF-κB, inflammation, immunity and cancer: coming of age. Nat Rev Immunol 18:309–324
90. Taube JM, Anders RA, Young GD, Xu H, Sharma R, Mcmiller TL, Chen S, Klein AP, Pardoll DM, Topalian SL, Chen L (2012) Colocalization of inflammatory response with B7-h1 expression in human melanocytic lesions supports an adaptive resistance mechanism of immune escape. Sci Transl Med 4:127ra37
91. Vanpouille-Box C, Alard A, Aryankalayil MJ, Sarfraz Y, Diamond JM, Schneider RJ, Inghirami G, Coleman CN, Formenti SC, Demaria S (2017) DNA exonuclease Trex1 regulates radiotherapy-induced tumour immunogenicity. Nat Commun 8:15618
92. Wang H, Hu S, Chen X, Shi H, Chen C, Sun L, Chen ZJ (2017) cGAS is essential for the antitumor effect of immune checkpoint blockade. Proc Natl Acad Sci U S A 114:1637–1642
93. Wang X, Schoenhals JE, Li A, Valdecanas DR, Ye H, Zang F, Tang C, Tang M, Liu CG, Liu X, Krishnan S, Allison JP, Sharma P, Hwu P, Komaki R, Overwijk WW, Gomez DR, Chang JY, Hahn SM, Cortez MA, Welsh JW (2017) Suppression of type I IFN signaling in tumors mediates resistance to anti-PD-1 treatment that can be overcome by radiotherapy. Cancer Res 77:839–850
94. Weichselbaum RR, Ishwaran H, Yoon T, Nuyten DS, Baker SW, Khodarev N, Su AW, Shaikh AY, Roach P, Kreike B, Roizman B, Bergh J, Pawitan Y, Van De Vijver MJ, Minn AJ (2008) An interferon-related gene signature for DNA damage resistance is a predictive marker for chemotherapy and radiation for breast cancer. Proc Natl Acad Sci U S A 105:18490–18495
95. Wherry EJ, Kurachi M (2015) Molecular and cellular insights into T cell exhaustion. Nat Rev Immunol 15:486–499

96. Wilson JE, Petrucelli AS, Chen L, Koblansky AA, Truax AD, Oyama Y, Rogers AB, Brickey WJ, Wang Y, Schneider M, Mühlbauer M, Chou WC, Barker BR, Jobin C, Allbritton NL, Ramsden DA, Davis BK, Ting JP (2015) Inflammasome-independent role of AIM2 in suppressing colon tumorigenesis via DNA-PK and Akt. Nat Med 21:906–913

97. Yang X, Zhang X, Fu ML, Weichselbaum RR, Gajewski TF, Guo Y, Fu YX (2014) Targeting the tumor microenvironment with interferon-β bridges innate and adaptive immune responses. Cancer Cell 25:37–48

98. Yasmin-Karim S, Bruck PT, Moreau M, Kunjachan S, Chen GZ, Kumar R, Grabow S, Dougan SK, Ngwa W (2018) Radiation and local anti-CD40 generate an effective. Front Immunol 9:2030

99. Yoneyama M, Kikuchi M, Natsukawa T, Shinobu N, Imaizumi T, Miyagishi M, Taira K, Akira S, Fujita T (2004) The RNA helicase RIG-I has an essential function in double-stranded RNA-induced innate antiviral responses. Nat Immunol 5:730–737

100. Zhang X, Brann TW, Zhou M, Yang J, Oguariri RM, Lidie KB, Imamichi H, Huang DW, Lempicki RA, Baseler MW, Veenstra TD, Young HA, Lane HC, Imamichi T (2011) Cutting edge: Ku70 is a novel cytosolic DNA sensor that induces type III rather than type I IFN. J Immunol 186:4541–4545

Chapter 11
Ultimate Precision: Targeting Cancer But Not Normal Self-Replication

Vamsidhar Velcheti, David Schrump, and Yogen Saunthararajah

Abstract Self-replication is the engine that drives all biological evolution, including neoplastic evolution. A key oncotherapy challenge is to target this, the heart of malignancy, while sparing the normal self-replication mandatory for health and life. Self-replication can be demystified: it is an activation of replication, the most ancient of cell programs, uncoupled from activation of lineage-differentiation, metazoan programs more recent in origin. The uncoupling can be physiologic, as in normal tissue stem cells, or pathologic, as in cancer. Neoplastic evolution selects to disengage replication from forward-differentiation where intrinsic replication rates are the highest – in committed progenitors that have division times measured in hours versus weeks for tissue stem cells - via partial loss-of-function in master transcription factors that activate terminal-differentiation programs (e.g., *GATA4*) or in the coactivators they use for this purpose (e.g., *ARID1A*). These loss-of-function mutations bias master transcription factor circuits, which normally regulate corepressor versus coactivator recruitment, towards corepressors (e.g., DNMT1) that repress rather than activate terminal-differentiation genes. Pharmacologic inhibition of the corepressors re-balances to coactivator function, activating lineage-differentiation genes that dominantly antagonize MYC (the master transcription factor coordinator of replication) to terminate malignant self-replication. Physiologic self-replication continues because the master transcription factors in tissue stem cells activate stem cell, not terminal-differentiation, programs. Druggable corepressor proteins are thus the barriers between self-replicating cancer cells and the terminal-differentiation fates intended by their master transcription factor content. This final common pathway to oncogenic self-replication, being separate and

V. Velcheti (✉)
Hematology and Oncology, New York University School of Medicine,
New York City, NY, USA
e-mail: vamsidhar.velcheti@nyulangone.org

D. Schrump
Thoracic Oncology, National Cancer Institute, Bethesda, MD, USA

Y. Saunthararajah
Department of Translational Hematology & Oncology Research, Taussig Cancer Institute,
Cleveland Clinic, Cleveland, OH, USA

© Springer Nature Switzerland AG 2021
A. C. Chiang, R. S. Herbst (eds.), *Lung Cancer*, Current Cancer Research,
https://doi.org/10.1007/978-3-030-74028-3_11

distinct from the normal, offers the favorable therapeutic indices needed for clinical progress.

Keywords Lung Cancer · Epigenetics · Therapy

1 Introduction

Reproduction/self-replication propels all biological evolution, including neoplastic evolution. Multi-billion dollar public and private efforts have focused on investigating and targeting cancer self-replication as the heart of malignancy [1]. For meaningful clinical translation, however, normal tissue stem cell self-replication, necessary for a healthy natural life-span, should be simultaneously spared. The quest can therefore be framed as a search for differences between malignant and normal self-replication that can be used for therapy. Fortunately, such differences have been found, although as a matter of course drug development and clinical evaluation lag.

2 Replication and Lineage-Differentiation Are Linked

Cellular replication, the orchestrated duplication and partitioning of cellular components in all their forms and quantity, is a staggeringly complex process coordinated for millennia by the ancient transcription factor MYC [2, 3]. That is, MYC is a master transcription factor – only a few of the ~100 transcription factors expressed in cells are masters, collaborating in combinations to powerfully regulate the expression of other transcription factors and hundreds to thousands of genes, thereby governing cell fates and functions, illustrated by their remarkable capacity to convert cells of one lineage into another [6, 7, 46–48], or to reverse cells to earlier stages of their ontogeny in a lineage [4], even into embryonic stem cells [5]. As canonical a master transcription factor as MYC is, it is nevertheless subordinate to other master transcription factors, that activate programs emblematic of metazoan (multicellular) physiology: apoptosis (cell suicide), activated by p53 and its key co-factor p16/CDKN2A, and lineage-differentiation programs (cell specialization), activated by various master transcription factor combinations. Apoptosis dominantly antagonizes MYC to temporarily or permanently prevent cell replication. Lineage-differentiation programs, however, regulate MYC in dramatically different ways depending on phases of advance of cells along lineage-differentiation axes (Fig. 11.1):

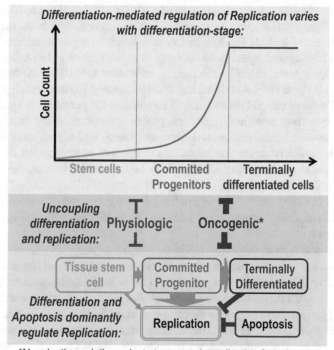

Fig. 11.1 Differentiation dominantly regulates replication, but in different ways, depending on the stage of advance of cells along lineage-differentiation axes - neoplastic evolution selects to uncouple replication from forward-differentiation where intrinsic replication rates are highest, in lineage-committed progenitors. Apoptosis also dominantly regulates replication

1. *Tissue stem cells.* Underpinning tissue homeostasis are stem cells, the cells in normal adult physiology inherently capable of both self-replication and multi-potency. The self-replication is, however, severely restricted in its rate, certainly as documented for hematopoietic stem cells: upregulation of MYC is limited, intervals between cell divisions extend to weeks or months, and overall proliferation kinetics are quiescent or linear [6–8] (reviewed in [9]). In fact, the master transcription factor HLF simultaneously produces hematopoietic stem cells and imposes quiescence - knock-out of HLF both increased replication and released forward-differentiation, eventually eliminating the hematopoietic stem cell pool [10]. Transcription factors activating stem cell programs in other tissues have also been shown to concurrently dampen replication: SOX9 in the case of intestinal stem cells [11]; RBPJ for muscle stem cells [12, 13]; Notch in neural stem cells [14]; and LHX1 and hair follicle stem cells [15].

   Why do stem cell programs go with restricted replication? Stem cells must preserve the integrity of their genomes if they are to replenish tissues through the life-span of an organism. Although quiescence does not provide complete protection to the genome, replication carries with it additional risks, from mistakes by DNA polymerase, breakage of elongating strands, and from errors in the repair of such damage [16]. The reality and danger of replication errors to physiology is highlighted by inherited defects in repair capacity: DNA double strand breaks are a form of replication error, estimated at ~10 DNA double strand breaks/cell cycle [17]. Ataxia telangiectasia mutated (*ATM*), which participates in DNA double-strand break repair, is mutated in the germline in ataxia telangiectasia syndrome, producing phenotypes of premature aging in skin, bones, small intestine, blood and central nervous system, and higher risks for cancers [18–20]. Similarly, germ line mutations in Fanconi anemia genes that repair of DNA double-strand breaks also produce bone marrow failure, developmental abnormalities, and higher risks for cancers.

If not in tissue stem cells, where then does the volume of replication needed to withstand daily entropy and attrition, estimated at >100 billion cells per day, occur?

2. *Lineage-committed progenitors.* Tissue stem cell daughters that commit to differentiate towards specific lineage fates (lineage-committed progenitors, transit amplifying cells) activate and stabilize MYC to high levels, producing intervals between cell divisions measured in hours [6–8] and exponential growth kinetics [21–25] (reviewed in [9]). The biochemical basis for this augmentation of MYC has been shown for myeloid differentiation: master transcription factor drivers of granulo-monocytic lineage-fates, PU.1, CEBPA, RUNX1, localize enhancers for *MYC* [26], and co-localize with MYC at proliferation genes [27]. This partnership produces replications that are rapid in rate but restricted in number, because of eventual activation of terminal-differentiation programs that antagonize MYC and force cell cycle exits [28–35] (Fig. 11.1).

3. *Terminally-differentiated cells.* These do not actively divide but focus instead on performing the specialized functions needed by the overall multi-cellular aggregate.

3   Dis-Engaging Replication from Advances Along a Lineage

Hence, oncogenesis necessarily uncouples replication from forward-differentiation, which would otherwise eventually terminate replication. Accordingly, Hansemann, upon the first histological examinations of cancer in 1890, remarked on 'anaplasia' (loss-of-differentiation) and 'dedifferentiation' [36], and today, clinical pathologists routinely use differentiation-failure to distinguish malignant from benign tumors, e.g., adenocarcinoma from adenoma, and more from less aggressive transformation, e.g., acute myeloid leukemia (AML) from myelodysplastic syndromes (MDS). Even when loss-of-differentiation is not obvious by light microscopy it is evident by gene expression analyses. For example, Grade 1 hepatocellular carcinomas (HCC), although 'well-differentiated' by light microscopy, demonstrate suppression of hundreds of hepatocyte epithelial-differentiation genes relative to normal liver cells [37].

At which phase of lineage-differentiation, and how, does oncogenic disengagement of replication from forward-differentiation occur?

1. *Gain-of-function in tissue stem cells (cancer 'stem' cell model)* [38]: Since normal tissue stem cells naturally permit replication without forward-differentiation, gain-of-function events, for example, *RAS* mutations that stabilize MYC, or copy number gains of *MYC* [39, 40], might upregulate replication without triggering forward-differentiation. Caveats are that the gain-of-function mutations would need to originate in the stem cell compartment, which has been found not to be the case for *RAS* mutations in AML, since they were detected only in downstream lineage-committed progenitors but not hematopoietic stem cells [41–43]. Also, this model assumes that high grade MYC upregulation does not promote forward-differentiation, but experimentally, MYC introduction into epidermal or hematopoietic stem cells promoted differentiation into epidermal/sebaceous and myeloid lineages respectively [21, 25, 44].

   A variation of this model, proposed for leukemia fusion proteins containing truncated MLL (KMT2A), is that key genes linked with tissue stem cells, e.g., *HOXA9*, are aberrantly activated in lineage-progenitors, for stem cell-like delinking of replication from forward-differentiation [45]. We have found, however, that key *HOX* genes including *HOXA9* are dominantly regulated by lineage-differentiation activating master transcription factors, not vice-versa (HOXA9 does not regulate master transcription factors but is regulated by them) [27].

2. *Loss-of-function in lineage-committed progenitors (cancer initiating cell model)*: Loss-of-function alterations, for example, deletion of coactivators that lineage master transcription factors need to activate terminal-differentiation, might allow replication without forward-differentiation (self-replication) to emerge (Fig. 11.1) [46, 47]. The guilty genetic alterations may originate, however, in compartments preceding lineage-committed progenitors, e.g., in tissue stem cells or germ line, discussed below in 'Cell-of-Origin versus Cell-of-Transformation'.

4   The Importance of Reconciling These Different Models

Conceptual frameworks can profoundly influence selection of hypotheses. As an example, the gain-of-function model, when applied to potently oncogenic MLL (KMT2A) fusion proteins, emphasizes their interactions with coactivators e.g. DOT1L, that by activating stem cell genes (e.g., HOXA9) might delink replication from forward-differentiation [45], and therefore seeks to inhibit DOT1L [48]. The loss-of-function model looks for ways in which MLL leukemia fusion proteins might, via deletion of the MLL SET domain (the SET domain generates an epigenetic activation mark, H3K4me3), repress terminal-differentiation (Fig. 11.2), and seeks to inhibit this aberrant repression, e.g., by inhibiting DNA methyltransferase 1 (DNMT1) [49, 50]. Starting from the same empiric observations, therefore,

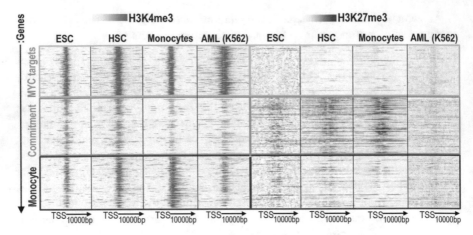

Fig. 11.2 Acquisition of the H3K4me3 epigenetic activation ('on') mark, is needed at monocyte terminal-differentiation genes in particular during monocyte ontogeny – replication genes are 'on' to begin within the earliest tissue precursors of embryonic stem cells (ESC), while commitment genes acquire the H3K27me3 repression ('off') mark during monocyte ontogeny. Notably, potently leukemogenic MLL leukemia fusion proteins invariably lose the SET domain that creates the H3K4me3 'on' mark. Comparative Marker Selection (Morpheus, Broad) identified ~200 myeloid commitment and ~300 terminal monocytic differentiation genes by analysis of gene expression in hematopoietic stem cells (HSC), common myeloid progenitors (CMP), granulocyte-monocyte progenitors (GMP), colony forming unit monocytes (CFUM) and monocytes from GSE24759, we then validated these gene sets in a separate gene expression database of normal hematopoiesis as we describe in a manuscript in press, that includes the gene lists [74] and GEO database numbers for the ChIP-Seq values analyzed. MYC target genes were identified by others using ChIP-Seq [61]. Rows = genes centered on transcription start sites [TSS]) in ESC, HSC and CD14+ monocytes

different models drive to drugs aiming at quite different molecular targets and goals: inhibiting coactivators to turn genes 'off', versus inhibiting corepressors to turn genes 'on'.

5 Cell-of-Origin Versus Cell-of-Transformation

To reconcile or choose between these models, examination for the cell-of-origin, the cell in which founding mutations originate ('first hits' in multi-hit oncogenesis) does not provide an automatic answer. *RUNX1* loss-of-function mutations in the germ line are the most frequently identified cause of familial AML. Cellular expansion and transformation, however, is several commitment decisions removed from the germ line cell-of-origin, in lineage-committed myeloid progenitors, via disruption to the PU.1/RUNX1 master transcription factor circuit which normally activates terminal granulo-monocytic lineage-fates, shown both *in vitro* and *in vivo* [50–54]. Another illustrative example is the recurrent AML mutation *DNMT3A-R882H*, detected in hematopoietic stem cells in patients' bone marrows

[41–43] – despite the mutation, these cells yield normal multi-lineage hematopoie-sis upon engraftment in immune-compromised mice [41–43]. On the other hand, lineage-progenitors from the same patient bone marrows, to which the *DNMT3A* mutations are propagated, additionally acquire mutations in *NPM1* and *FLT3* (the most highly recurrent mutations in human AML), and produce leukemic hemato-poiesis, wherein the cells replicate without forward-differentiation [41–43]. As would be expected from these observations, bone marrow replacement in AML patients is by cells that phenocopy granulocyte-monocyte progenitors [55]. Similarly, germline *Dnmt3a* haploinsufficient and *Dnmt3a* hematopoiesis-condi-tional knockout mice (Mx1-CRE crossed with *Dnmt3a*$^{fl/fl}$) demonstrate bone mar-row and spleen replacement by lineage-committed myeloid progenitors (e.g., granulocyte-monocyte progenitors), accumulating at the expense of hematopoietic stem cells and mature cells [56, 57]. In short, several studies of AML, previously reviewed by us in detail [38], have indicated that malignant transformation – the emergence of uncontrolled self-replication - occurs in lineage-committed progeni-tors, remote from germ line or stem 'cell-of-origin' of founder mutations.

6   Master Transcription Factor Alterations in Cancer Cells

Cancers of the same histology, despite profound diversity in genomic alterations, consistently have hundreds of genes similarly suppressed, and similarly up-regulated, versus their normal tissue counterparts [37, 50, 58–60]. Amongst sup-pressed genes, there is consistent high representation of terminal-differentiation genes [37, 50, 58, 59], whilst amongst upregulated genes, there is consistent high representation of replication genes (MYC-target genes) [60, 61]. Such broad and consistent programmatic changes suggest altered function of the master transcrip-tion factor circuits that regulate the expression of these hundreds of genes – what is the pattern of expression, and of genetic alteration, of these master transcription factors and their key cofactors in cancer?

1. **Master transcription factors expressed by self-replicating cancer cells**: Cancer cell lines self-replicate indefinitely ex vivo in plastic bottles and plates, so long as media and conditions meet basic metabolic needs. In cancer cell lines repre-senting the different cancer histologies afflicting humankind, the master tran-scription factor MYC, or its paralogue MYCN, are consistently highly expressed [60]. Also highly expressed are master transcription factors known to drive tissue lineage-differentiation [60]. This is also true of primary cancer tissues: the mas-ter transcription factors expressed resemble those in their normally terminally-differentiated tissue counterparts (Fig. 11.3) [60]. Thus, malignant melanoma cells express high levels of the melanocyte differentiation drivers MITF and SOX10 [62, 63], rhabdomyosarcomas express high levels of the muscle specify-ing transcription factor MYOD [64], clear cell renal cell cancers (RCC) express

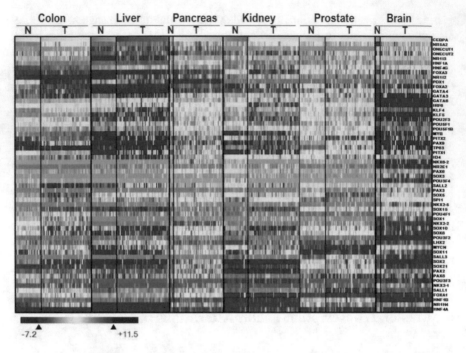

Fig. 11.3 Master transcription factors highly expressed in cancers are that of the corresponding normal differentiated lineage. TCGA Pan-Cancer RNA sequencing, N = normal tissue, T = tumor tissue, 50 cases randomly selected for each cancer, and up to 25 of available normals (total n = 412)

very high levels of the renal epithelial-fate driving transcription factors PAX2 and PAX8, HCCs express very high levels of hepatocyte fate transcription factors FOXA1, FOXA3, and to some extent, GATA4, and AML cells, including AML cells that can overcome inter-species barriers to initiate leukemia in immune-compromised mice (called leukemia 'stem' cells or leukemia initiating cells), express PU.1, CEBPA and RUNX1 at levels similar to or exceeding that observed in normal terminally differentiated granulocytes and monocytes, with miniscule levels of hematopoietic stem cell master transcription factors (reviewed in [38, 47]). Underscoring that such expression is not epi-phenomena, suppression by RNA interference of expressed lineage-differentiation driving master transcription factors is lethal – cancer cells, being committed to lineage, depend for their existence on lineage master transcription factors [51, 65–72].

2. *Master transcription factor alterations in cancer cells*: Yet, by gene expression analyses, hundreds of target terminal-differentiation genes of these lineage master transcription factors are suppressed, not activated [60] (reviewed in [47]), suggesting at a minimum, partial loss-of-function. Accordingly, *GATA4* and *GATA3*, master transcription factors essential for producing several tissue lineages, are haploinsufficient in ~50% of all cancers (Fig. 11.4). *RUNX1*, *CEBPA*, *RARA*, *IKZF1*, *EBF1*, and *PAX5*, necessary for several hematopoietic lineages,

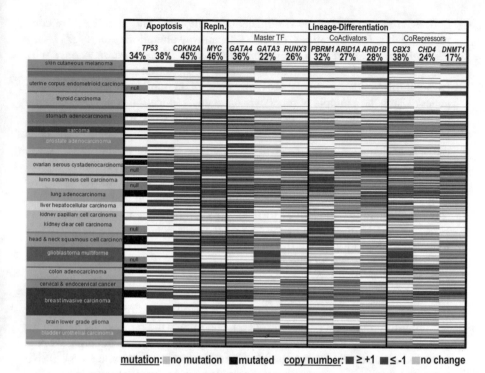

mutation: no mutation ■mutated   copy number: ■ ≥ +1 ■ ≤ -1 no change

Fig. 11.4 Master transcription that activate major metazoan programs, or their key cofactors, are recurrently altered in cancer; p53 (*TP53*) and its co-factor p16 (*CDKN2A*) that activate apoptosis are frequently bi-allelicaly inactivated; *MYC* that coordinates replication is frequently amplified; lineage master transcription factors with 'pioneer' function (able to access closed chromatin to initiate the remodeling needed for subsequent activation), or the key coactivators they use for this purpose are recurrently inactivated by deletion or mutation, while the corepressors they recruit are frequently amplified. Apoptosis and proliferation are activated by the same master transcription factors across histologies and species (p53 and MYC respectively) while lineage-differentiation has various master transcription factors/preferred coactivators. Percentages are the frequency of mutations or deletions (copy number ≤−1), or gains (copy number ≥+1) for MYC and corepressors (TCGA pan-cancer n = 10,845, data from Xena browser)

are recurrently mutated, deleted or translocated (reviewed in [38, 73]), or aberrantly dislocated into cytoplasm [74], in hematopoietic malignancies. It is worth emphasizing, however, that the loss-of-function is necessarily partial, since differentiation is a continuum along which all cells exist – suppression or inactivation of surviving alleles of an expressed lineage master transcription factor circuit is incompatible with cancer cell existence, shown for both liquid [51, 65–70, 75–77] and solid tumor malignancies [37, 71, 72] (Fig. 11.4).

This partial loss-of-function in differentiation circuits contrasts with bi-allelic inactivation, in ~80% of cancers, of *TP53* and/or *p16/CDKN2A* that regulate apoptosis (Fig. 11.4) - in common with terminal-differentiation, apoptosis dominantly suppresses MYC-coordinated replication, requiring p53-system inactivation, even as MYC may be simultaneously amplified and stabilized by copy number gains, *RAS* mutations, PI3K/AKT pathway alterations etc. (Fig. 11.4).

3. ***The epigenetic gradient to activation of terminal-differentiation genes***: Why does partial loss-of-function in lineage master transcription factor circuits repress terminal-differentiation but spare activation of commitment and replication genes? Using the example of monocyte ontogeny, replication genes (MYC target genes) are already 'poised' or 'on', that is, DNA CpG hypomethylated and H3K4me3 enriched, in the earliest tissue precursors, embryonic stem cells through to hematopoietic stem cells (Fig. 11.2). Myeloid commitment genes, although less poised to begin with, interestingly acquire the H3K27me3 repression ('off') mark rather than the activation mark during monocyte ontogeny (Fig. 11.2). By contrast, monocyte terminal-differentiation genes undergo substantial chromatin remodeling, to lose CpG methylation marks and increase H3K4me3 marks, during ontogeny, and AML is characterized by a failure of this remodeling (Fig. 11.2) [37, 47]. Thus, terminal-differentiation genes are particularly vulnerable to loss of chromatin-remodeling function [37, 50]:

4. ***Genomic alterations in the coactivators needed to activate terminal-differentiation***: Several lineage master transcription factors have been shown to be 'pioneers': they enter chromatin closed to lessor transcription factors, e.g., at terminal-differentiation genes (Fig. 11.2), and initiate the remodeling needed for access by the basal transcription factor machinery [78]. The remodeling work is executed by coactivators recruited by the transcription factors, e.g., SWI/SNF proteins, that use the energy from ATP hydrolysis to move obstructing nucleosomes away from transcription start sites [79] – these coactivators are inactivated by deletion and/or mutation in >60% of cancers (Fig. 11.4). Lineage master transcription factors are particular in the coactivators they use [80, 81], and accordingly, different SWI/SNF coactivators are inactivated in different cancers [82] (Fig. 11.4). For example, PBRM1 coactivates for the PAX2/PAX8 master transcription factor circuit (our observations in review) that activates the kidney epithelial-differentiation program, and *PBRM1* is universally at least haploinsufficient in clear cell renal cell cancers, with bi-allelic inactivation in ~40% of cases; and ARID1A coactivates for the GATA4/FOXA1 master transcription factor hub that activates hepatocyte epithelial-differentiation, and *ARID1A* is deleted or mutated (inactivating mutations) in ~40% of HCCs [37]. Recurrently inactivated coactivators include members of the mediator, splicing, cohesion and trithorax families (Fig. 11.5) [53].

Coactivators can also be inactivated indirectly, e.g., gain-of-function mutations in isocitrate dehydrogenases (IDHs) in gliomas and AMLs produce an oncometabolite (R-enantiomer of 2-hydroxyglutarate) that inhibits coactivator components TET2, KDM4A and KDM4C that use α-ketoglutarate as a cofactor [83], and phosphorylation of master transcription factors belonging to the CEBP family, by the RAS and FLT3 pathways that are constitutively activated by oncogenic mutations, has been shown to decrease their coactivator recruitment and repress rather than activate target differentiation genes [84, 85].

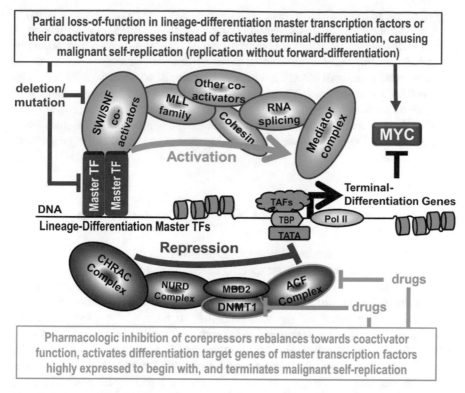

Fig. 11.5 An empirically observable property of cancers is high expression of lineage master transcription factors, yet anomalously, suppression of terminal-differentiation target genes of these commanders. Transcription factors integrate signaling inputs via dynamic interchange of opposing coactivators and corepressors - coactivators create the chromatin modifications that facilitate gene activation, while corepressors execute the opposite function. A common final pathway of oncogenesis is a shift in coactivator/corepressor stoichiometry at lineage master transcription factor hubs toward *corepressors and away from coactivators*. Onco-genetically induced corepressor/coactivator imbalance can be corrected pharmacologically

5. ***Mathematics***: The tissue compartments in which mutations originate, and the order in which they occur, has been documented in exquisitely for leukemogenesis. The picture painted is that tissue stem cells are crucial for neoplastic evolution, since their natural self-replication confers the long lives, high total number of cell divisions, and high volume of progeny (via committed daughter cells) necessary for random, multi-hit neoplastic evolution. For all this, these cells are still only pre-leukemic: transformation is of lineage-committed daughters to which founding mutations are propagated, shown by (i) master transcription factor expression of cancer cells, (ii) the programs consistently suppressed and upregulated versus normal tissue counterparts, (iii) surface and gene expression phenotypes of demonstrably self-replicating cells, (iv) surface and gene expression phenotypes of cells that accumulate, (v) inactivating mutation and/or haplo-insufficiency of lineage master transcription factors and their key coactivators,

(vi) origin of key transforming mutations (e.g., RAS, NPM1, FLT3 mutations) in lineage-committed progenitors, and (vii) the epigenetic gradient to activation of terminal-differentiation but not commitment genes [38, 47]. With intrinsic replication rates naturally so skewed in favor of lineage-progenitors versus tissue stem cells, even small advantages here can be amplified tremendously [86]. The corollary is that any advantage accrued to stem cells would have to be massive to compete with normally maximally replicative lineage-progenitors [86]. By way of analogy, committed progenitors are already speeding down the highway, and only need to disable the brakes, while tissue stem cells sit still in the garage with the engine off.

7 Targeting Cancer, But Not Normal, Self-Replication

Thus, cancer cells are destined for terminal-differentiation by overall master transcription factor content, and rely on specific corepressors to forestall these fates and create malignant self-replication (Fig. 11.5). Inhibiting these corepressors relinks replication to forward-differentiation, activates terminal-differentiation programs, and terminates malignant self-replication [29, 49, 50, 52, 53, 58, 87, 88] (Fig. 11.5). Since MYC is subservient to terminal-differentiation, replication is terminated even if MYC is stabilized and/or amplified by other genetic alterations typical of cancer including *RAS* mutations and *MYC* amplifications [29, 49, 50, 52, 53, 58, 87, 88]. Since this pathway of cell cycle exits does not require p53/p16, it can cytoreduce even p53/p16-null cancers that are resistant to standard apoptosis-intending (cytotoxic) chemotherapy and radiation [29, 47, 49, 50, 58]. Normal committed progenitors, like the lineage-committed cancer and leukemia cells (including leukemia/cancer 'stem' cells), also differentiate [50, 87, 89]. The same treatments increase self-renewal of normal tissue stem cells since these express high levels of master stem cell transcription factors, not differentiation-drivers [50, 87, 89–96]. In short, effecting corepressor/coactivator exchange in lineage master transcription factor hubs is sound in the overall genetic and clinical context of cancer.

1. *Effecting corepressor/coactivator exchange (specific clinical indications)*: The retinoic acid receptor (RARA) exchanges corepressors for coactivators upon binding of its cognate ligand retinoic acid (ATRA), to thereby activate granulocyte terminal-differentiation genes. In acute promyelocytic leukemia (APL), the PML gene is fused with RARA, to create the fusion protein PML-RARA: physiologic concentrations of ATRA cannot trigger corepressor/coactivator exchange at PML-RARA, and thus granulocyte terminal-differentiation genes are repressed instead of activated. Treatment of APL patients with pharmacologic doses of ATRA, however, forces the corepressor/coactivator exchange and activates granulocyte terminal-differentiation. Arsenic that degrades PML-RARA, via an interaction with PML, also corrects corepressor/coactivator imbalance to activate granulocytic fates [97]. The combination of just these two drugs produces

>95% 2 year survival in APL, compared with <30% 2 year survival with conventional cytotoxic chemotherapy [98–100].

Inhibition of kinases that phosphorylate master transcription factors is another indirect method of actuating corepressor/coactivator exchange and terminal-differentiation [85, 101], as is inhibition of mutant IDH2 that generates an oncometabolite that inhibits coactivator components TET2, KDM4A and KDM4C [102]. We have found that low concentrations of nuclear export inhibitors, sufficient to inhibit mutant-NPM1 mediated nuclear-export of the master transcription factor PU.1, restore terminal-differentiation in *NPM1*-mutated AML cells, observations we hope to translate into clinical therapy for chemorefractory disease [74].

2. *Inhibiting corepressors directly (multiple clinical indications)*: The methods of effecting corepressor/coactivator exchange above are for very specific oncogenetic contexts. An alternative is to inhibit corepressors directly, an approach that has been scientifically validated for broad application (Fig. 11.4). The challenge is to develop specific and potent small molecule inhibitors that do not have off-target anti-metabolite effects that undermine therapeutic indices:

DNMT1: The maintenance methyltransferase and corepressor component DNMT1 is enriched in highly expressed master transcription factor hubs of multiple cancer types, and has been scientifically validated as a pan-cancer target for differentiation-restoring therapy [29, 49, 50, 52, 53, 58, 88, 103–129] (reviewed in [46]) (Figs. 11.4 and 11.5). The clinical drug decitabine can be administered by dosages and schedules that deplete DNMT1 without cytotoxicity [49, 50, 58, 59, 88]. Non-cytotoxic treatments are especially needed to treat myeloid malignancies in the elderly, since the cause of morbidity and death is low blood counts. We therefore treated such patients with a decitabine regimen documented to deplete DNMT1 without cytotoxicity [130, 131]: 0.1–0.2 mg/kg/day compared to the FDA-approved 20-45 mg/m^2/day (a 75–90% reduction), administered 1–3 days/week nonstop to increase probabilities that cancer S-phase entries coincide with drug presence in cells, which is required because DNMT1-depletion by decitabine is S-phase dependent. The treated patients were mostly elderly, and many had disease that was relapsed/refractory to initial treatments. Responses meeting International Working Group criteria occurred in 44% of subjects and were highly durable, with treatment-induced freedom from transfusion lasting a median of 1025 days with 20% of the subjects treated for more than 3 years, including several patients >80 years old [88]. Consistent with DNMT1-depletion targeting a final common pathway of transformation, hematologic and cytogenetic responses occurred across the diverse genetic spectrum of disease, including in cases with complex chromosome abnormalities and *TP53* mutations [88, 128, 132, 133]. Non-cytotoxic DNMT1-depletion was confirmed by serial bone marrow γ-H2AX and DNMT1 analyses. MYC master oncoprotein levels were markedly decreased by treatment [88].

This therapy could not be simply extended to patients with solid tumor malignancies, since decitabine is rapidly deaminated (inactivated) by the enzyme cytidine deaminase (CDA) that is highly expressed in solid tissues (this is why decitabine and other cytidine analogues have severely limited oral bioavailability) [103, 134, 135]. CDA upregulation within cancer cells is moreover a well-documented mechanism of resistance to cytidine analogues (reviewed in [136]). We have thus combined decitabine with a CDA-inhibitor (tetrahydrouridine) for orally administered, non-cytotoxic DNMT1-depleting treatment of *TP53*-mutated solid and liquid cancers, trials that are ongoing at this time (clinical trials.gov NCT02664181; NCT02847000; NCT02846935) [135].

Histone deacetylases (HDAC): HDACs, that are key components of several multiprotein corepressor complexes, are also enriched in lineage master transcription factor hubs in cancer cells [37, 52, 137], and have been pre-clinically validated repeatedly as molecular targets for the induction of terminal-differentiation of liquid and solid tumor cancer cells [138–148], with several HDAC inhibitors FDA approved to treat peripheral T-cell malignancies. Clinical application of HDAC inhibitors has been limited unfortunately by pleiotropic roles of HDACs outside of chromatin, rendering it difficult to separate anti-metabolite/cytotoxicity from epigenetic effects [149–153]: the unintended effects limit achievement of intended epigenetic effect *in vivo*. Since the side-effects reflect the widespread roles of HDAC in normal physiology, it is not immediately clear if this problem will be solved with newer HDAC inhibitors.

Lysine demethylase 1 (LSD1, KDM1A): KDM1A, a flavine adenine dinucleotide (FAD)-dependent monoamine oxidase, is another corepressor component highly enriched in lineage master transcription factor hubs in cancer cells, and genetic or pharmacologic inhibition of KDM1A has been shown to induce terminal maturation in a number of liquid and solid cancer models [154–158]. Several KDM1A inhibitors are in clinical trials for cancer indications (EudraCT number: 2013-002447-29; ClinicalTrials.gov identifiers: NCT02177812, NCT02034123, NCT01344707). At least two of the compounds in trials (ORY-1001, GSK2879552) are built around a tranylcypromine warhead that inhibits brain monoamine oxidases that metabolize catecholamine neurotransmitters, a potential source of side-effects that might limit realization of intended epigenetic effects.

CHD4 and SMARCA5: Nucleosomes (histone octamers) proximal to gene transcription start sites are physical barriers to gene activation. Repositioning these obstructions is energetically expensive work executed by SWI/SNF or ISWI family chromatin remodeling proteins containing the HELICc-DExx ATP-ase domain [80, 159, 160]. We have noted enrichment for CHD4 and SMARCA5 HELICc-DExx containing corepressors in the master transcription factor protein hubs of both liquid and solid cancers [37, 137], and we therefore screened for and identified a drug-like compound series that inhibits the HELICc-DExx domains of SMARCA5 and CHD4 to activate terminal-differentiation in liquid and solid cancer cell lines (our unpublished data).

Since nucleosome positioning is the crux of the obstruction to gene activation, inhibition of this action could in principle offer corresponding potency.

In sum, validated targets for inhibition have been identified, but there are few drugs for their inhibition, all with limitations (as to be expected). This is a target space crying for new non-cytotoxic drugs.

3. *Resistance*: Targeting malignant self-replication is not expected to be curative per se, since all drugs are metabolized, must distribute into all target cells, and successfully engage molecular targets to produce intended molecular pharmacodynamic effects - several opportunities for evasion. In other words, resistance will need to be addressed, e.g., with rational combinations of corepressor targeting drugs, for the worthy aspiration of extending broadly the extraordinary results seen with just two non-cytotoxic drugs in APL.

8 Conclusion

Consistent with corepressor/coactivator imbalance being at the heart of malignant, but not normal, self-replication, effecting corepressor/coactivator exchange, indirectly or directly, is clinically proven therapy for some indications - in fact, the best overall survival for any disseminated malignancy is for APL treated by this non-cytotoxic modality (~95%) [88, 98–100, 128, 132, 133]. Unleashing the activity of lineage master transcription factors already highly expressed contrasts with the intent of most conventional oncotherapy, which applies stress upstream of p53 in the hope of upregulating it for apoptosis, a toxic and futile intent when p53 is absent/non-functional (reviewed in [47]). In short, actuating corepressor/coactivator exchange releases terminal-differentiation fates intended by the master transcription factors most abundantly contained in self-replicating cancer cells, per the Hippocratic dictum: "Natural forces within us are the true healers of disease".

References

1. Kaiser J (2015) The cancer stem cell gamble. Science 347:226–229
2. Domazet-Loso T, Tautz D (2010) Phylostratigraphic tracking of cancer genes suggests a link to the emergence of multicellularity in metazoa. BMC Biol 8:66
3. Srivastava M, Simakov O, Chapman J et al (2010) The Amphimedon queenslandica genome and the evolution of animal complexity. Nature 466:720–726
4. Riddell J, Gazit R, Garrison BS et al (2014) Reprogramming committed murine blood cells to induced hematopoietic stem cells with defined factors. Cell 157:549–564
5. Takahashi K, Yamanaka S (2006) Induction of pluripotent stem cells from mouse embryonic and adult fibroblast cultures by defined factors. Cell 126:663–676
6. Nygren JM, Bryder D, Jacobsen SE (2006) Prolonged cell cycle transit is a defining and developmentally conserved hemopoietic stem cell property. J Immunol 177:201–208

7. Schwartz GN, Vance BA, Levine BM et al (2003) Proliferation kinetics of subpopulations of human marrow cells determined by quantifying in vivo incorporation of [2H2]-glucose into DNA of S-phase cells. Blood 102:2068–2073

8. van der Wath RC, Wilson A, Laurenti E et al (2009) Estimating dormant and active hematopoietic stem cell kinetics through extensive modeling of bromodeoxyuridine label-retaining cell dynamics. PLoS One 4:e6972

9. Li J (2011) Quiescence regulators for hematopoietic stem cell. Exp Hematol 39:511

10. Komorowska K, Doyle A, Wahlestedt M et al (2017) Hepatic leukemia factor maintains quiescence of hematopoietic stem cells and protects the stem cell pool during regeneration. Cell Rep 21:3514–3523

11. Roche KC, Gracz AD, Liu XF et al (2015) SOX9 maintains reserve stem cells and preserves radioresistance in mouse small intestine. Gastroenterology 149:1553–1563 e10

12. Bjornson CR, Cheung TH, Liu L et al (2012) Notch signaling is necessary to maintain quiescence in adult muscle stem cells. Stem Cells 30:232–242

13. Mourikis P, Sambasivan R, Castel D et al (2012) A critical requirement for notch signaling in maintenance of the quiescent skeletal muscle stem cell state. Stem Cells 30:243–252

14. Chapouton P, Skupien P, Hesl B et al (2010) Notch activity levels control the balance between quiescence and recruitment of adult neural stem cells. J Neurosci 30:7961–7974

15. Mardaryev AN, Meier N, Poterlowicz K et al (2011) Lhx2 differentially regulates Sox9, Tcf4 and Lgr5 in hair follicle stem cells to promote epidermal regeneration after injury. Development 138:4843–4852

16. Zeman MK, Cimprich KA (2014) Causes and consequences of replication stress. Nat Cell Biol 16:2–9

17. Haber JE (1999) DNA recombination: the replication connection. Trends Biochem Sci 24:271–275

18. Burkhalter MD, Rudolph KL, Sperka T (2015) Genome instability of ageing stem cells-induction and defence mechanisms. Ageing Res Rev 23:29–36

19. Ruzankina Y, Pinzon-Guzman C, Asare A et al (2007) Deletion of the developmentally essential gene ATR in adult mice leads to age-related phenotypes and stem cell loss. Cell Stem Cell 1:113–126

20. Choi M, Kipps T, Kurzrock R (2016) ATM mutations in cancer: therapeutic implications. Mol Cancer Ther 15:1781–1791

21. Wilson A, Murphy MJ, Oskarsson T et al (2004) c-Myc controls the balance between hematopoietic stem cell self-renewal and differentiation. Genes Dev 18:2747–2763

22. Reavie L, Della Gatta G, Crusio K et al (2010) Regulation of hematopoietic stem cell differentiation by a single ubiquitin ligase-substrate complex. Nat Immunol 11:207–215

23. Laurenti E, Varnum-Finney B, Wilson A et al (2008) Hematopoietic stem cell function and survival depend on c-Myc and N-Myc activity. Cell Stem Cell 3:611–624

24. Zhang J, Xiao Y, Guo Y et al (2011) Differential requirements for c-Myc in chronic hematopoietic hyperplasia and acute hematopoietic malignancies in Pten-null mice. Leukemia 25:1857–1868

25. Arnold I (2001) Watt FM: c-Myc activation in transgenic mouse epidermis results in mobilization of stem cells and differentiation of their progeny. Curr Biol 11:558–568

26. Bahr C, von Paleske L, Uslu VV et al (2018) A Myc enhancer cluster regulates normal and leukaemic haematopoietic stem cell hierarchies. Nature 553:515

27. Gu X, Mahfouz R, Zhang J et al (2016) Cytoplasmic localization of PU.1 with mutated NPM1 causes myeloid differentiation arrest. Cancer Res 76:2872

28. Acosta JC, Ferrandiz N, Bretones G et al (2008) Myc inhibits p27-induced erythroid differentiation of leukemia cells by repressing erythroid master genes without reversing p27-mediated cell cycle arrest. Mol Cell Biol 28:7286–7295

29. Negrotto S, Hu Z, Alcazar O et al (2011) Noncytotoxic differentiation treatment of renal cell cancer. Cancer Res 71:1431–1441

30. Grote D, Souabni A, Busslinger M et al (2006) Pax 2/8-regulated Gata 3 expression is necessary for morphogenesis and guidance of the nephric duct in the developing kidney. Development 133:53–61
31. Green LM, Wagner KJ, Campbell HA et al (2009) Dynamic interaction between WT1 and BASP1 in transcriptional regulation during differentiation. Nucleic Acids Res 37:431–440
32. Lucas B, Grigo K, Erdmann S et al (2005) HNF4alpha reduces proliferation of kidney cells and affects genes deregulated in renal cell carcinoma. Oncogene 24:6418–6431
33. Ramaswamy S, Nakamura N, Sansal I et al (2002) A novel mechanism of gene regulation and tumor suppression by the transcription factor FKHR. Cancer Cell 2:81–91
34. Aschauer L, Gruber LN, Pfaller W et al (2013) Delineation of the key aspects in the regulation of epithelial monolayer formation. Mol Cell Biol 33:2535–2550
35. Kojima T, Shimazui T, Horie R et al (2010) FOXO1 and TCF7L2 genes involved in metastasis and poor prognosis in clear cell renal cell carcinoma. Genes Chromosomes Cancer 49:379–389
36. Bignold LP, Coghlan B, Jersmann H (2009) David Paul Hansemann: chromosomes and the origin of the cancerous features of tumor cells. Cell Oncol 31:61
37. Enane FO, Shuen WH, Gu X et al (2017) GATA4 loss of function in liver cancer impedes precursor to hepatocyte transition. J Clin Invest 127:3527
38. Saunthararajah Y (2016) Chapter 4 - critical updates to the leukemia stem cell model A2 - Liu, Huiping. In: Lathia JD (ed) Cancer stem cells. Academic, Boston, pp 101–119
39. Lapidot T, Sirard C, Vormoor J et al (1994) A cell initiating human acute myeloid leukaemia after transplantation into SCID mice. Nature 367:645–648
40. Dick JE (2008) Stem cell concepts renew cancer research. Blood 112:4793–4807
41. Jan M, Snyder TM, Corces-Zimmerman MR et al (2012) Clonal evolution of preleukemic hematopoietic stem cells precedes human acute myeloid leukemia. Sci Transl Med 4:149ra118
42. Corces-Zimmerman MR, Hong WJ, Weissman IL et al (2014) Preleukemic mutations in human acute myeloid leukemia affect epigenetic regulators and persist in remission. Proc Natl Acad Sci U S A 111:2548–2553
43. Shlush LI, Zandi S, Mitchell A et al (2014) Identification of pre-leukaemic haematopoietic stem cells in acute leukaemia. Nature 506:328–333
44. Watt FM, Frye M, Benitah SA (2008) MYC in mammalian epidermis: how can an oncogene stimulate differentiation? Nat Rev Cancer 8:234–242
45. Bernt KM, Zhu N, Sinha AU et al (2011) MLL-rearranged leukemia is dependent on Aberrant H3K79 methylation by DOT1L. Cancer Cell 20:66–78
46. Saunthararajah Y, Triozzi P, Rini B et al (2012) p53-independent, normal stem cell sparing epigenetic differentiation therapy for myeloid and other malignancies. Semin Oncol 39:97–108
47. Velcheti V, Radivoyevitch T, Saunthararajah Y (2017) Higher-level pathway objectives of epigenetic therapy: a solution to the p53 problem in cancer. Am Soc Clin Oncol Educ Book 37:812–824
48. Stein EM, Garcia-Manero G, Rizzieri DA et al (2014) The DOT1L inhibitor EPZ-5676: safety and activity in relapsed/refractory patients with MLL-rearranged leukemia. Blood 124:387
49. Ng KP, Ebrahem Q, Negrotto S et al (2011) p53 independent epigenetic-differentiation treatment in xenotransplant models of acute myeloid leukemia. Leukemia 25:1739–1750
50. Negrotto S, Ng KP, Jankowska AM et al (2012) CpG methylation patterns and decitabine treatment response in acute myeloid leukemia cells and normal hematopoietic precursors. Leukemia 26:244–254
51. Ng KP, Hu Z, Ebrahem Q et al (2013) Runx1 deficiency permits granulocyte lineage commitment but impairs subsequent maturation. Oncogenesis 2:e78
52. Hu Z, Gu X, Baraoidan K et al (2011) RUNX1 regulates corepressor interactions of PU.1. Blood 117:6498–6508

53. Gu X, Hu Z, Ebrahem Q et al (2014) Runx1 regulation of Pu.1 corepressor/coactivator exchange identifies specific molecular targets for leukemia differentiation therapy. J Biol Chem 289:14881–14895
54. Sun W, Downing JR (2004) Haploinsufficiency of AML1 results in a decrease in the number of LTR-HSCs while simultaneously inducing an increase in more mature progenitors. Blood 104:3565–3572
55. Quek L, Otto GW, Garnett C et al (2016) Genetically distinct leukemic stem cells in human CD34- acute myeloid leukemia are arrested at a hemopoietic precursor-like stage. J Exp Med 213:1513
56. Celik H, Mallaney C, Kothari A et al (2015) Enforced differentiation of Dnmt3a-null bone marrow leads to failure with c-Kit mutations driving leukemic transformation. Blood 125:619–628
57. Cole CB, Russler-Germain DA, Ketkar S et al (2017) Haploinsufficiency for DNA methyltransferase 3A predisposes hematopoietic cells to myeloid malignancies. J Clin Invest 127:3657–3674
58. Alcazar O, Achberger S, Aldrich W et al (2012) Epigenetic regulation by decitabine of melanoma differentiation in vitro and in vivo. Int J Cancer 131:18–29
59. Negrotto S, Hu ZB, Alcazar O et al (2011) Noncytotoxic differentiation treatment of renal cell cancer. Cancer Res 71:1431–1441
60. Garcia-Alonso L, Iorio F, Matchan A et al (2018) Transcription factor activities enhance markers of drug sensitivity in cancer. Cancer Res 78:769–780
61. Kim J, Woo AJ, Chu J et al (2010) A Myc network accounts for similarities between embryonic stem and cancer cell transcription programs. Cell 143:313–324
62. McGill GG, Horstmann M, Widlund HR et al (2002) Bcl2 regulation by the melanocyte master regulator Mitf modulates lineage survival and melanoma cell viability. Cell 109:707–718
63. Cronin JC, Wunderlich J, Loftus SK et al (2009) Frequent mutations in the MITF pathway in melanoma. Pigment Cell Melanoma Res 22:435–444
64. Yang Z, MacQuarrie KL, Analau E et al (2009) MyoD and E-protein heterodimers switch rhabdomyosarcoma cells from an arrested myoblast phase to a differentiated state. Genes Dev 23:694–707
65. Goyama S, Schibler J, Cunningham L et al (2013) Transcription factor RUNX1 promotes survival of acute myeloid leukemia cells. J Clin Invest 123:3876–3888
66. Ohlsson E, Hasemann MS, Willer A et al (2014) Initiation of MLL-rearranged AML is dependent on C/EBPalpha. J Exp Med 211:5–13
67. Rosenbauer F, Wagner K, Kutok JL et al (2004) Acute myeloid leukemia induced by graded reduction of a lineage-specific transcription factor, PU.1. Nat Genet 36:624–630
68. Aikawa Y, Yamagata K, Katsumoto T et al (2015) Essential role of PU.1 in maintenance of mixed lineage leukemia-associated leukemic stem cells. Cancer Sci 106:227–236
69. Zhou J, Wu J, Li B et al (2013) PU.1 is essential for MLL leukemia partially via crosstalk with the MEIS/HOX pathway. Leukemia 28:1436
70. Will B, Vogler TO, Narayanagari S et al (2015) Minimal PU.1 reduction induces a preleukemic state and promotes development of acute myeloid leukemia. Nat Med 21:1172–1181
71. Tsherniak A, Vazquez F, Montgomery PG et al (2017) Defining a cancer dependency map. Cell 170:564–576 e16
72. McDonald ER 3rd, de Weck A, Schlabach MR et al (2017) Project DRIVE: a compendium of cancer dependencies and synthetic lethal relationships uncovered by large-scale, deep RNAi screening. Cell 170:577–592 e10
73. Somasundaram R, Prasad MA, Ungerback J et al (2015) Transcription factor networks in B-cell differentiation link development to acute lymphoid leukemia. Blood 126:144–152
74. Gu XR, Mahfouz RZ, Ebrahem Q et al (2016) The mechanism by which mutant Nucleophosmin (NPM1) creates leukemic self-renewal is readily reversed. Blood 128:444

75. Mendler JH, Maharry K, Radmacher MD et al (2012) RUNX1 mutations are associated with poor outcome in younger and older patients with cytogenetically normal acute myeloid leukemia and with distinct gene and MicroRNA expression signatures. J Clin Oncol 30:3109–3118
76. Alpermann T, Schnittger S, Eder C et al (2016) Molecular subtypes of NPM1 mutations have different clinical profiles, specific patterns of accompanying molecular mutations and varying outcomes in intermediate risk acute myeloid leukemia. Haematologica 101:e55–e58
77. Dufour A, Schneider F, Metzeler KH et al (2010) Acute myeloid leukemia with biallelic CEBPA gene mutations and normal karyotype represents a distinct genetic entity associated with a favorable clinical outcome. J Clin Oncol 28:570–577
78. Suzuki T, Maeda S, Furuhata E et al (2017) A screening system to identify transcription factors that induce binding site-directed DNA demethylation. Epigenetics Chromatin 10:60
79. Lai WKM, Pugh BF (2017) Understanding nucleosome dynamics and their links to gene expression and DNA replication. Nat Rev Mol Cell Biol 18:548–562
80. Lemon B, Inouye C, King DS et al (2001) Selectivity of chromatin-remodelling cofactors for ligand-activated transcription. Nature 414:924–928
81. Ho L, Jothi R, Ronan JL et al (2009) An embryonic stem cell chromatin remodeling complex, esBAF, is an essential component of the core pluripotency transcriptional network. Proc Natl Acad Sci U S A 106:5187–5191
82. Shain AH, Pollack JR (2013) The spectrum of SWI/SNF mutations, ubiquitous in human cancers. PLoS One 8:e55119
83. Chowdhury R, Yeoh KK, Tian YM et al (2011) The oncometabolite 2-hydroxyglutarate inhibits histone lysine demethylases. EMBO Rep 12:463–469
84. Kowenz-Leutz E, Pless O, Dittmar G et al (2010) Crosstalk between C/EBPbeta phosphorylation, arginine methylation, and SWI/SNF/mediator implies an indexing transcription factor code. EMBO J 29:1105–1115
85. Radomska HS, Basseres DS, Zheng R et al (2006) Block of C/EBP alpha function by phosphorylation in acute myeloid leukemia with FLT3 activating mutations. J Exp Med 203:371–381
86. Ashkenazi R, Gentry SN, Jackson TL (2008) Pathways to tumorigenesis--modeling mutation acquisition in stem cells and their progeny. Neoplasia 10:1170–1182
87. Hu Z, Negrotto S, Gu X et al (2010) Decitabine maintains hematopoietic precursor self-renewal by preventing repression of stem cell genes by a differentiation-inducing stimulus. Mol Cancer Ther 9:1536–1543
88. Saunthararajah Y, Sekeres M, Advani A et al (2015) Evaluation of noncytotoxic DNMT1-depleting therapy in patients with myelodysplastic syndromes. J Clin Invest 125:1043–1055
89. Milhem M, Mahmud N, Lavelle D et al (2004) Modification of hematopoietic stem cell fate by 5aza 2 ' deoxycytidine and trichostatin A. Blood 103:4102–4110
90. De Felice L, Tatarelli C, Mascolo MG et al (2005) Histone deacetylase inhibitor valproic acid enhances the cytokine-induced expansion of human hematopoietic stem cells. Cancer Res 65:1505–1513
91. Bug G, Gul H, Schwarz K et al (2005) Valproic acid stimulates proliferation and self-renewal of hematopoietic stem cells. Cancer Res 65:2537–2541
92. Young JC, Wu S, Hansteen G et al (2004) Inhibitors of histone deacetylases promote hematopoietic stem cell self-renewal. Cytotherapy 6:328–336
93. Lee JH, Hart SR, Skalnik DG (2004) Histone deacetylase activity is required for embryonic stem cell differentiation. Genesis 38:32–38
94. Araki H, Mahmud N, Milhem M et al (2006) Expansion of human umbilical cord blood SCID-repopulating cells using chromatin-modifying agents. Exp Hematol 34:140–149
95. Suzuki M, Harashima A, Okochi A et al (2004) 5-Azacytidine supports the long-term repopulating activity of cord blood CD34(+) cells. Am J Hematol 77:313–315
96. Chung YS, Kim HJ, Kim TM et al (2009) Undifferentiated hematopoietic cells are characterized by a genome-wide undermethylation dip around the transcription start site and a hierarchical epigenetic plasticity. Blood 114:4968–4978

97. Hu Z, Saunthararajah Y (2012) CEBPE activation in PML-RARA cells by arsenic. Blood 119:2177–2179
98. Smith ML, Hills RK, Grimwade D (2011) Independent prognostic variables in acute myeloid leukaemia. Blood Rev 25:39–51
99. Lo-Coco F, Avvisati G, Vignetti M et al (2013) Retinoic acid and arsenic trioxide for acute promyelocytic leukemia. N Engl J Med 369:111–121
100. Huang ME, Ye YC, Chen SR et al (1987) All-trans retinoic acid with or without low dose cytosine arabinoside in acute promyelocytic leukemia. Report of 6 cases. Chin Med J (Engl) 100:949–953
101. Sexauer A, Perl A, Yang X et al (2012) Terminal myeloid differentiation in vivo is induced by FLT3 inhibition in FLT3/ITD AML. Blood 120:4205–4214
102. Stein EM, DiNardo CD, Pollyea DA et al (2017) Enasidenib in mutant IDH2 relapsed or refractory acute myeloid leukemia. Blood 130:722–731
103. Ebrahem Q, Mahfouz R, Ng KP et al (2012) High cytidine deaminase expression in the liver provides sanctuary for cancer cells from decitabine treatment effects. Oncotarget 3:1137–1145
104. Shakya R, Gonda T, Quante M et al (2013) Hypomethylating therapy in an aggressive stroma-rich model of pancreatic carcinoma. Cancer Res 73:885–896
105. Cecconi D, Astner H, Donadelli M et al (2003) Proteomic analysis of pancreatic ductal carcinoma cells treated with 5-aza-2′-deoxycytidine. Electrophoresis 24:4291–4303
106. Kumagai T, Wakimoto N, Yin D et al (2007) Histone deacetylase inhibitor, suberoylanilide hydroxamic acid (Vorinostat, SAHA) profoundly inhibits the growth of human pancreatic cancer cells. Int J Cancer 121:656–665
107. Yamada T, Ohwada S, Saitoh F et al (1996) Induction of Ley antigen by 5-aza-2′-deoxycytidine in association with differentiation and apoptosis in human pancreatic cancer cells. Anticancer Res 16:735–740
108. Belinsky SA, Klinge DM, Stidley CA et al (2003) Inhibition of DNA methylation and histone deacetylation prevents murine lung cancer. Cancer Res 63:7089–7093
109. Belinsky SA, Grimes MJ, Picchi MA et al (2011) Combination therapy with vidaza and entinostat suppresses tumor growth and reprograms the epigenome in an orthotopic lung cancer model. Cancer Res 71:454–462
110. Zochbauer-Muller S, Minna JD, Gazdar AF (2002) Aberrant DNA methylation in lung cancer: biological and clinical implications. Oncologist 7:451–457
111. Liu CC, Lin JH, Hsu TW et al (2015) IL-6 enriched lung cancer stem-like cell population by inhibition of cell cycle regulators via DNMT1 upregulation. Int J Cancer 136:547–559
112. Kim HJ, Kim JH, Chie EK et al (2012) DNMT (DNA methyltransferase) inhibitors radiosensitize human cancer cells by suppressing DNA repair activity. Radiat Oncol 7:39
113. Rauch T, Wang Z, Zhang X et al (2007) Homeobox gene methylation in lung cancer studied by genome-wide analysis with a microarray-based methylated CpG island recovery assay. Proc Natl Acad Sci U S A 104:5527–5532
114. Peters SL, Hlady RA, Opavska J et al (2013) Essential role for Dnmt1 in the prevention and maintenance of MYC-induced T-cell lymphomas. Mol Cell Biol 33:4321–4333
115. Hoglund A, Nilsson LM, Forshell LP et al (2009) Myc sensitizes p53-deficient cancer cells to the DNA-damaging effects of the DNA methyltransferase inhibitor decitabine. Blood 113:4281–4288
116. Guan H, Xie L, Klapproth K et al (2013) Decitabine represses translocated MYC oncogene in Burkitt lymphoma. J Pathol 229:775–783
117. Hassler MR, Klisaroska A, Kollmann K et al (2012) Antineoplastic activity of the DNA methyltransferase inhibitor 5-aza-2′-deoxycytidine in anaplastic large cell lymphoma. Biochimie 94:2297–2307
118. Kalac M, Scotto L, Marchi E et al (2011) HDAC inhibitors and decitabine are highly synergistic and associated with unique gene-expression and epigenetic profiles in models of DLBCL. Blood 118:5506–5516

119. Leshchenko VV, Kuo PY, Jiang Z et al (2014) Integrative genomic analysis of temozolomide resistance in diffuse large B-cell lymphoma. Clin Cancer Res 20:382–392
120. Iqbal J, Kucuk C, Deleeuw RJ et al (2009) Genomic analyses reveal global functional alterations that promote tumor growth and novel tumor suppressor genes in natural killer-cell malignancies. Leukemia 23:1139–1151
121. Kozlowska A, Jagodzinski PP (2008) Inhibition of DNA methyltransferase activity upregulates Fyn tyrosine kinase expression in Hut-78 T-lymphoma cells. Biomed Pharmacother 62:672–676
122. Ripperger T, von Neuhoff N, Kamphues K et al (2007) Promoter methylation of PARG1, a novel candidate tumor suppressor gene in mantle-cell lymphomas. Haematologica 92:460–468
123. Han Y, Amin HM, Frantz C et al (2006) Restoration of shp1 expression by 5-AZA-2′-deoxycytidine is associated with downregulation of JAK3/STAT3 signaling in ALK-positive anaplastic large cell lymphoma. Leukemia 20:1602–1609
124. Ushmorov A, Leithauser F, Sakk O et al (2006) Epigenetic processes play a major role in B-cell-specific gene silencing in classical Hodgkin lymphoma. Blood 107:2493–2500
125. Tsai HC, Li H, Van Neste L et al (2012) Transient low doses of DNA-Demethylating agents exert durable antitumor effects on hematological and epithelial tumor cells. Cancer Cell 21:430–446
126. Momparler RL, Cote S, Momparler LF (2013) Epigenetic action of decitabine (5-aza-2′-deoxycytidine) is more effective against acute myeloid leukemia than cytotoxic action of cytarabine (ARA-C). Leuk Res 37:980
127. Chaurasia P, Gajzer DC, Schaniel C et al (2014) Epigenetic reprogramming induces the expansion of cord blood stem cells. J Clin Invest 124:2378
128. Liu Y, Tabarroki A, Billings S et al (2014) Successful use of very low dose subcutaneous decitabine to treat high-risk myelofibrosis with Sweet syndrome that was refractory to 5-azacitidine. Leuk Lymphoma 55:447–449
129. Tabarroki A, Saunthararajah Y, Visconte V et al (2014) Ruxolitinib in combination with DNA methyltransferase inhibitors; clinical responses in symptomatic myelofibrosis patients with cytopenias and elevated blasts counts. Leuk Lymphoma 56:497
130. Saunthararajah Y, Hillery CA, Lavelle D et al (2003) Effects of 5-aza-2 '-deoxycytidine on fetal hemoglobin levels, red cell adhesion, and hematopoietic differentiation in patients with sickle cell disease. Blood 102:3865–3870
131. Olivieri NF, Saunthararajah Y, Thayalasuthan V et al (2011) A pilot study of subcutaneous decitabine in beta-thalassemia intermedia. Blood 118:2708–2711
132. Saleh MFM, Saunthararajah Y (2017) Severe pyoderma gangrenosum caused by myelodysplastic syndrome successfully treated with decitabine administered by a noncytotoxic regimen. Clin Case Rep 5:2025–2027
133. Tabarroki A, Saunthararajah Y, Visconte V et al (2015) Ruxolitinib in combination with DNA methyltransferase inhibitors: clinical responses in patients with symptomatic myelofibrosis with cytopenias and elevated blast(s) counts. Leuk Lymphoma 56:497–499
134. Lavelle D, Vaitkus K, Ling Y et al (2012) Effects of tetrahydrouridine on pharmacokinetics and pharmacodynamics of oral decitabine. Blood 119:1240–1247
135. Molokie R, Lavelle D, Gowhari M et al (2017) Oral tetrahydrouridine and decitabine for noncytotoxic epigenetic gene regulation in sickle cell disease: a randomized phase 1 study. PLoS Med 14:e1002382
136. Saunthararajah Y (2013) Key clinical observations after 5-azacytidine and decitabine treatment of myelodysplastic syndromes suggest practical solutions for better outcomes. Hematology Am Soc Hematol Educ Program 2013:511–521
137. Gu XR, Hu ZB, Ebrahem Q et al (2014) Runx1 regulation of Pu.1 corepressor/coactivator exchange identifies specific molecular targets for leukemia differentiation therapy. J Biol Chem 289:14881–14895

138. Gozzini A, Rovida E, Dello SP et al (2003) Butyrates, as a single drug, induce histone acety-lation and granulocytic maturation: possible selectivity on core binding factor-acute myeloid leukemia blasts. Cancer Res 63:8955–8961

139. Kosugi H, Towatari M, Hatano S et al (1999) Histone deacetylase inhibitors are the potent inducer/enhancer of differentiation in acute myeloid leukemia: a new approach to anti-leukemia therapy. Leukemia 13:1316–1324

140. Nowak D, Stewart D, Koeffler HP (2009) Differentiation therapy of leukemia: 3 decades of development. Blood 113:3655–3665

141. Spira AI, Carducci MA (2003) Differentiation therapy. Curr Opin Pharmacol 3:338–343

142. Gore SD, Samid D, Weng LJ (1997) Impact of the putative differentiating agents sodium phenylbutyrate and sodium phenylacetate on proliferation, differentiation, and apoptosis of primary neoplastic myeloid cells. Clin Cancer Res 3:1755–1762

143. Wang J, Saunthararajah Y, Redner RL et al (1999) Inhibitors of histone deacetylase relieve ETO-mediated repression and induce differentiation of AML1-ETO leukemia cells. Cancer Res 59:2766–2769

144. Moldenhauer A, Frank RC, Pinilla-Ibarz J et al (2004) Histone deacetylase inhibition improves dendritic cell differentiation of leukemic blasts with AML1-containing fusion pro-teins. J Leukoc Biol 76:623–633

145. Jones PA, Taylor SM (1980) Cellular differentiation, cytidine analogs and DNA methylation. Cell 20:85–93

146. Pinto A, Attadia V, Fusco A et al (1984) 5-Aza-2′-deoxycytidine induces terminal differentia-tion of leukemic blasts from patients with acute myeloid leukemias. Blood 64:922–929

147. Creusot F, Acs G, Christman JK (1982) Inhibition of DNA methyltransferase and induction of Friend erythroleukemia cell differentiation by 5-azacytidine and 5-aza-2′-deoxycytidine. J Biol Chem 257:2041–2048

148. Niitsu N, Hayashi Y, Sugita K et al (2001) Sensitization by 5-aza-2′-deoxycytidine of leukae-mia cells with MLL abnormalities to induction of differentiation by all-trans retinoic acid and 1alpha,25-dihydroxyvitamin D3. Br J Haematol 112:315–326

149. Scuto A, Kirschbaum M, Kowolik C et al (2008) The novel histone deacetylase inhibitor, LBH589, induces expression of DNA damage response genes and apoptosis in Ph- acute lymphoblastic leukemia cells. Blood 111:5093–5100

150. Lee JH, Choy ML, Ngo L et al (2010) Histone deacetylase inhibitor induces DNA damage, which normal but not transformed cells can repair. Proc Natl Acad Sci USA 107:14639–14644

151. Conti C, Leo E, Eichler GS et al (2010) Inhibition of histone deacetylase in cancer cells slows down replication forks, activates dormant origins, and induces DNA damage. Cancer Res 70:4470–4480

152. Gaymes TJ, Padua RA, Pla M et al (2006) Histone deacetylase inhibitors (HDI) cause DNA damage in leukemia cells: a mechanism for leukemia-specific HDI-dependent apoptosis? Mol Cancer Res 4:563–573

153. Minucci S, Pelicci PG (2006) Histone deacetylase inhibitors and the promise of epigenetic (and more) treatments for cancer. Nat Rev Cancer 6:38–51

154. Komura S, Semi K, Itakura F et al (2016) An EWS-FLI1-induced osteosarcoma model unveiled a crucial role of impaired osteogenic differentiation on osteosarcoma development. Stem Cell Rep 6:592–606

155. Mohammad HP, Smitheman KN, Kamat CD et al (2015) A DNA Hypomethylation signature predicts antitumor activity of LSD1 inhibitors in SCLC. Cancer Cell 28:57–69

156. Mould DP, McGonagle AE, Wiseman DH et al (2015) Reversible inhibitors of LSD1 as thera-peutic agents in acute myeloid leukemia: clinical significance and progress to date. Med Res Rev 35:586–618

157. Schenk T, Chen WC, Gollner S et al (2012) Inhibition of the LSD1 (KDM1A) demethylase reactivates the all-trans-retinoic acid differentiation pathway in acute myeloid leukemia. Nat Med 18:605–611

158. Harris WJ, Huang X, Lynch JT et al (2012) The histone demethylase KDM1A sustains the oncogenic potential of MLL-AF9 leukemia stem cells. Cancer Cell 21:473–487
159. Hartley PD, Madhani HD (2009) Mechanisms that specify promoter nucleosome location and identity. Cell 137:445–458
160. Parnell TJ, Huff JT, Cairns BR (2008) RSC regulates nucleosome positioning at Pol II genes and density at Pol III genes. EMBO J 27:100–110

Index

© Springer Nature Switzerland AG 2021
A. C. Chiang, R. S. Herbst (eds.), *Lung Cancer*, Current Cancer Research,
https://doi.org/10.1007/978-3-030-74028-3

Printed in the United States
by Baker & Taylor Publisher Services